# Praise for *The AFib Cure*

"*The AFib Cure* provides clear step-by-step information that AFib patients can use to cure their AFib. The book contains valuable information about AFib causes, triggers, medications, supplements, diet, biomarkers, and lifestyle changes that you may not have seen anywhere else and probably have not heard from any doctor. Of particular value in the Treatment Section is the tool for determining your Tipping Point for when to have an ablation and the list of Twelve Questions to Ask Your EP. This book provides a complete compendium of what AFib patients need to know. It just might help you stop, or even cure, your AFib."

—Mellanie True Hills, founder and CEO, StopAFib.org and author of *A Woman's Guide to Saving Her Own Life*

"*The AFib Cure* is an outstanding and up-to-date tour-de-force patient guide for effectively managing—and even eliminating—the bane that is atrial fibrillation, penned by world-renowned electrophysiologists, Dr. John Day and Dr. T. Jared Bunch. As editor of AFibbers.org, the longest running AFib-centric patient education/advocacy resource online, I enthusiastically salute *The AFib Cure* for setting a new standard! Written with in-depth yet accessible and easy-to-digest insights into this often-complex topic, the authors offer a comprehensive road map for combining the best of lifestyle optimization protocols plus cutting-edge discoveries from the front lines of electrophysiology. Highly recommended with five stars!"

—Shannon W. Dickson, editor of The AFib Report at AFibbers.org

"*The AFib Cure* is a thorough, evidence-based guide to help patients with atrial fibrillation. Any patient living with AFib will find inspiration for their own treatment within this book. A must-have book for every patient!"

—Percy F. Morales MD, author of *Your Complete Guide to AFib*

"Dr. John Day, Dr. T. Jared Bunch, and Matthew D. LaPlante present a credible, easy-to-read, and engaging resource for anyone affected by the electrical epidemic of AFib. With years of experience, knowledge, and research, the authors provide a truly integrative step-by-step plan using science, storytelling, and actionable information. *The AFib Cure* is a must-read guide for anyone who wants to overcome this major health challenge."

—Aseem Desai, MD, FHRS, codirector of Mission Heritage Heart Rhythm Specialists and author of *Restart Your Heart: The Playbook for Thriving with AFib*

"A book for AFib patients that includes all of us, especially the concerns and challenges of the emerging younger female population that are often overlooked. Drs. Day and Bunch have taken the current research and explained it into our language. With this book, you will have step-by-step options and end-of-chapter summaries to guide you."

—Debbe McCall, BS, MBA, cardiovascular patient PI, DSMB, researcher, and moderator of the Atrial Fibrillation Support Forum

# THE
# AFIB
# CURE

**Also by John D. Day**

*The Longevity Plan: Seven Life-Transforming Lessons from Ancient China*
(with Jane Ann Day and Matthew D. LaPlante)

**Also by Matthew D. LaPlante**

*Superlative: The Biology of Extremes*

*Lifespan: Why We Age—and Why We Don't Have To*
(with David A. Sinclair, PhD)

*The Longevity Plan: Seven Life-Transforming Lessons from Ancient China*
(with John D. Day, MD, and Jane Ann Day)

# THE AFIB CURE

## Get Off Your Medications, Take Control of Your Health, and Add Years to Your Life

JOHN D. DAY, MD
T. JARED BUNCH, MD
WITH MATTHEW D. LaPLANTE

BENBELLA

BenBella Books, Inc.
Dallas, TX

This book is for informational purposes only. It is not intended to serve as a substitute for professional medical advice. The author and publisher specifically disclaim any and all liability arising directly or indirectly from the use of any information contained in this book. A health care professional should be consulted regarding your specific medical situation. Any product mentioned in this book does not imply endorsement of that product by the author or publisher.

*The AFib Cure* copyright © 2021 by John Day

All rights reserved. No part of this book may be used or reproduced in any manner whatsoever without written permission of the publisher, except in the case of brief quotations embodied in critical articles or reviews.

BenBella Books, Inc.
10440 N. Central Expressway
Suite 800
Dallas, TX 75231
www.benbellabooks.com
Send feedback to feedback@benbellabooks.com

*BenBella* is a federally registered trademark.

Printed in the United States of America
10 9 8 7 6 5 4 3 2 1

Library of Congress Control Number: 2020042978

ISBN 9781950665426 (trade paper)
ISBN 9781950665648 (electronic)

Editing by Leah Wilson and Greg Brown
Copyediting by James Fraleigh
Proofreading by Karen Wise and Dylan Julian
Indexing by IndexBusters
Text design and composition by PerfecType, Nashville, TN
Cover design by Ty Nowicki
Printed by Lake Book Manufacturing

Distributed to the trade by Two Rivers Distribution, an Ingram brand
www.tworiversdistribution.com

**Special discounts for bulk sales are available. Please contact
bulkorders@benbellabooks.com.**

*To our families*

# CONTENTS

## Introduction

---

# ∿ THE PROMISE ∿

---

**Much of what you've heard about AFib is true.
Much isn't. Here's the real story.**

The first time you experience atrial fibrillation is likely to be the scariest moment of your life.

Everything is fine. And then, just like that, it's not. All of a sudden your heart is pounding away.

One hundred and forty beats a minute.

Then one hundred and sixty.

Then one hundred and eighty.

That's two or three times faster than it should be going. Just like that, something you've taken for granted your entire life instantly becomes the only thing that matters. You can feel it throbbing in your neck. You can hear it pounding in your ears. Your chest hurts. You become lightheaded.

If you're standing, you sit down. If you're sitting, you lie down. You think you're dying.

What is going on?

*Oh no, I'm having a heart attack!* you think, and the sound of that thought seems to be screaming in your head.

You reach for the phone. Your hands are shaking, but you manage to call.

"911. What's your emergency?"

"I . . . don't know . . . my heart . . . it's . . . out of control."

"Stay calm," the emergency dispatcher says. "Help is on its way."

The dispatcher stays on the line and tries to collect some additional information. Your name. Your address. Your location inside your home. But you're having trouble answering basic questions. Your thoughts turn to your family.

*Will I ever see them again?*

If you're a praying person, this is when you pray. And sometimes even if you're *not* a praying person, this is when you pray.

The operator asks if you can make it to the front door. You say that you'll try. Everything seems like it's happening in slow motion. Everything, that is, except your heart; it seems like it's beating even *faster* now.

*How is that even possible?!*

You make it to the door. You unlock the deadbolt. Somehow, that simple act feels like a victory. You slide to the floor. There's nothing to do now but wait.

If you've had an experience like this, or know someone who has, you're in good company. Atrial fibrillation (AFib) is a condition characterized by unpredictable episodes of chaotic electrical activity in the heart's upper chambers, causing rapid and irregular heartbeats that just get worse with time if not treated. It is the world's most commonly diagnosed arrhythmia (a condition in which the heart beats abnormally). Former presidents George H. W. Bush and Richard Nixon both had it. So have former vice presidents Joe Biden and Dick Cheney. So have singers Barry Manilow and Elton John. So have comedians Ellen DeGeneres and Howie Mandel. So have basketball Hall of Famers Larry Bird and Bill Bradley. The list goes on and on.

One in four American adults will suffer from atrial fibrillation at some point in their lives,[1] and some studies suggest that, for some groups in the United States, the risk of developing AFib might be as high as one in three.[2] All told, more than sixty million adult Americans are likely to suffer at least one AFib episode in their lives. And that's *just* in the United States; the global population is also growing and aging, and the incidence of AFib appears to be increasing. Worldwide, sixty-five million people over the age of thirty-five have *already* been diagnosed with AFib.[3] Many, many more simply haven't been diagnosed yet.

These people do not suffer from this condition alone. Their partners suffer, too. So do their parents, siblings, children, and friends. And because the average cost for treating atrial fibrillation hovers around $20,000—often much more[4]—even people who are fortunate to not have had personal experience with AFib are indirectly impacted by higher insurance rates that support others in the pool, or higher taxes to support those who are uninsured, underinsured, or insured through government programs. That's not to mention the costs attributed to lost productivity.[5]

If you're reading this book, though, chances are that you've had a *direct* experience like the one described previously or know someone who has.

This book is for you.

## A WORLD OF CHANGE

What's covered in the rest of this book represents more than twenty years of our research and clinical experience in treating thousands of AFib patients around the world.

Cardiologists who specialize in arrhythmias are called electrophysiologists, or EPs for short. John is an EP at St. Mark's Hospital, where he leads the cardiac and vascular services for the mountain states division hospitals for HCA Healthcare, the largest healthcare provider in the United States. Jared is the chief EP at University of Utah Health, one of the nation's top academic healthcare systems. In other words, we lead the two biggest heart rhythm programs in our region for healthcare providers that, at least in a market sense, compete against each other— but we've come together to write this book because most AFib patients aren't offered a full picture of their medical options. Worse, they're often painted a picture that is very grim.

But that's not the picture we paint for our patients, because it's simply not backed by the emerging research. We should know: between the two of us, and often in collaboration, we have authored more than one hundred peer-reviewed scientific articles, served as editors-in-chief of medical journals, and led our medical society in the heart rhythm field.

We're also both practitioners: we have treated thousands of AFib patients over the years—during a time of immense changes in this field.

One of the biggest changes is the type of patient who comes through our clinics' doors. Back in the 1990s, a newly minted EP, fresh out of residency, likely would have been very surprised to meet an AFib patient under the age of fifty. Just a few decades later, though, the patient demographic landscape has changed. Now, doctors regularly see patients who are seeking treatment for AFib in their forties, thirties, and sometimes even their twenties. That's in no small part because of our dreadfully poor diet and exercise habits, ever-increasing waistlines, lack of restorative sleep, and overstressed lives—a perfect storm for premature aging and AFib (as we'll come to see quite well in chapter one). Indeed, AFib may be a warning sign that you are aging too fast and that you may be wearing out your heart long before its time.

In fact, you may be wearing out everything, right down to your chromosomes. For example, our study of more than 3,500 patients demonstrated that people with AFib tend to have shorter telomeres—the deterioration-protective caps at the ends of each chromosome—which is a sign of premature aging.[6] So, if you have been diagnosed with AFib, it's not just your heart that is at risk; your whole body may be aging faster.

Another reason why we are seeing so many more young people with AFib is a positive one. We now have myriad consumer technologies that can detect AFib easier and earlier than ever before. Many smartwatches can now detect signs of potential AFib even before an arrhythmia episode occurs. As tech giants eagerly promote consumer "wearables" that can easily diagnose this condition without a doctor's help, what was once a rarely talked-about heart condition is now a common topic in consumer technology spaces. These devices are a big part of the reason why more than two million Americans who are *under* age sixty-five are now diagnosed with atrial fibrillation each year.[7]

There is one more reason for the increase in people seeking information about atrial fibrillation—a reason exemplified by the experience of a twenty-seven-year-old patient named Gavrilo.[8] His story begins during the holidays.

"For Christmas, my fiancée offered to pay for a pretty extensive DNA test for both of us, and I was excited for several reasons, both of which were related to the fact that I am adopted," the software engineer from San Francisco explained. "First, I really wanted to better understand where my family came from. I'd always been told that part of my family came from Serbia, but I didn't know anything more than that. Second, because I don't know my birth parents, I can't ask them about my family health history. Does cancer run in our family? Does heart disease? I have no idea. So, I wanted to know as much as I can to fill in all those blank spots."

Gavrilo's DNA test showed he had inherited one copy of each of the two atrial fibrillation SNPs (which stands for single-nucleotide polymorphisms and is pronounced "snips"). This genetic abnormality upped his lifetime risk of AFib to nearly one in two.

"Honestly, up until that point, I don't think I'd ever even heard of atrial fibrillation," he said, "but the test sent me into 'research mode,' and I was pretty surprised to learn how common it actually is."

He was also surprised to learn how much it could impact his life if it wasn't addressed. Not only were his chances of getting AFib higher, but so was his risk of blood clots and strokes.

"I was about to be married," he said. "We were already talking about having children, and obviously I wanted to make sure I would be around for all that, but also that I would be able to do all of the things I never got to do with my own birth father—wrestling around, playing soccer, going on hikes, all that sort of stuff."

Gavrilo had never had an episode of AFib, and he was determined to do everything he could to make sure he never would—thus his scramble for answers about what he could do to prevent this condition from ruining his life. In doing so, Gavrilo joined other "proactive preventers" who have seen the destruction AFib has brought into the lives of their parents, grandparents, or siblings, and are committed to keeping it from striking them in the way it did their loved ones.

Although it is exceptionally common, AFib doesn't get much attention in the media. It's not a well-known disease. Like Gavrilo, most people haven't even heard of it until they have been diagnosed with it, have had a loved one who had it, or have learned they have a genetic predisposition for it. But once a diagnosis is made—whether in the emergency room, prompted by an EKG-enabled smartwatch, or precipitated by a genetic test—*everyone* wants to know as much as they can.

That's probably why you're here. You've been looking for answers. And, if you're like many people, much if not most of what you've learned so far is likely quite disheartening.

## THE BAD NEWS

You might already have run across the statistic that 14 percent of people diagnosed with AFib will pass away within one month of diagnosis.[9] That's a scary fact, and it's one based on research, but it's also important to put this number into context: the vast majority of people diagnosed are over sixty-five. Still, sixty-five is hardly "old." Or it shouldn't be, at least. Today, our mid-sixties are a time in which most people should be able to live a healthy and active life, confident that they have decades more to come.

You've probably also learned—either from experience, from a doctor, or by doing your own research—that this arrhythmia often comes with palpitations, rapid heart rate, dizziness, chest pain, shortness of breath, lightheadedness, and sometimes fainting spells. You've also likely discovered that the drug options for treatment come with a long list of side effects, increased risks for other debilitating conditions, and a substantially reduced quality of life. You may have found out that AFib drastically increases the risk of strokes, heart failure, cognitive decline, and dementia. In fact, every time a person's heart shifts into AFib, the blood flow to their brain is compromised, meaning their brains are *constantly* being starved of oxygen.[10] As a result, their brain may actually shrink, potentially putting them at risk of suffering from memory deficits, difficulties in language use, challenges in how their brains process visual images, and trouble paying attention.[11] In fact, our research team has discovered that many of the same biomarkers of brain injury that are elevated after a concussion are also chronically high in atrial fibrillation patients—a reflection of the persistent insult of the abnormal heart rhythm on the brain.[12] Indeed, one study showed that 40 percent of people with AFib have visible brain damage on an MRI, even if they have no prior neurologic symptoms.[13] And all of these brain changes may help explain why so many people who have always felt quite intelligent and "high functioning" come to us for help; their brains are no longer capable of functioning at these high levels when their heart is out of rhythm.

Indeed, the outlook sure seems bleak. So it's no wonder that researchers have found that people who have been diagnosed with AFib are more likely to report declines in their satisfaction at work and home, a decrease in enjoyment of leisure time, a reduction of social activities, and a drop in their satisfaction with their sex lives.

But it's time for a change in perspective. Yes, AFib can be the worst thing that ever happens to you—but it can also be the best.

No, *really*.

## THE GOOD NEWS

AFib is a warning—a literal heart-felt warning—that something is amiss and even more is likely to go wrong very soon. Because of this, the health optimization strategies offered in this book won't just help you prevent and reduce the occurrence of dangerous arrhythmias; they will help you live a longer, healthier, and happier life in every way.

And so . . .

. . . if you don't want to take handful upon handful of medications for the rest of your life . . .

. . . if you don't want to go from one doctor to the next . . .

. . . if you don't want to be a prisoner to your condition . . .

. . . if you don't want "the healthy part" of your life to be over . . .

. . . if you don't just want hope, but direction . . .

. . . and if, indeed, you'd like to start working toward a life that is better than it was before the words "atrial fibrillation" were part of your vocabulary . . .

. . . then this book is for you. Because what this book offers is a path to a cure.

Your doctor may scoff at that word. They might tell you there is no such thing as an "AFib cure." So be it. Respectfully, we disagree.

According to the National Cancer Institute, most doctors consider cancer to be "cured" when a patient goes five years without a recurrence. If you apply the same standard to AFib, then we can tell you the stories of many people who have been diagnosed with AFib and have indeed been cured.

Now, to be fair and frank, the people we see who achieve this goal are those who are highly motivated—committed people who recognize that this is the fight of their lives. But we believe that most people can indeed achieve this goal if they adhere to the treatment strategies detailed in this book.

Feeling a bit skeptical? Maybe *a lot* skeptical? That's good. We live in a world in which it's often far easier to find snake oil than real science, where people throw words like "cure" around without regard for the damage they cause to patients who get their hopes up, only to have them dashed on the rocks of reality. In this journey, your skepticism will serve you well.

But skepticism and optimism are not mutually exclusive ideas. And the science suggests that there's plenty of room for people with AFib to feel hopeful and confident about the future, especially if those people are willing to ask questions and seek answers.

## SOME COMMON QUESTIONS

At this point, you probably have a lot of questions related to the path we will explain in this book. Some of the common ones include:

*Do I have to quit my doctor?*

Do you like your doctor? And does your doctor want you to be well? If so, then you should very much keep that doctor on your team. And, to be clear, this book is absolutely *not* a replacement for a doctor. This book is intended to help educate you about AFib. It is not intended to be a substitute for professional medical advice, diagnosis, or treatment! If you *don't* have a doctor, what you're going to learn in this book is that you really need to find one. In particular, you need to find a great electrophysiologist—a doctor who specializes in arrhythmia care and can help you understand your heart by helping you understand what it's trying to tell you. (More on that later.)

*Do I have to be a risk taker?*

Absolutely not. The risks are greater—so much greater—for those who stick to the status quo of a lifetime of medications and increasingly debilitating symptoms. Studies show that not only can the lessons in this book extend your life, but also that following the guidelines offered here will likely, and quite dramatically, improve the *quality* of your life.

*Is this something only for young people?*

By young, do you mean eighty? Patients in their late eighties have used the lessons in this book to beat back their AFib by taking advantage of transformational procedures, getting off medications, and making lifestyle choices that help them optimize their lives.

*What if I'm not even sure if I have AFib?*

For some people, palpitations can feel like a fluttering. For this reason, atrial fibrillation is often confused with another arrhythmia in the upper chambers of the heart, atrial flutter. This typically features a fast and regular rhythm as opposed to AFib, in which the heartbeat is usually fast and irregular.

But while the rhythm is often regular with atrial flutter, it can still do all the same bad things that AFib can do, like cause strokes, heart failure, and the like. And the same things that trigger AFib can also trigger flutter. Likewise, the treatments for AFib also treat flutter. So while you will see "AFib" used predominantly in this book, please know that everything we discuss applies to both of these arrhythmias. If you suspect that you might have AFib or atrial flutter, please check with your doctor immediately, as only your doctor can tell you if you have either condition.

*Will I have to get a procedure or surgery?*
A catheter ablation is a minimally invasive procedure in which an EP moves a thin, flexible tube through a patient's blood vessels and into their heart, where one of several techniques is used to repair the abnormal electrical pathways that lead to AFib. Ablations are a vital part of many patients' treatment, but they are not a foregone conclusion. Using the practices detailed in this book, many patients are able to put their AFib into remission without procedures.

*Do I have to be into technology?*
No, but you should be willing to collect some very basic data about your life—tracking your meals and workouts—as well as wear an EKG-enabled smartwatch. If you're tech-savvy, all the better, but the basic tech that makes the AFib Cure possible is so simple a toddler could use it.

This isn't speculative. It's true that the idea of a "cure" for atrial fibrillation doesn't align with the traditional view of this condition and can still, for now, rightly be called an "alternative" course of treatment. But it's also a course of treatment backed by published medical studies—lots of them.

It's also backed by a lot of people's experiences. There's a quickly growing group of people who have resolved to reject the traditional views that atrial fibrillation is best treated with daily handfuls of medications and that, even with drugs, it always gets worse over time.

## THIS BOOK ISN'T FOR EVERYONE

The AFib Cure can work for anyone.

That doesn't make it *right* for everyone, though, for there's a big difference between people who *can* succeed on this plan and those who would be better off just sticking to the traditional way of dealing with this condition.

The traditional treatment regimen is good for people who

- accept atrial fibrillation as a lifelong medical problem,
- don't mind taking medications for the rest of their lives, or
- believe that atrial fibrillation is just part of getting older.

The AFib Cure requires people who

- are 100 percent committed to seeing an immediate improvement in their lives,
- believe it's important to do everything they can to put AFib into remission by prioritizing natural interventions, and
- believe that age doesn't need to be an indicator of health.

There are a lot of people in that latter group. In this book, you're going to meet some of them. Their stories are inspiring. More importantly, their experiences provide a road map for those who want to slow, stop, and even reverse their AFib.

To do that, though, we can't just give you a "do this" and "don't do that" checklist. To take full advantage of the transformative power of this guide, you'll need to develop a better understanding of the mysteries of this condition. Indeed, you're going to need to understand what's happening in your heart and in your body, and why. You don't need to go to medical school to "get it," however. Once explained in the right way, *anyone* can learn what they need to know to mount a sophisticated attack on their atrial fibrillation.

Are you ready for that? If so, there is absolutely no time to lose.

None of us knows how much time we have left on this planet. But those with an AFib diagnosis can be assured that, if they're not willing to make some pretty big changes to their lives, their time is even more limited. Even if AFib doesn't kill you, if you don't address it—and soon—it is only the *start* of your problems.

We recognize that's not the most cheerful way to begin a book about fighting AFib. But this is the reality of the disease we're fighting, and of the world in which we live. It's important that we talk openly and honestly about what atrial fibrillation is and what it can take from us. It's important that we don't talk about this like it's no big deal.

This isn't a condition that simply makes life harder, more painful, or more frustrating. This is a disease that can do all of that *and* takes lives, too. And it can take them in tragic ways.

Yet, all over the world, people are learning that it's possible to fight this disease. They're learning that they can change its impact on their lives. Some have beaten it into complete remission and will never be impacted by it again.

Indeed, they've *cured* their AFib.

## Chapter One

# ~PROBABLE CAUSES~

*Everyone gets into AFib a different way.*
*Most get out the same way.*

Most people think atrial fibrillation is a heart problem. It's not.

To understand this, it's helpful to think about the last time you had a fever—because while not everyone has had AFib, there aren't many people who don't know what it's like to have a fever. When you have a fever, the root of the problem isn't the fact that you have an abnormally high body temperature—although that *is* a problem, and a potentially deadly one. But if our treatment only focused on lowering the high temperature, whatever gave you a fever in the first place would still be present. That's because fever is a marker of infection in the body, much the same way that AFib is a marker of a systemic bodily disease.

This is why, when you're going to battle against atrial fibrillation, you can't just fight the arrhythmia alone. If you're going to beat this thing long term, you've got to figure out what caused it in the first place.

There's an important distinction to make here between causes and triggers. You'll need to understand both, but the long-term factors that put people at greater risk of AFib, also known as substrate causes, aren't always the same things that prompt a specific incident of AFib. Here, a wildfire analogy might be helpful. Any spark can trigger a single blaze, but the chances of having lots of fires in a season are greatly increased by conditions that accumulate over time, including drought, insect infestation, and the growth of underbrush. So while we'll talk a lot about triggers in this book, and we want to limit those as much as possible, it's extremely important that we also identify the long-term substrate causes of AFib.

When doctors talk to their patients about substrate causes, they're often met with surprise—and even anger.

"I know I've made bad health and food decisions," a middle-school history teacher named Paula said as she recalled her first visit to a doctor after her AFib diagnosis, "but it seemed like my doctor was dead-set on forcing me to talk about those things. And I felt guilty enough as it was. All I wanted was to get whatever medicine I needed, or get whatever procedure I needed, and then to not have to think about the terrible things I may have done to myself and my family."

It's impossible to know if Paula's doctor approached her new patient with the correct—and exceptionally elusive—combination of confidence and compassion that we often call a physician's "bedside manner." What we can say is that if your intention is to fight your AFib, rather than just treat it and wait for it to get worse over time, you absolutely must engage in the process of understanding what factors led to the disease in the first place.

In fact, Paula was pretty lucky to have the doctor she had. Even today, with plenty of science to refute the conventional wisdom that AFib is a heart condition that, for many people, is little more than another inevitable consequence of aging, many doctors still tell their patients that there's nothing they could have done about it—and that there's not much they can do now but make it "less bad." They prescribe some drugs, or order up a procedure, and that is that.

But rather than reflexively throwing pharmaceutical drugs at the condition, or addressing only the most obvious symptom with a procedure, the better course of action is to search for the unique and specific underlying cause to keep it from coming back—especially because that cause is almost always, in fact, a *combination* of causes. And the "this plus this and also that" equation that adds up to atrial fibrillation is subtly and sometimes significantly different for everyone. No two people come to have AFib for the exact same reasons.

Paula understands that, now.

"Now that I know more about AFib, I see that first visit to my doctor in a very different light," Paula said. "If I'd just taken whatever medications she gave me, and never did anything about the underlying issues that led me to get AFib in the first place, nothing would have changed. I might have felt better for a while, and then things likely would have gotten worse."

We have all made potentially bad health and lifestyle decisions. Even physicians, who generally have easy access to the research literature and the training to understand it, frequently make life choices that lead to AFib. It's not unusual at all to meet a doctor, even a cardiologist, who has had to battle this disease.

And so, with that in mind, please understand that the following exercise, in which we'll ask you to assess all the potential causes of your AFib, isn't a guilt trip. Not at all. Rather, it's a vital part of developing a treatment plan that's right for you.

## WHY DO I HAVE AFIB?

So, why did you get atrial fibrillation? There are a lot of possible substrate causes—some of which you can control and some of which you cannot.

### You Inherited the Wrong Gene

Like Gavrilo in our introduction, some people inherit a genetic predisposition that makes AFib more likely. Up to a third of all people who have atrial fibrillation without another identified cause have a familial history of the condition.[1]

Often, this association has to do with a gene named *KCNQ1*, which acts as a sort of instruction book for building important components of heart muscle cells for transporting potassium ions. At least fifteen different "potassium channel" mutations have been linked to AFib.

Another gene on which heart researchers are increasingly focused, *SCNA5*, impacts the body's ability to move sodium ions. At least seven "sodium channel" mutations are associated with AFib.

Potassium and sodium ions are atoms that carry electric charges and thus are essential to the signaling system that tells parts of the heart to contract in rhythm. But a lot of non–ion-channel mutations have been linked to AFib, too. These include mutations in a protein-coding gene called *NUP155*; a gene known as *LMNA* that is linked to many heart disorders; a gene called *NPPA* that encodes a vital hormone created in the heart; and a set of genes known as *GATA4*, *GATA5*, and *GATA6* that are key to the development of new heart tissue.

Those aren't the only genes that have been linked to AFib, though—there are actually more than one hundred. Even if we were to create an exhaustive list, it would soon be outdated. Emerging research is revealing other "candidate genes" that may have links to AFib. For now, however, there isn't a test that can scan for all of the known and potential "AFib genes." While over-the-counter commercial DNA tests can scan for some, you're really just scratching the surface with these products.

What's important to note is that while it can be very helpful to know whether you've inherited a genetic predisposition to AFib, there's nothing you can do about the genes you were dealt.

However, it is equally important to understand that research conducted over the past few decades in the field of epigenetics has conclusively demonstrated that we do have the power to *influence* which genes are "expressed" and which genes are "silenced" based on the hundreds of little health decisions we make every day. Indeed, health outcomes among the individuals who have inherited any of these genes vary greatly based on factors that extend far beyond that inheritance.

## You Have Another Heart Problem

If you were to round up all of the people with AFib in the world, you would find that somewhere close to half of them have also been diagnosed with another cardiovascular condition. Of these, the three most common culprits are heart failure, cardiac valve problems, and coronary artery disease.

Mark was in a very tough situation when he came to see us. Not only did he have AFib that had probably been going on for months, but he was also suffering from coronary artery disease and heart failure as well. Years ago he'd been stented for an arterial blockage. But more recently he developed very rapid AFib, causing his heart to be stuck at 130 beats per minute—a rate that would be considered normal for a healthy person engaged in strenuous exercise.

"I knew things were pretty grim," Mark said. "I had everything. Chest pain. Shortness of breath. Palpitations. You name it."

The fact that Mark was battling multiple problems made it all the more important for him to avoid long-term AFib medications, the reported side effects of which could potentially increase the risk of adverse outcomes related to other heart conditions.

There wasn't much Mark could do at that time for the damage his other conditions had inflicted upon his heart. The good news, though, was that a commitment to putting his AFib into remission—using the strategies you'll read about in this book—had the potential to work wonders for his other heart challenges, too.

## You've Got a Few Years Under Your Belt

Margaret had been a picture of health for most of her life. She had followed a mostly plant-based diet free of fried, processed, and fast foods.

She didn't eat sugar. She'd never been overweight. She did aerobics every day at the gym and attended a yoga class three times a week. She practiced deep-breathing exercises whenever stress levels were getting too high. She slept well at night. She even volunteered as a crosswalk guard at the elementary school across the street from her house.

And since no one in her family had ever been diagnosed with AFib, she was more than a little irritated when her doctor told her she had that arrhythmia.

But here's the thing: Margaret was ninety-four years old. And the truth is that even if your genes are perfect and you do just about everything right, you can still get AFib as a result of age. Just as your skin will wrinkle over the years, the simple act of living life will put some wear and tear on your heart cells over time.

But there's a big difference between being ninety-four and fifty-four—between AFib that results from natural aging and AFib that comes about due to *premature* aging. Most of the AFib cases we see are due to the latter kind of aging.[2] And while there is nothing we can do to stop how many candles are on our birthday cakes—that's *chronological* age—there is plenty we can do to slow the process of *biological* aging.

The steps in this book won't just help you go to battle with AFib. What you do to change your life could actually help you slow or even reverse your biological age.

## Your Blood Pressure Is Too High

Hypertension occurs when the force of a person's blood against the walls of their arteries is high enough that it puts a person at risk of health problems. Within the heart, this means that, with every heartbeat, the organ is working harder to pump blood through more restrictive arteries. And all of this strain on the heart can cause the muscle to thicken and enlarge, disrupting electrical pathways and causing AFib. Indeed, of all the factors that have been associated with atrial fibrillation, none may be stronger than hypertension. High blood pressure is the most commonly encountered condition in AFib patients, and research has shown that it nearly doubles the risk of developing atrial fibrillation.[3] Studies show that 90 percent of Americans are hypertensive by age fifty-five,[4] so it's little wonder why AFib is so common.

It doesn't have to be this way. Only 4 percent of the centenarians living in southern China's famed "Longevity Village" of Bapan had high blood pressure. That finding is similar to studies of hunter-gatherers living in the Amazon rain forest or elsewhere in the world consistently showing a natural blood pressure of about 110/70 that doesn't increase much, if any, with age.[5] Indeed, it appears from many studies that our genes are designed to keep our blood pressure naturally in this 110/70 range without medication as long as we don't mess things up with our modern lifestyle. Low body weight, a mostly plant-based diet devoid of sugar and processed foods, daily physical exercise, rejuvenating sleep, and low perceived stress levels protected these people from the scourge of hypertension.[6] It might seem like it's impossible in a modern context to live as these people do, and that's true. But the lessons we can draw from these elders are virtually endless, and your ability to apply these lessons to your own life are limited only by your imagination, as we will discuss further in chapter ten.

## It's One of the Medications You Are On

Sakari was in his mid-forties. He had a good job at a local airport, a daughter who brought him great joy, and a love of performing in musicals with his local community theater group. A regular runner and occasional participant in charity 5K and 10K races, he was fit, followed a natural and mostly plant-based diet, and almost always got a good night's sleep. And, because an uncle with whom he was quite close had recently been diagnosed with atrial fibrillation, Sakari already knew a lot more about AFib than most people.

"So I was pretty confused," he said, "because I had learned that having a healthy lifestyle was a really effective preventative measure, even for those of us who drew a bad genetic card. But then one day my heart started going crazy, and I was just flabbergasted, because I was pretty sure I knew what was happening, and it just didn't make any sense."

Except, as Sakari would later learn, it *did* make sense. That's because, ever since being diagnosed with hypertension in his late thirties, he had been taking a regular dose of hydrochlorothiazide, often known as HCTZ, which is a common diuretic that doctors often prescribe to help their patients address high blood pressure. Further testing would later show that Sakari's body was indeed greatly depleted of the minerals potassium and magnesium due to HCTZ.

HCTZ comes from a class of drugs called thiazides that are known to cause mineral depletion in the body. Reduction of those key minerals, especially potassium and magnesium, is often enough to trigger atrial fibrillation.[7]

Was it Sakari's high blood pressure, his hypertension medication, or something else that caused his AFib? While high blood pressure is one of the most significant AFib risk factors, it's quite possible that the HCTZ also contributed as a trigger by lowering his potassium and magnesium. In our experience, cases of drug-induced AFib are usually the result of taking one or two offending drugs on top of other AFib risk factors. But given how healthy he appeared to be in other ways, it was likely playing a role in the arrhythmias he was experiencing.

"It felt like a good dose of irony, that's for sure," he said. "A big part of the reason why I have been so focused on healthy living is because of my experience with hypertension. Other than the occasional aspirin for a headache, this was literally the only drug I was taking, and there's a good chance it was contributing to my AFib."

The further irony was that Sakari likely didn't need to be taking HCTZ anymore. His blood pressure had long since dropped to very healthy levels. And while the drugs initially might have helped get him there, it was his diet, lean body weight, exercise, sleep habits, and low-stress lifestyle that was keeping him there.

Thiazide diuretics like HCTZ aren't the only medications that have been linked to atrial fibrillation. Nonsteroidal anti-inflammatory drugs, or

NSAIDs, can also induce AFib; these are relatively common drugs like ibuprofen and naproxen that are often used to fight pain. NSAIDs are particularly troublesome for AFib patients because they increase the risk of heart and kidney failure. For those who are also on a blood thinner, NSAIDs also raise the risk of an emergency room visit for a life-threatening gastrointestinal bleed.

Proton-pump inhibitors, which suppress stomach acid, can also induce an arrhythmia by blocking magnesium absorption or possibly by changing a person's gut microbiome. These drugs include omeprazole, lansoprazole, and pantoprazole, often sold under the brand names Prilosec, Prevacid, and Protonix, respectively.

Steroids, like prednisone and methylprednisolone, can cause atrial fibrillation, too, by pushing blood glucose levels very high and increasing blood pressure through fluid retention and weight gain.

That's not all. Back in the early 2000s, a team led by epidemiologist Bruno Stricker began to pore over the research and case studies linking various drugs to AFib. They noted that cardiac stimulant medications had been associated with AFib. Even over-the-counter decongestants such as pseudoephedrine, which is sold as Sudafed,[8] or medications for attention-deficit/hyperactivity disorder[9] can trigger an AFib attack.

Perhaps a bit counterintuitively, some classic drugs used to treat abnormal heart rhythms (digoxin and calcium channel blockers such as verapamil and diltiazem) can trigger attacks as well.[10] Stricker's group noted that many asthma and emphysema medications have also been linked to AFib. This includes stimulant inhalers like albuterol, as well as xanthine derivatives like theophylline.

Less common drugs, including cytostatics used to treat cancer, some skin diseases, and infections, can also induce AFib, according to the group's work. So can central nervous system drugs, including some antidepressants like fluoxetine (much more commonly known by the brand name Prozac); antimigraine drugs like sumatriptan (commonly sold as Imitrex); anticholinergics, which are sometimes used as antipsychotics and also to treat Parkinson's disease; and dopamine agonists, such as apomorphine, which is also used to treat Parkinson's. We've even seen beta-blockers, which are often prescribed for AFib, linked to AFib episodes due to associated weight gain, particularly in women.

Stricker and his team found reports and case studies connecting atrial fibrillation to more than sixty-five different prescription drugs—and this was back in 2004. Each year since, more medications that might be linked to AFib have been added to the list.

A few years back, for instance, reports began to surface that certain osteoporosis-preventing drugs, like Fosamax, could be linked to atrial fibrillation. These reports caused concerns for millions of women on them. Fortunately, in our study of more than 47,000 people, we did not find any association between atrial fibrillation and these medications, known as bisphosphonates.[11] But every medication deserves to be evaluated in the same way, and not all of them have been.

Even when there is a clear cause for concern, a medication's possible AFib association doesn't mean you shouldn't take it. All drugs have potential side effects, after all. The best way to make decisions about the medications you have been prescribed is to consult your doctor. Under no circumstances should you decide on your own volition to come off a drug you have been prescribed; you should always do so with a physician's guidance. If you have an atrial fibrillation diagnosis, or if you have concerns that AFib might be on your horizon, you should immediately inform your doctor about all of the medications you are taking, both regular prescriptions and once-in-a-while over-the-counters.

You don't have to wait for an appointment to start gathering the information you need, though. Both the common and less frequently known side effects of all medications are available from a variety of reputable sources, including the US Food and Drug Administration. A simple internet search for "AFib" and the name of the drug you're taking can tell you whether there is a possible connection.

Also, when you do talk to your doctor, be sure to mention any supplements you're taking. People don't always think of vitamins and supplements as drugs, but just like any form of therapy, these substances should only be taken for the right reasons and at the right doses. One of our studies, for example, found that the risk of developing AFib was two and a half times greater among individuals who were taking too much vitamin D.[12]

| Top 10 Drugs Causing Atrial Fibrillation | Mechanism of Action |
| --- | --- |
| 1.  Some antiarrhythmics | Electrical conduction changes in the heart |
| 2.  Stimulants of any kind | Adrenaline release, blood pressure increase |
| 3.  Steroids | Fluid retention, blood pressure increase |
| 4.  Nonsteroidal anti-inflammatory drugs like ibuprofen, naproxen, etc. | Fluid retention, blood pressure increase |
| 5.  Diuretics of any kind | Electrolyte depletion, dehydration |
| 6.  Thyroid hormone or medications that can cause thyroid hormone to be released, like amiodarone | Excessive thyroid hormone is a stimulant |
| 7.  Proton-pump inhibitors like Prilosec, Prevacid, Protonix, etc. | Blocks magnesium absorption in the gut |
| 8.  Nicotine | Cardiac toxicity, stimulant, inflammation from vaping |
| 9.  Alcohol | Cardiac toxicity, weight gain, blood pressure increase, sleep apnea |
| 10. Marijuana/THC | Cardiac toxicity, autonomic nervous system changes, inadequate blood flow to the heart, inflammation from vapors |

## The Amount of Exercise You're Getting Is Out of Balance with Your Body's Needs

When we learned Sakari was a regular runner, the first thing we wanted to know about was the kind of running Sakari did.

"Marathons? Ultras? Endurance stuff?" we asked.

"Well, I did a marathon in my late twenties," Sakari said, "and I did my first triathlon a few years ago, but honestly, I didn't like those events so much, and now I stick to shorter races. But if it helps, I can totally—"

"Oh no," we interjected, "our concern isn't that you aren't running enough. Believe it or not, it's actually possible that too much running can put you at risk of AFib."

Over the years, we explained, we have noticed a particularly increased risk of atrial fibrillation in patients who regularly compete in ultra-endurance events, including running, biking, and cross-country skiing. Sakari was shocked, as are many people when they learn that people who run marathons, competitively cycle, or do Ironman Triathlons are five times more likely to develop atrial fibrillation.[13] What is particularly perplexing, however, is that studies have not tended to show higher rates of arrhythmias in athletes who participate in other strenuous forms of exercise, such as boxing, wrestling, and weightlifting.[14] There is something particular about *endurance* sports that increases the risk of AFib. (One exception to this may be football. Among former NFL athletes, the risk of AFib is six times higher, although this may be due to the use of performance-enhancing substances or the weight these athletes put on to compete at a professional level.[15])

Also, it bears noting that while aggressively competing in endurance sports might put you at a greater *risk* of AFib, participation in these activities certainly does not *guarantee* you'll get AFib. It is reassuring to note that recreational participation in endurance sports, even if it is a marathon or triathlon, doesn't seem to increase this risk. And regular exercise in general isn't risky at all—in fact, it's exceptionally protective. To put things into perspective, for every thousand patients we see with atrial fibrillation, perhaps one may be at risk for atrial fibrillation due to overexercising. The biggest problem, by far, is that most patients aren't exercising enough.

There is far greater risk from not exercising enough than from exercising too much. People who live sedentary lifestyles are at significant risk of AFib,[16] not to mention all of the other health consequences of not getting enough exercise.

## Your Metabolism Is Out of Sync

Amita didn't need her doctor to tell her that she was overweight. Although she was an active golfer and tried to make healthy food choices, she had always been a bit on the high end of the healthy weight spectrum for a woman of her height.

She certainly isn't alone in that respect. The United States accounts for about 5 percent of the world's population, but it includes 13 percent of the global total of overweight and obese people. Nearly three-quarters of American men and nearly two-thirds of American women are overweight, if not obese. The share of people across the planet who are at risk of health conditions because of their elevated weight has increased rapidly, too, from 20 percent in 1980 to 30 percent in 2013. Today more than two billion people worldwide are overweight or obese.[17]

Just about everyone knows that obesity puts people at risk of lots of other health challenges, especially diabetes. And it stands to reason that diabetes and obesity have been shown to be associated with an elevated risk of AFib, too. In fact, the scientific data connecting weight and AFib are so compelling that many electrophysiologists (EPs) specializing in heart rhythm disorders feel that carrying extra weight is a primary *cause* of AFib. Our research has shown that even a few extra pounds can make a big difference in a person's AFib risk and how they respond to treatments.[18] Other studies have shown that carrying too much weight is the main cause of an enlarged left atrium and premature heart aging—two critical components in the development of AFib, as we'll discuss further in the next chapter.[19]

If you don't know whether you're overweight, a good place to start is the Centers for Disease Control and Prevention Adult Body Mass Index (BMI) Calculator. While not a perfect metric, this basic weight-divided-by-height tool can be a good starting place for understanding where you're at relative to where you probably should be. Even if it's only by a few extra pounds, being overweight can significantly raise your risk of AFib.

And maybe it's *not* just a few pounds. Perhaps you are obese. That word has a lot of negative baggage attached to it, which may be one of the reasons why people are reluctant to even check their BMI. Consciously or subconsciously, they simply don't want to know. But when people do check, many are surprised to learn that they might indeed be obese, which *substantially* increases the risk of atrial fibrillation.

The risk increases even more if you have diabetes or prediabetes. If that's the case, not only is your risk of AFib substantially increased, but your experience with that disease is likely to be a lot worse, as people with diabetes have worse AFib symptoms, report a lower quality of life, are more likely to spend time in a hospital, and experience higher mortality rates.[20] There is good news in this regard, though: type 2 diabetes (also known as adult-onset diabetes, although children are increasingly affected) is usually reversible through weight control and carbohydrate reduction. That makes it manageable.

Manageable doesn't mean "easy." We live in a world that is constantly conspiring against us when it comes to the food choices that drive so many of our metabolic challenges. It's also a world in which we're constantly being told there are shortcuts to just about everything. But we'll go to battle against those forces very soon. And we'll do it together. It is something that even we, as cardiologists, have to battle every day. But, again, the important thing, at this moment, is to understand if this is one of the challenges you are facing. If so, the first step is to acknowledge that challenge, and accept its connection to AFib.

## You're Eating Too Much Sugar and Too Many Processed Carbohydrates

Food is good medicine. A diet that respects what our bodies need to thrive might be the best way to prevent atrial fibrillation, or to beat it back once it starts.

A bad diet does the exact opposite. In fact, there isn't much that is worse for you, when it comes to AFib, than eating foods loaded with sugar and other simple carbohydrates.

The Standard American Diet (the acronym "SAD" is tragically telling) has *way* more sugar than anyone needs, and it's a veritable mass-delivery system for other simple carbs, which your body breaks down to create fast energy.

Most people know that if they're trying to eat healthy, they should avoid sugar-filled foods like pastries, confections, and candies, along with sodas. What many people fail to recognize is that many of the foods we often think of as "healthy" are also packed with sugar. This is in no small part because the thing we generally call "sugar"—the tiny white or brown granules we use for baking or add to our morning coffee—is actually just one type of sugar: sucrose. There are five other types of sugar: glucose, fructose, galactose, lactose, and maltose. As a result, even conscientious "label readers" can miss the fact that the food they're purchasing, and putting in their bodies, has added sugar that has been hidden in healthy-sounding ingredients like fruit juice, honey, nectar, agave, barley malt, and rice syrup. But regardless of their name, they cause our bodies to respond in roughly the same way: a sudden shockwave of sugar courses through our blood, and these blood-sugar fluctuations may cause cardiac scarring, which, over time, can cause atrial fibrillation.[21]

Another bulk supplier of simple carbs in many people's diets is refined grains like white flour and white rice, which have been stripped of most of their natural nutrients and fibers. The more processed a grain is, the faster it will be digested to make sugar. That has the added consequence of making these foods less filling, so when you eat a white rice dish or a piece of white toast, you're bound to be hungry again very soon. Sadly, even whole wheat bread isn't much better. A single slice can spike your blood glucose higher than a Snickers bar.

That doesn't mean you should avoid carbs altogether. Not at all. In fact, some researchers believe that while working to limit carbs in general might be a good idea, exceptionally low-carb diets may actually lead to a *greater* risk of AFib.[22] The key is making sure that, to the greatest extent possible, the carbohydrates you're getting are complex carbs, including fruits and especially vegetables. (We'll talk a lot more about these complex carb–rich, high-fiber foods in chapter nine.)

For now, though, it's important to do a realistic assessment of your habits related to sugars and processed carbs. Anyone who isn't actively avoiding foods with any and all types of added sugar, and limiting their carbohydrate intake to those foods that are packed with complex carbohydrates (think vegetables and fruit), may be at an increased risk of AFib.

## Your Electrolytes Are Out of Balance

Scientists aren't yet certain why competitive endurance athletes are so prone to atrial fibrillation, but one of the potential reasons is that long-distance athletic endeavors tax the body's balance of electrolytes.

But you definitely don't have to be a marathon runner for your electrolytes to be thrown out of whack. A sudden change in eating habits, some medications like diuretics (as Sakari discovered), and even simple incidences of dehydration can tip the balance of the electrically charged ions potassium, sodium, calcium, and magnesium, which play critical roles in ensuring your body holds onto enough water to function and help direct the electrical impulses that keep your heart beating. That, of course, makes electrolyte levels that are too high or too low potentially dangerous—especially to people who might already be prone to atrial fibrillation for other reasons.

One study from researchers in the Netherlands showed that low levels of potassium could quadruple the chances of AFib in some individuals.[23] Those experiencing magnesium deficiency are also at considerable risk.[24]

Most people can't simply "feel" an electrolyte imbalance, other than the occasional muscle cramp. However, if you're an endurance athlete, are prone to dehydration, are fighting kidney disease, have a hormonal or endocrine disorder, or have been taking chemotherapy drugs, diuretics, antibiotics, or corticosteroids, you may be at greater risk of an electrolyte imbalance that can increase your risk of AFib.

How can you know if your electrolytes are out of balance? A comprehensive metabolic panel—one of the many biomarker tests we'll discuss in chapter four—is the easiest way.

## Your Vitamin D or Thyroid Hormone Levels Are Out of Whack

A little thyroxine goes a long way. That's what Ayano, a veteran park ranger with the US National Park Service, discovered when she was forty-six years old.

Thyroxine is the main hormone created by the thyroid gland, and people suffering from hyperthyroidism have bodies that make way too much of it. That's a big problem because thyroxine is a potent cardiac stimulant. In a way, having hyperthyroidism is like having a little energy-drink factory in your neck. So, you can see why people who have hyperthyroidism might experience increased heart rates, palpitations, and arrhythmias such as atrial fibrillation.

The scary thing is it doesn't take full-blown hyperthyroidism to increase the risk of AFib. As Ayano learned, it doesn't take a lot of thyroxine to give our bodies and our hearts a jolt.

"One of the first things the doctors checked when I came into the hospital, after my first experience with AFib, was my thyroid hormone levels," she said. "I was within what they called 'the normal range,' but I was on the high side of that range."

That makes it likely that Ayano's AFib came in part because of a "high normal" thyroxine level. Our research showed that when people had thyroid hormone levels in the higher end of normal, they were 40 percent more likely to develop AFib.[25]

Another factor may have been at play in Ayano's case. For most of her career, she had been an interpretive park ranger in Arizona, where she spent most of her working hours outside, talking to visitors from around the world. About a year before her first experience with AFib, though, she had accepted a promotion to a management position in Montana. That meant a lot less sunlight.

"Like quite a few people of Asian descent, I'm lactose intolerant," she said, "so I wasn't getting any vitamin D that way, either. But honestly, until my doctor asked about it, I'd never even considered it might be a problem."

Most people know about vitamin D's role in bone health, but in recent years its other roles have come into better focus—including its association with thyroid diseases and, as you might have guessed by now, atrial fibrillation. More work is needed to understand the relationship between vitamin D levels and AFib, but the weight of the evidence so far suggests that too little or too much vitamin D may put you at risk.[26]

If you suspect that your thyroid hormone levels are too high (either from a thyroid disease or from taking thyroid hormone pills) or you recognize that you don't get a lot of vitamin D, it's likely these factors might increase your risk of AFib. But since even slightly higher-than-average levels of thyroid hormones can impact AFib rates, and since a little shift this way or that can matter when it comes to vitamin D, it's a good idea to get these biomarkers checked—we'll talk more about that soon.

## You're Relying Too Much on Energy Drinks or Alcohol

Cassandra was the proud "supermom" of three adorable elementary schoolers. She was also a full-time accountant, a part-time soccer coach, and the president of the parent-teacher association at her children's school. Staying on top of all that meant some late nights and early mornings.

Energy drinks were a big help. But, after a while, they started to take their toll.

For most people with AFib, caffeine isn't a problem. Indeed, studies have shown that the caffeine from chocolate, coffee, and tea doesn't trigger AFib for most people.[27] And while sugar-sweetened soda pop has clearly been linked to weight gain, diabetes, and hypertension (and even artificially sweetened soda pop can be a problem[28]), the good news is that these drinks don't appear to be causally related to atrial fibrillation.[29] But when caffeine is combined with other stimulants, such as those found in energy drinks, they may wreak havoc on your AFib, or even cause premature death, as their mingled effects make the drink more potent.[30] And if your caffeine intake is keeping you up at night and also harming your sleep, as it was in Cassandra's case, then it may further aggravate your atrial fibrillation.

Another complicating factor: genetics. Like about 50 percent of the population, Cassandra had a variant in the *CYP1A2* gene that slows the rate at which her body metabolizes caffeine.[31] The result was that even after a long and exhausting day, she often could not fall asleep. Her body simply couldn't process all those stimulating methylxanthine chemicals fast enough.

Eventually she developed heart palpitations. These palpitations often kept her up at night, which made matters even worse. She tried to ignore them at first, but, over time, they got worse, and she decided to go to the doctor to figure out what was wrong. Within a matter of days she had been diagnosed with paroxysmal atrial fibrillation, which is also known as intermittent AFib.

Remarkably, even after being told that her energy drink consumption was likely one of the aggravating factors for her AFib, Cassandra found it difficult to quit "cold turkey." And she's not alone. More than half of Americans have a persistent desire for caffeine or have failed at efforts to cut back, according to a study led by researchers at the Johns Hopkins University School of Medicine. Strikingly, the researchers found that one in seven Americans continues to use caffeine even after concluding it was harming their health in other ways, including stoking anxiety, worsening insomnia, and aggravating hypertension.[32] And that's just when it comes to caffeine. In most of those drinks, caffeine is mixed with taurine, glucuronolactone, guarana, ginseng, and ginkgo biloba, among other ingredients.

The good news is that energy drinks were the only chemicals Cassandra was regularly putting into her body. She didn't drink alcohol, which can significantly increase a person's risk of developing atrial fibrillation, even in quantities as small as a single serving of beer or wine per day,[33] which can cause scar tissue to form in the heart or directly damage its electrical pathways.[34]

Alcohol use doesn't just increase the risk of AFib. It also increases the risk of countless other diseases, including cancer. And while some studies have demonstrated that a small amount of alcohol can offer a few health benefits, when it comes to all-cause mortality those benefits are outweighed by the increased risk of other health-related harms, according to a 2018 study in the prestigious British medical journal, *The Lancet*, that pulled no punches. "The conclusions of the study are clear and unambiguous: alcohol is a colossal global health issue," the authors wrote, adding that there was strong support for a guideline published by the chief medical officer of the United Kingdom, who found there is "no safe level of alcohol consumption."[35]

None of this means you have to quit alcohol entirely. There is clearly a difference in health outcomes between people who drink the occasional alcoholic beverage and those who down a six-pack a day.

But if you're trying to take stock of the reasons you developed atrial fibrillation, or trying to understand your future risk, this much is clear: energy drinks are not your friend. And alcohol in any quantity can increase your risk.

## Your Sleep Is Off

Whenever people try to get healthier, and no matter what the underlying reason for that effort, they almost always start with diet and exercise. Those are two very important factors, but without addressing a third factor— sleep—people are almost assuredly doomed to fail in their efforts to eat better and exercise more.

Nonetheless, most of us are *really* bad at sleep. And as a global community, it would appear, we're actually getting worse at it, even as the science that demonstrates its importance to our lives has gotten more and more compelling. The World Health Organization has raised the possibility that sleep problems are an emerging global epidemic.[36] In the United States, 70 percent of adults report insufficient sleep at least once a month, and 11 percent report insufficient sleep every night.[37]

For a while, it did seem like we were getting the message about the importance of sleep to our health. After a century of consistently diminishing sleep, researchers who study the way we slumber noticed something promising. From 2004 to 2012, the number of people who were getting less than six hours of sleep each night finally started to level out. Maybe, some thought, we were finally getting the message. Or maybe, others argued, we'd simply hit rock bottom. Either way, it seemed, we could finally start working to move the needle in the other direction.

But when demographic sociologist Connor Sheehan and his collaborators dove into the subject in the late 2010s, they were dismayed by what they found. Yes, there had been a leveling out starting in 2004, but between 2013 and 2017 there was a significant shift. Far more people were reporting far less sleep. We hadn't hit rock bottom after all.

What changed? Among the most important factors are the devices we increasingly carry in our pockets and purses, and on our person. Closely coinciding with the plummeting rate of adequate sleep was the acceleration of smartphone ownership, which went from 35 percent in 2011 to 77 percent in 2016. "Americans now spend more time looking at a screen," Sheehan and his collaborators wrote, "and, due to the mobile nature of these devices, technology has increasingly entered the bedroom."[38]

This isn't just happening in the United States. More than five billion people around the world now have mobile devices, and more than half of those devices are smartphones. Leading the way in the adoption of tiny, glowing screens is South Korea, where 95 percent of adults have a smartphone and where, perhaps not coincidentally, adults get nearly forty minutes less sleep each night, on average, than their global counterparts.[39] Because smartphones may be a cause of poor sleep—and as these devices have become increasingly equipped to detect the health consequences that result from poor sleep—it should come as no surprise that atrial fibrillation diagnoses in Korea have been skyrocketing.[40]

The impact of poor sleep on AFib has been well documented. Even small interruptions of sleep quality and duration can increase the risk of atrial fibrillation by 47 percent,[41] and people who experience insomnia are 36 percent more likely to develop AFib.[42] People who do not reach deep levels of sleep—the sort of sleep that is key to recovery—have at least an 18 percent increased risk of atrial fibrillation, and it worsens each time they wake up at night. It's even worse for people with sleep disorders such as sleep apnea; they have a 200 to 400 percent increased risk of AFib over individuals without a sleep breathing disorder.[43] And the problem is compounded once AFib actually develops; the presence of an abnormal rhythm can increase the risk of poor sleep quality, or short sleep, by three to four times.[44] It's a vicious cycle.

That makes complete sense. In addition to the miserable experience of simply not feeling well rested, sleep deprivation causes the release of excess cortisol and adrenaline. Cortisol causes you to retain water, lose potassium, and have higher blood sugar and blood pressure. Adrenaline also increases your blood pressure, forcing your heart to work harder. In fact, when we want to trigger an atrial fibrillation episode during procedures intended to identify the trouble spots within a patient's heart, we give our patients a form of intravenous adrenaline.

As it turns out, sleep was indeed one of the key underlying issues that likely led to Paula's diagnosis.

"I'd always thought that getting less sleep was sort of something to be proud of," she said. "I was a highly effective teacher, I did a lot of volunteer work for my church, I was a pretty good tennis player, and I definitely like to think that I was a good mom for my three kids, too. People would say, 'You must not get much sleep' and I would sort of proudly say, 'Well, that's a sacrifice that is worth it to me.'"

What Paula has learned, though, is that her habitual lack of sleep was almost certainly related to her development of atrial fibrillation when she was just forty-seven years old.

"Once my heart started giving me such trouble, the irony was really clear to me," she said. "It was a lot harder to be a good teacher. I had to cut way back on my volunteer work. I couldn't play tennis anymore. I still think I'm a good mom, but part of being a good mom is being around, isn't it? And I'd put myself at greater risk for stroke, heart attacks, and all sorts of other potential medical problems that could have cut my life short."

Sleep didn't just contribute to Paula's AFib: it was also fundamental to her recovery. We'll come back to that part of her story in chapter five—and we'll also talk more at that time about how anyone can get more sleep and better sleep.

## You're Too Stressed

Angelica was fifty-seven years old when she was diagnosed with atrial fibrillation. It had been two years since her husband passed away suddenly of a heart attack and, while she missed him desperately, life was finally starting to feel as though it was returning to normal.

At the time, Angelica had been working for nearly twenty years as a manager at a grocery store that had recently been taken over by a new corporate owner. With one of her three children in college and another about to start, she was hopeful the new owner might be able to give her a raise—it had been years since she'd had one, after all. "But when I asked about that, they told me that my salary was actually higher than the equivalent for people in other stores in the chain, and while they were going to honor that level of pay, I shouldn't expect a raise any time soon," she said.

Angelica began driving for a rideshare company to make some extra money. "I actually enjoyed getting to meet so many new people all the time," she said, "but the driving part itself could be hard. The traffic in my city seems like it gets worse every day, and there is construction everywhere. Even though people are very nice, they're also very concerned about getting where they need to be as fast as possible, especially when they are trying to get to a meeting or to catch a plane."

Meanwhile, her youngest child had just started middle school. Like many children in that phase of life, he was having a rough time navigating the complexities of social groups and avoiding bullies. His anxiety about school got so bad that, for a few weeks, he refused to go at all, and it took an all-hands-on-deck meeting involving Angelica, the school counselor, the principal, and a private therapist to create the conditions that made the boy feel comfortable going back to school again.

As if all of that wasn't enough, Angelica had recently been told by her regular doctor that she was prediabetic and had hypertension.

"I guess it goes without saying that things were really stressful for me at that time," Angelica said.

When Angelica experienced her first episode of AFib, she panicked, thinking she was having a heart attack just like her husband. Her thoughts immediately turned to her children. When she learned at the hospital that what she actually had experienced was an arrhythmia, it came as a relief, at least at first.

"Pretty soon, though, AFib just felt like one more stress in my life," she said.

But this wasn't just another stressor. It was a stressor that was likely caused, at least in part, by the other stressors in her life—a real "double whammy."

Psychological stress has long been thought to be a possible trigger of atrial fibrillation,[45] and the association appears to be strong among women.[46] But men aren't immune.

Neither are cardiologists—who, it can be said, have one of the most stressful jobs in the world. That's what Dr. Damien Legallois learned when he was just twenty-eight years old.

"I was on call when a cardiac arrest call came from our cardiac intensive care unit, pulling me from my sleep," he wrote of his experience in a letter to the *International Journal of Cardiology*. "It was a false alert and I went back to bed when I noticed some palpitations. My pulse was rapid and seemed irregular."

An electrocardiogram (EKG) of Legallois's heart showed atrial fibrillation with a ventricular rate of more than 180 beats per minute.[47] And Legallois isn't alone. We have treated countless doctors over the years with AFib as well as innumerable CEOs, lawyers, accountants, politicians, athletes, celebrities, and others who have come to see us for treatment largely because of the enormous stresses they are under.

If a stressful incident can push a young cardiologist with no history of heart problems—or any major medical issues for that matter—into atrial fibrillation, imagine what it can do to someone like Angelica, who was already facing some health challenges and many other life stressors.

What kinds of challenges can create stress that triggers AFib? A research group in Denmark concluded that the severely stressful experience of losing a partner increased the risk of atrial fibrillation for an entire year.[48] Another international group of researchers found that divorced men had a higher incidence of death associated with atrial fibrillation.[49] And a group from Sweden revealed a potential dose-response relationship between work-related stress, like getting fired from a job, and atrial fibrillation.[50] In fact, the Swedish researchers found that just the experience of having a job with high psychological demands and with little control over your work situation could increase your AFib risk by 50 percent.[51]

When Yale University researcher and electrophysiologist Dr. Rachel Lampert surveyed the way her patients were feeling emotionally to see if she could predict whether or not they would go into AFib that day, the results were absolutely startling. In a 2014 study published in the *Journal of the American College of Cardiology*, she noted that feelings of sadness, anger, stress, impatience, and anxiety increase the risk of an AFib attack up to 500 percent in the same day. Happiness, meanwhile, appears to be protective. If you are feeling happy, you are 85 percent less likely to have your heart go out of rhythm that day, according to Lampert's research.[52]

Thus, it is no surprise that those who deal with deep and abiding feelings of sadness and disengagement might be even more at risk. Depression is simply not good for the heart, especially when it comes to AFib. One study showed that depression increases the risk of AFib by up to 700 percent.[53] Fortunately, this same study showed that getting your depression treated dramatically reduces your risk. But with more than sixteen million Americans, and hundreds of millions of others around the world, dealing with depression, there are a lot of people who have a significant risk factor for AFib and don't even know it.

But emotional and mental stress aren't the only things that can send your body into a state of chaos. Researchers have connected AFib episodes to physical stressors caused by events like surgery, bad infections, and car crashes.[54] In the case of irregular, singular events like those, there is a chance that after the stressor has passed, the AFib will go away. More likely, though, this is a harbinger of things to come. Our hearts are remarkably resilient, but if an incident of great stress pushed you into AFib, something else has likely been pushing you toward that precipice a long time before that incident occurred.

## You're a Smoker or Live in a Polluted City

If you haven't been to Salt Lake City, it's worth a trip. It's nestled into the foothills of the splendid Wasatch Mountains, and there are few cities in the world that boast such immediate access to the outdoors. In the summer, it's a paradise for hikers and mountain bikers. For skiers and snowboarders, the winters are simply legendary.

Sounds nice, right? Well, before calling the moving company, there's another thing you should know about Utah's capital city. Because it rests in a valley, nearly surrounded by mountains, it suffers from lengthy inversions: weather events in which cold, polluted air gets trapped under a blanket of warmer air. During these periods, studies show, the air can get more harmful with each passing hour and can even increase the incidence of deadly diseases.[55] Among these diseases is atrial fibrillation; researchers have demonstrated a significant association between the development of AFib and the gaseous pollutants most often found in toxic air.[56]

Can bad air trigger individual AFib events? That question was at the heart of one of our early studies to assess the risks of short-term elevations in exposure to fine-particulate air pollution. Fortunately, our study failed to identify any measurable risk, so an occasional trip to a place where the air is bad isn't likely to trigger an AFib episode, particularly if it's brief.[57]

In the long term, however, bad air can be a very bad thing.

While not everyone has a choice about where they live, everyone *can* choose what they voluntarily put into their bodies. Yet across the globe, more than one billion people smoke or vape tobacco products, according to the World Health Organization. You won't be surprised to learn that people who smoke have a substantially increased risk of developing atrial fibrillation,[58] not to mention all of the other health problems smoking causes, from cancer to emphysema. Even living with or being around a smoker can increase your AFib risk. Every pack of cigarettes an adult smokes on an average day increases their children's risk of getting AFib by 18 percent.[59] That's a legacy no parent wants to leave.

Regardless of how toxic air gets into your lungs, if it's there, there's a good chance it has increased your risk of AFib.

## TRIGGERS

Now that we've discussed the most common substrate causes, it's time to talk about triggers.

Remember: causes are what lead a person to get AFib, while triggers are the things that incite specific incidents of arrhythmia. Sometimes, triggers are very obvious. Other times, they're subtle or impossible to determine.

A few years ago, researchers from the University of California at San Francisco tried to better understand the diversity of perceived triggers that exist for people with AFib. What they found in their investigation was that people who are healthier usually have definitive triggers, while people who are less healthy might not even require a trigger to push their heart out of rhythm.[60] They also found that while just about everyone has different perceived triggers, some are far more common than others.

The top three? Alcohol, caffeine, and exercise—in that order. While all of these factors may be part of the combination of causes that push people toward AFib, it would be very rare for any of these factors alone to be the sole cause. But once someone is at that precipice, alcohol, caffeine, and exercise can be powerful inciting triggers that can send their heart out of control.

Alcohol as an AFib trigger shouldn't come as a big surprise. Any emergency room doctor can share many stories of high school or college students who have presented with AFib after binge drinking. Caffeine is a powerful stimulant that can have a significant impact on our hearts. And because exercise is the most natural way in the world to shift our hearts into higher gear, it's no shock that, if your heart is already prone to beating erratically, a quick burst of exercise could push it over the edge.

After alcohol, caffeine, and exercise, the second tier of AFib triggers include lack of sleep, dehydration, large meals, and stress or anxiety. That last one is particularly interesting, because it wasn't one of the choices provided in the survey. Respondents had to proactively write it on their questionnaire. Thus, it is quite possible that stress and anxiety could be an even bigger AFib trigger than alcohol.

The third tier of AFib triggers from this study included lying on the left side of the body (a position in which gravity pulls your heart against your chest wall), cold beverages and foods, salty foods, and other specific food triggers, in addition to not exercising at all.

Why would food be a trigger? Perhaps because gastrointestinal (GI) problems are known to stimulate the vagus nerve, which connects your gut, heart, and brain. We don't understand this connection in depth, but our research has shown that GI diseases are associated with atrial fibrillation.[61] Also, when those GI issues have resolved, the AFib usually settles down as well. We also know that GI triggers may be far more prevalent than this study indicated—as was the case with stress and anxiety, problems like bloating, nausea, or constipation weren't among the preprinted triggers on the survey and thus had to be handwritten in.

## PUTTING IT ALL TOGETHER

Very few people have all of the attributes we've discussed so far in this chapter. But most people who develop atrial fibrillation have *many* of these substrate causes working against them. It's exceptionally rare to find an AFib patient who doesn't have several of these situations in their lives.

And, among those with genetic risk factors for AFib, any *one* of these conditions can be all it takes to push an otherwise healthy person into a dangerous arrhythmia.

But, as you might have noticed, all of these factors are characteristic of *many* other diseases. AFib just happens to be the disease that often comes first.

In this way, atrial fibrillation is the canary in the coalmine. And like the little yellow birds coal miners used to take deep underground with them to warn of potentially deadly gases, AFib could be the thing that saves your life. Because if you're ready, willing, and able to make some pretty big decisions about the way you live your life, AFib is almost always very treatable.

We can't say the same about stroke, one of the most common and feared complications of AFib; a first bout of atrial fibrillation is rarely the last thing that will happen to you, while a stroke is the final mortal experience for millions of people across the globe each year.

We also can't say the same thing for Alzheimer's disease, dementia, and vascular disease; our study, published in 2010 by the journal *Heart Rhythm*, established that all of those diseases, which are hard or impossible to reverse, are independently associated with atrial fibrillation.[62]

And we can't say the same thing about cancer; atrial fibrillation, researchers believe, is a "risk marker" for a future diagnosis of cancer,[63] which ultimately kills about half of the people it besets.[64] AFib has also been connected in peer-reviewed studies to heart attacks, heart failure, chronic kidney disease, and venous thromboembolism.[65]

What AFib offers is an opportunity to get ahead of *all* of that. To hear and heed the call of the canary in the coalmine. To recognize that something is off. To take stock of the rhythm of our lives in such a way as to ensure that the beat goes on.

And on.

And on.

And *that's* the good news. Whether you have every one of these risk factors or just one (and even if you have none at all), you can take control of your life in such a way that can cure your AFib or avert it altogether. And, in doing so, you can take a tremendously important step toward preventing all of those other diseases, too.

Yes, this is going to take some hard work. But if you've come this far, you've already taken the first step: you've identified the potential causes for an increased risk of AFib.

"Potential" is an important word here. Perhaps you drink a little more alcohol than you probably should, or you don't sleep as much as you should. That doesn't mean you'll get AFib. Likewise, if you've already been diagnosed, those aren't necessarily the reasons why you developed this arrhythmia. It also doesn't mean that, if you allow those situations to persist, you won't be able to put your AFib into remission.

But please don't forget that this is a battle for a better quality of life—if not life itself. In such a fight, isn't it best to target as many of the potential causes of AFib as possible?

It is. It absolutely is. And that's something that becomes crystal clear when we dive into the physiology of a human body suffering from atrial fibrillation.

## AFIB CAUSES CHECKLIST
### (CHECK ALL THAT APPLY TO YOU)

### Possible or known genetic predisposition

❑   A genetic test has confirmed a mutation in one or more genes associated with AFib

❑   You or a family member developed AFib before age fifty

❑   You have a close family member with AFib

### Other prior or current heart problems

❑   Heart blockages

❑   Heart attack

❑   Heart failure

❑   Heart valve problems

## Age

- ❑ Over sixty
- ❑ Over seventy
- ❑ Over eighty
- ❑ Over ninety

## Blood pressure

- ❑ Over 130/80

## Medications

- ❑ Antiarrhythmics
- ❑ Stimulants
- ❑ Steroids
- ❑ Nonsteroidal anti-inflammatory drugs (ibuprofen, naproxen, etc.)
- ❑ Diuretics
- ❑ Thyroid hormone
- ❑ Proton-pump inhibitors (Prilosec, Prevacid, Protonix, etc.)
- ❑ Marijuana/THC

## Exercise

- ❑ No regular exercise program
- ❑ Endurance athlete

## Metabolism

- ❑ Overweight
- ❑ Obese

## Sugar and processed carbohydrates

- ❑ Regular sugar consumption
- ❑ Regular processed carbohydrate consumption

## Electrolytes

- ❑ Low potassium (below 3.5 mEq/L)
- ❑ Low magnesium (below 1.8 mg/dL)

### Vitamin D and thyroid hormone

- ❑ Low vitamin D (below 20 ng/mL)
- ❑ High vitamin D (above 100 ng/mL)

### Energy drinks or alcohol

- ❑ Energy drink consumption
- ❑ Alcohol consumption

### Sleep

- ❑ Less or more than seven to nine hours per night
- ❑ Sleep apnea

### Mental and emotional stress

- ❑ Sadness
- ❑ Anger
- ❑ Stress
- ❑ Impatience
- ❑ Anxiety
- ❑ Depression

### Smoking and pollution

- ❑ Smoking and tobacco use of any kind
- ❑ Poor air quality in your home city

This is not an exhaustive checklist of substrate causes, nor do any of these causes present the same risk for AFib. The more of these boxes you have checked, however, the more work you may have to do to put your AFib into remission. But please don't be discouraged—no matter how many boxes you've checked, there's almost certainly someone else out there who has started from a similar place and tremendously improved their life by following the practices in this book.

## Chapter Two

# ⎯⎯⎯⎯⎯⎯⎯ ⩊ INSIDE OUT ⩊ ⎯⎯⎯⎯⎯⎯⎯

Why understanding what is happening in your body is
vital to building your mindset for the battle ahead

When Lucas was diagnosed with atrial fibrillation in the late 2000s, his doctor told him there probably wasn't much he could do about it.

"Believe it or not, my doc sort of had me convinced it was the beginning of the end," said Lucas, who was in his mid-sixties and had been running a general construction business for more than forty years at the time of his diagnosis. "He said, 'Just get used to feeling this way because once AFib starts, it just keeps getting worse.'"

While most doctors will tell you that atrial fibrillation gets worse as you get older, most are unaware of how bad "worse" is. Duke University's Jonathan Piccini has demonstrated that for people sixty-five or older, an atrial fibrillation diagnosis means there is a one-in-four chance of dying within the next year.[1]

That statistic—which Lucas found online—was a wake-up call. "And man-oh-man," he recalled, "I just figured, if I'm going out, I want to make sure whatever time I had left was as good as possible."

It's important to note here that Lucas's wake-up call wasn't to get *healthier*. It was simply to enjoy the time he thought he had left. He left the doctor's office on that day with a feeling of despair and resolve to make the best of a bad situation, rather than a feeling of hope and determination to improve his life.

Lucas sold his business, and his house, and moved to a cabin on the edge of the Flathead National Forest in Montana. He took his AFib medications regularly, figuring that was as much as he could do to keep things from getting even worse.

Almost every weekend one set of grandkids or another would come to visit him, "but on the weekdays, to tell you the truth, it did get a little bit boring," he said, "so one day I just decided that I was going to set off for a hike, and I just walked until I was as far as I thought it was safe to go, and then turned around and walked back." The hikes became a daily habit, and they got longer and longer every day. By the end of the year, Lucas was regularly hiking fifteen miles almost every day.

He'd never been obese, but he nonetheless began to drop a lot of excess weight. "I attribute that as much to the way I was eating as to the hikes," he said. "When I was working, a drive-through burger on a big bun, fries, and a soda was lunch just about every day. Once I started hiking, I'd just pack in some nuts and dried fruits for lunch."

Having retired from the day-to-day headaches of running a business, he was also feeling a lot less stressed. "And then one day I just realized—it had been a long time since I had an AFib episode, and it suddenly dawned on me that maybe I had more time left than I thought I did."

Almost by accident, Lucas had found hope.

A decade after his first AFib episode, Lucas was a model of health. He was still hiking every day, and he was no longer taking AFib medications. Not only had he proven that atrial fibrillation isn't anything like a death sentence, he showed that life can actually get *better* after the diagnosis.

While not everyone can send their AFib into remission without meaning to, the truth is that the 25 percent one-year mortality rate revealed by the study Lucas stumbled across on the internet should *never* have been that high. Over the years, a lot of people have died from diseases and medical events associated with atrial fibrillation who could have been helped if their doctors had only told them to make some of the same simple changes Lucas discovered on his own.

It's not like AFib is new to us, after all. The first known description of a condition that's most likely AFib can be found in a Chinese text that's at least 2,000 years old, the origins of which might date back *another* 2,000 years.[2] The *Huangdi Neijing,* also known as *The Yellow Emperor's Classic of Medicine,* says, "When the pulse is irregular and tremulous . . . then the impulse of life fades." Think about that! Even before the advent of the Qin Dynasty, which marks the beginning of Imperial China, doctors appeared to be associating AFib with age, and using it to mark the beginning of the end. For most of the years since then we've stuck quite closely to that approach.

Now, as the years went by, there were almost certainly some doctors who recognized that atrial fibrillation could be addressed through diet and exercise—it's too obvious to have been missed for that long. Those doctors, however, don't appear to have gotten the attention of the medical establishment, for the historical medical literature on atrial fibrillation is rather lacking until the late 1700s, when the English physician William Withering, who had come upon a traditional herbal remedy made with foxglove, first reported that the plant seemed to be effective at making an irregular heartbeat "more full and more regular."[3] The active chemical compound that was later isolated from foxglove is now known as digoxin. (Note that while digoxin has gradually been falling out of favor as a modern-day treatment strategy for AFib, most pharmacies still carry it.)

Withering's discovery ushered in the era of modern therapeutics—including and perhaps especially for the condition Withering had first tried to treat with foxglove. For centuries to come, researchers remained on the hunt for better and better pharmaceutical treatments to what many physicians continued to believe was an inevitable condition of old age.

These ideas about atrial fibrillation can perhaps be forgiven by those who had no way of knowing what was actually happening inside a person's heart during an episode of AFib. Theories abounded, but it wasn't until the 1990s that an "explosion of research" into the mechanisms of AFib, including studies in which scientists induced AFib in model organisms, and technology that allowed us to peek inside the human body, "greatly modified our perspective and had a significant impact on therapeutic approaches."[4] By that time, though, thousands of years of conventional wisdom about the inevitability of AFib, and hundreds of years of using drugs to treat it, had metastasized. Thus it's not at all surprising that Lucas's physician's advice was to prepare for a fast decline en route to the cemetery. Patients were getting advice like that all the time back then. Sadly, they still do today.

But now we know better. Or we should. Because while there are still certain mysteries about *why* atrial fibrillation occurs—it's different in every-one, as you know—we no longer have to guess about what is happening inside the human body *when* AFib occurs.

These days, we know a lot.

## THE INSIDE STORY

Having already read chapter one, you now have a grasp of what factors in your life either played a role in the development of your atrial fibrillation or put you at greater risk for developing AFib, as well as those that are likely to trigger your arrhythmia. And now, at this point in this chapter, you also have a good understanding of how it came to be that so many patients have been told that their best option for dealing with AFib is to take handfuls of drugs in an increasingly futile attempt to make things "less bad." But before we can truly dive into all of the ways to address the risk factors, and before we can undo centuries of conventional wisdom about this disease, there is one more thing we need to know: what exactly is happening *inside* the body of someone with atrial fibrillation?

Atrial fibrillation, as you know, isn't *only* a disease of the heart. But we can start there, because that's where the symptoms are most pronounced and usually the place where we first notice the problem.

To get there, it's helpful to picture one of those zany Rube Goldberg machines. You know these things—they are the sorts of contraptions that are both ridiculously and charmingly designed to link together a bunch of common items, each one kinetically acting upon the next to complete a simple task in a complicated way. A marble is rolled down a track and bumps into a spring. The spring is sprung and strikes a Matchbox car. The car rolls down a ramp and knocks a pin out of place. And since the pin was holding down one end of a rope on a pulley, and the other end was attached to a weight, the pulley is set into action, raising a flag. Ta-da!

These are the sorts of ways in which each of the stressors we discussed in chapter one may ultimately lead you down the AFib path—things like smoking, high blood pressure, diabetes, and prediabetes; failing to achieve moderate levels of daily exercise; too much stress; not getting enough quality sleep; and other stressors.

Take body fat, for instance. We've all got some. We need it, in fact. But most of us have too much of it. And while we might not particularly like the way it looks, that's really the least of our concerns, because fat doesn't just sit along our bellies. If there is fat around your waist, then odds are that your heart is encased in fat as well, and that's making your heart work harder by increasing needed pumping pressure. It's also releasing immune system chemicals called cytokines, among other damaging substances, right into your heart.

Fat is just one of many stressors. Each one sets into motion a very different kind of physiological chain reaction leading to a premature beat from one of four veins that lead from the lungs to the heart, known as pulmonary veins, in the left atrium, one of the two upper cavities of the heart.

If you were to look at these veins under a microscope, you would see cardiac muscle cells line a portion of these veins. The tissues composed of these cells are very sensitive to any physical stress, including stress from elevated pumping pressure in the left atrium, inflammation, adrenaline and other hormonal changes, and vagus nerve stimulation. Sometimes the heart muscle tissue in your pulmonary veins becomes diseased, through either poor lifestyle choices or bad genetics. Either way, this is most often the point at which AFib begins within the heart—a spark that can light a fire. If the heart is perfectly healthy, the blaze won't go far. But if the cardiac muscle cell is repeatedly injured, either through lifestyle or other medical conditions that result in inflammation, there's plenty of kindling in the form of fibrosis.

*Fibrosis* is a fancy term for scar tissue, which is made up of dead heart cells. If there's no fibrosis in your atria, then a spark from the pulmonary veins probably won't trigger an AFib episode. However, the more fibrosis you develop, the more likely it is that one randomly occurring premature beat from the pulmonary veins, or elsewhere in the atria, is all you need for a full-blown AFib attack, and a resulting visit to the emergency room. That's why, if your goal is to stop AFib from getting worse, you absolutely have to stop the ongoing process of scarring. And if your goal is to make things better, you can't just stop fibrosis—you have to reverse it.

Before you can fight fibrosis, though, you've got to understand what it is.

Fibrosis occurs naturally with aging—particularly after age sixty. But natural scarring usually isn't enough to sustain an AFib episode from a pulmonary vein–initiated premature contraction. Excessive fibrosis, on the other hand, may disrupt how normal heart cells, called cardiomyocytes, look and move, just as the kind of scarring we're most familiar with—called dermal fibrosis—can make our scarred skin look and move differently from the rest of our skin. When we remember that every part of our heart is in constant movement, and all of those parts have been designed to work in harmony with the others, it becomes clear how this can become problematic. Imagine, for instance, what would happen if you were to replace a valve in your home plumbing with one that was ever-so-slightly different in shape, or that moved a little differently from the valve that came before. Everything downstream of that valve would be affected, right? The same

thing is happening in the hearts of people with atrial fibrillation when cardiomyocytes are transformed from their ever-supple natural state to the
tough and inflexible nature of scar tissue.

But unlike most home plumbing, our bloodstreams are part of a closed
circulatory system. In a manner of thinking, then, *everything* in our bodies
is downstream of our atria, at all times. (Like the drawings of never-ending
stairs by famous Dutch graphic artist M. C. Escher, even our atria are
downstream of our atria!) So when fibrosis impacts the very shape and
movement of our hearts—like when you see left atrial enlargement on an
cardiac ultrasound, also known as an echocardiogram—*everything* in the
system is affected. You can see this in the echocardiogram image below.
(By way of convention, cardiac ultrasound images like this are inverted—
left is right and top is bottom.) The key here is to note that the right and
left atria should be much smaller than the right and left ventricles. But, in
this case, both the right and left atria are massively enlarged. The result is
that there was little that could be done at this point to keep this patient's
heart in normal rhythm; the key is to intervene before changes like this
become permanent.

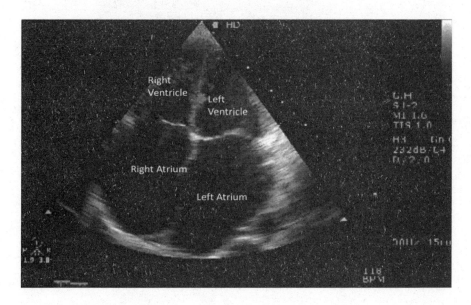

That, however, is not the worst of it. In heart tissue, fibrosis causes another problem: it changes the ways in which electrical impulses move through our hearts.

To understand this, it's helpful to get a look at a healthy heart. Below is a "fibrosis map" of the posterior (back) wall of the left atrium of a fit and healthy forty-two-year-old man. On this map, you can see four pulmonary veins entering into the left atrium, with a high-definition mapping catheter in the vicinity of the left lower pulmonary vein. Using this tool, we can read the electrical voltages that course through the heart.

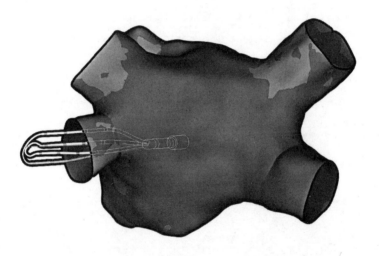

All of the darker areas on this map are places where there is a strong electrical signal—and, as you can see, the darker shading is everywhere, even a few centimeters up the shaft of each pulmonary vein. Thus, there is no detectable fibrosis. Every heart cell is electrically connected to its neighbors, contracting at once in response to electrical signals. This is how a healthy heart beats.

By contrast, the next image is a fibrosis map of a seventy-four-year-old woman suffering from obesity, high blood pressure, diabetes, and long-standing persistent AFib.

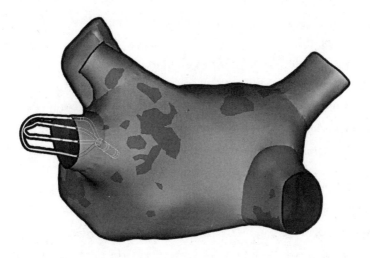

As you can see, there are only a few spotty areas in which electrical voltages are moving unimpeded through healthy heart tissue. The rest of the tissue is scarred.

Imagine what happens when an electrical signal courses through a heart like this. The disconnected healthy heart cells can't respond together. The result is chaos.

There is an old saying among cardiologists that "AFib begets AFib." What this means is that the more episodes of AFib your heart has, the easier it will be for the heart to go into AFib again. Think of this as negative cardiac muscle memory—a cycle that can add additional fibrosis to your heart independent of diabetes, high blood pressure, sleep apnea, excess body weight, and any other stressor. Eventually this may lead to your heart being stuck out of rhythm all the time. Studies have shown that just a thirty-minute episode of AFib is all your heart needs to start rewiring itself to make it *want* to go into AFib.[5] And five weeks of continuous AFib is all you need for the AFib alone to start adding more fibrosis to your heart, regardless of whether the other substrate causes are addressed.[6] Fortunately, studies also show that one good week of normal heart rhythm, also known as sinus rhythm, may be all you need to help break this downward spiral.[7] Once the AFib cycle begins, though, one good week might start to feel like a pipe dream.

In sum, cardiac fibrosis rewires the circuitry that controls the central machine in our circulatory system. It's as if the network of wires and fuses that keeps our homes lit has suddenly lost a few connection points.

This combination of pathology and electrophysiology results in a situation not unlike both the plumbing *and* the electricity in your home being thrown into disorder at the *same time*.

The result is an irregular heartbeat—a quiver—that materializes in the form of the four basic types of AFib.

The first type is known as *paroxysmal atrial fibrillation*. This is AFib that starts, then stops, all by itself. An episode of paroxysmal AFib might last thirty seconds. It can sometimes last a few hours. In some cases, it can stick around for days. The experience can be annoying or terrifying. Either way, though, it's potentially causing long-term damage to the rest of the body. In most of our patients with paroxysmal atrial fibrillation, however, only limited fibrosis has developed. These patients have the best chance of ultimately putting their AFib into remission.

The second type is *persistent atrial fibrillation*. As the name implies, this is AFib that doesn't stop, and the only way to get the heart back into a normal rhythm is through antiarrhythmic medications, an electrical shock (also known as a *cardioversion*), or an ablation procedure. There's no guarantee, however, that this will "fix" a quivering heart. When addressed by antiarrhythmic medications or cardioversion, the reset is usually just temporary; most people who have had their heart brought back into a normal rhythm through antiarrhythmic medications or cardioversion will develop atrial fibrillation again after some time. What's worse, studies show that antiarrhythmic medications and cardioversion don't increase life expectancy, nor are these measures protective against the medical conditions that are associated with atrial fibrillation, like stroke.[8] To put it another way: antiarrhythmic medications and cardioversion might buy you a little more rhythm, but not a little more life. If you have persistent AFib, you probably already have a fair amount of fibrosis in your atria.

The third type is *long-standing persistent atrial fibrillation.* This is unin-terrupted AFib—not a single beat of normal sinus rhythm—for more than a year. It would be shocking if this didn't leave a tremendous amount of fibrosis in the atria, and, indeed, patients with long-standing persistent atrial fibrillation usually have a lot of scarring. While all forms of AFib are bad news, this is the worst when it comes to the chances of restoring nor-mal sinus rhythm, because it usually can't be corrected with medication or cardioversion for any meaningful length of time. That doesn't mean things are hopeless, but it does mean it's time to be especially aggressive in the way you proceed if you want any chance of restoring normal rhythm again.

The last type of AFib is known as *permanent atrial fibrillation*, although this is a bit of a misnomer, because all "permanent" really means is that your doctor has given up on ever trying to get your heart back into normal sinus rhythm again. Sometimes this is justified; after many years of continuous AFib, without ever a beat of normal sinus rhythm, there is usually so much fibrosis that patients are in quite dire straits. But we've seen many cases—far too many, in fact—in which a patient's doctor simply gave up too early. There is always hope, if not for a complete cure, then for improvement in your quality of life.

No matter what type of atrial fibrillation a person might have, however, AFib itself usually doesn't kill people. That's important to know, although it also sort of hides the point, because the myriad conditions and diseases that AFib causes or aggravates can all be killers.

## THE THINGS THAT KILL

Since atrial fibrillation is caused when heart cells are damaged, it's probably not surprising to learn that most deaths among people with AFib are related to a cardiovascular problem, with heart failure accounting for more than half of those deaths.[9] This makes sense, of course. Heart failure occurs when the ventricles, the lower chambers of the heart, become either too weak or too stiff, making it difficult for them to fill with blood between beats. And what fills the ventricles? The atria, where AFib occurs.

Heart failure is caused by hearts that have become too weakened or too stiffened. Does that sound familiar? Indeed, the same conditions that cause atrial fibrosis can also induce ventricular fibrosis,[10] and ventricle remodeling, which can cause heart failure.[11]

Death by heart failure is a terrible fate, with pain that travels throughout the body, a futile struggle for breath, a body drowning from fluid retention, and, in so many very terrible cases, a final few moments spent in fear and panic. And so, if an increased risk of heart failure was *all* that AFib could do to us, it would be enough to do everything we can to battle this disease. The good news is that, as our research has shown, if atrial fibrillation is the cause of heart failure, then getting rid of AFib can also often get rid of heart failure.[12] The bad news is that heart failure isn't the only thing that gets AFib patients in the end.

The second most common cause of death among people who have been diagnosed with atrial fibrillation is infection. At first this might not seem to make sense—what does one have to do with the other? In many cases the association isn't directly causal. People who are unhealthy in any way are more likely to have trouble battling infections. And people who spend time in hospitals, for any reason, are more likely to pick up a healthcare-associated infection. Infections that come as a result of medical treatment kill nearly 100,000 people each year in the United States alone.[13] That's about three times the number of Americans who die in motor vehicle crashes each year, and yet we almost never hear about it. Atrial fibrillation more than doubles a person's risk of hospitalization,[14] which is one of the reasons why just having AFib adds a point to the "prediction score" for developing an infection while in a medical facility.[15]

It is possible that there is a more direct association, too. That's because atrial fibrillation is a disease caused by damaged cells, and the human immune system responds to damaged cells the same way it responds to irritants and pathogens—with inflammation. For example, we published a study a number of years ago showing that when a bacterium called *Helicobacter pylori* infects the GI tract, the result is a heightened inflammatory or immune response and increased rates of atrial fibrillation.[16] The "all hands on deck" immune response we know as inflammation is often beneficial. We can't fight infections or heal damaged tissue without it. But when it persists over time, the response can become troublesome. That can be particularly true when it comes to infections. If our immune system is already exhausted from being called into action by AFib, after all, what will we have left to fight new pathogens? This could be why our research has consistently linked chronic inflammation to an increased risk of atrial fibrillation.[17]

We cannot complete a conversation about AFib-associated killers without speaking of stroke, an event in which the flow of blood to part of the brain is cut off, causing downstream areas of the brain to die—sometimes all within seconds.

One of the world's most famous cases of an AFib-related stroke occurred on April 18, 1994. On that day, former US President Richard Nixon, while preparing to eat dinner in his home after a day spent preparing for an upcoming speech, suffered a massive stroke from an AFib-induced blood clot. Almost instantaneously, he couldn't speak and the right side of his body was paralyzed. And even though he was immediately rushed to New York Hospital–Cornell Medical Center in New York City, some of the world's best doctors couldn't save him. He passed away four days later, leaving behind a complicated legacy and also a warning for those with AFib.[18]

Strokes are common in AFib patients because the complete electrical chaos in the atria leads to loss of pumping. The result is stagnant blood flow, and stagnant blood clots easily, especially in the left atrial appendage. When these clots break off and enter the bloodstream, they are like missiles that can go anywhere in the body and do incredible damage. Clots that go to your gut, kidneys, or legs can all leave a trail of destruction. But when clots go to the brain, resulting in a stroke, the effect is immediate, devastating, and often deadly.

During a stroke, the brain is starved of oxygen and nutrients, a situation that almost immediately begins to kill brain cells. You'll also recall that AFib is usually associated with high blood pressure. That's a double disaster, since years of high blood pressure can damage the arteries in the brain long before the atrial fibrillation clot ever arrives. For all of these reasons, atrial fibrillation has been associated with a fivefold increase in the risk of stroke.[19] Those risks aren't uniform, of course. They increase with age, and also with other complicating medical conditions. But even among AFib patients who are young and relatively healthy in other ways, *no one* with AFib is safe from stroke. Strokes in patients with atrial fibrillation that do not kill often result in greater disability compared to strokes caused from other reasons. Even "small" strokes over time can impair cognition and greatly increase the risk of dementia.

Of course, AFib isn't only associated with death. Its impact on our lives is usually felt long before the end—in ways that sadly make some people feel as though the end wouldn't actually be so bad.

## A LIVING NIGHTMARE

Most people associate AFib with palpitations—a feeling that Lucas described as "like having a washing machine for a heart, putting a pair of steel-toe boots in it, and setting it on 'spin.'" Some say they feel that their heart is "flip-flopping" back and forth. Some say the sensation makes it seem as though their heart has "skipped a beat."

No matter how you perceive this feeling, it can, at a bare minimum, feel quite annoying. It can also be quite scary—even for people who have experienced it for years.

AFib patients often describe feeling as if they are "walking on egg-shells," always afraid that an unknown or unexpected trigger might spark an episode of AFib, requiring a cardioversion to get their hearts back into rhythm. Atrial fibrillation doesn't respect your schedule or plans; it can come in the middle of the night, while on an airplane, or in remote places far from medical help. As a result, for many AFib patients, the world gets smaller and smaller. They stop traveling and become reluctant to stray too far from the nearest hospital, where they become all too familiar with the sensation of being zapped with a low-voltage dose of electricity. (No, your body doesn't fly into the air when they put the paddles to your chest like you might see on TV. When done right, it is a quick and painless procedure without much, if any, drama.)

The problem with cardioversions, though, is that these procedures don't fix anything. They are just an electrical reset—kind of like rebooting your computer. In fact, our research shows that cardioversions just lead to more cardioversions.[20]

But even though a cardioversion doesn't fix anything long term, sometimes this short-term reprieve is necessary, particularly for those who are committed to fighting their AFib in other ways. It will be hard, if not impossible, to follow all of the steps in this book if you are stuck in a state of persistent AFib. Nonetheless, for many people, the thought of another cardioversion—never knowing when it might be needed—is enough to cause severe anxiety.

"Every time my heart would start racing, my mind would start racing, too," said Laura, a competitive cross-country skier who was first diagnosed with AFib when she was forty-four. "Intellectually, I knew what was going on and I knew it would pass, but emotionally it always sent me into such a sense of fear."

## THE COMMON AFIB SYMPTOMS

Once you know how AFib disrupts the flow of blood through the heart, and interferes with the electrical signals that command the heart to beat, it's not hard to understand why AFib causes many of its most common symptoms and, in particular, palpitations.

However, many of our patients mistakenly believe they don't have any AFib symptoms because they can't feel the palpitations that are commonly associated with this arrhythmia. In our experience, though, the most common symptom isn't palpitations but rather fatigue—and behind that symptom is shortness of breath. Palpitations are a distant third. That's a big problem: since so many people don't experience palpitations with their AFib, many times people who really need help don't get it.

It can, of course, be hard to pin feelings of being fatigued and breathless to one specific problem. These symptoms are side effects of many medications. They can also result from not exercising regularly, being overweight, or not sleeping well. But if you're feeling tired and breathless, and you can't figure out why, you need to find out.

Laura didn't do that, at first. "I've skied my whole life," she recalled. "Suddenly I couldn't anymore. I was always so tired—the way I used to feel after a race, except I wasn't racing."

That is likely because Laura's heart was beating much faster than normal and her body was struggling to keep up. It takes a lot of energy to keep a heart on overdrive, the same sort of energy it takes to engage in a heavy workout. But, like many people, Laura initially chalked up these symptoms as the consequences of "getting too old." (Which is why, when we help our patients get their hearts back into normal rhythm again, they often remark how much younger they feel.)

Lightheadedness, dizziness, and confusion are also very common symptoms of atrial fibrillation. "Brain fog," the feeling of not being able to think clearly, is another common symptom. And, again, once you understand what AFib does inside the body, these symptoms make perfect sense. Our brains are ravenous for oxygen, after all, and oxygen moves through our bodies via our circulatory system. In a healthy human body, this system is perfectly designed to deliver oxygen exactly where it is needed, when it is needed. But when the organ at the center of this closed system is malfunctioning, the entire system begins to falter. The oxygen molecules being transported by hemoglobin, a protein carried throughout our bodies by our red blood cells, may still arrive, but not at the same steady rate our brains are used to.

All of this helps explain why we, as well as other researchers, are coming to discover a long-term consequence of atrial fibrillation that is terrifying to a lot of people: brain damage. Our research team has discovered that many of the chemical signs of brain injury that are elevated after a concussion— like glial fibrillary acidic protein, stress response marker growth/differentiation factor 15, and tau protein—are chronically high in atrial fibrillation patients.[21] These proteins, which typically are elevated in response to an injury to the brain and its barrier from the rest of the body, are released very early in people who have atrial fibrillation, a reflection of the chronic insult of the abnormal heart rhythm on the brain.

It's not just molecules swimming around in our bodies that testify to the damage being done to our brains. When you use an MRI to look at the brains of people with AFib, nearly half have visible signs of brain damage in the form of brain lesions, even if they've never had a stroke.[22] Those who do not have brain lesions consistent with stroke often have volume loss, also known as "brain shrinkage," and small patterns of brain injury called "white matter disease." These changes reflect damage done to the brain from both atrial fibrillation and other medical problems, like hypertension and diabetes, that may have caused the AFib.

This might help explain why the rate of dementia and cognitive decline are so much higher among people with atrial fibrillation. We've known for nearly half a century that lesions are more common in the autopsied brains of people who suffered from dementia at the end of their lives, but it hasn't always been clear where these lesions came from.[23] More recently, our research has shown that atrial fibrillation is independently associated with all forms of dementia, including Alzheimer's disease. Not surprisingly, we saw that the presence of AFib was a strong predictor of which dementia patients are at highest risk of death. Also, and quite disconcertingly, these findings suggested that the risk of Alzheimer's, in particular, was increased even among younger AFib patients.[24]

Will the bad news ever end? As long as researchers are looking for connections between AFib and ways in which human lives become more miserable—and, alas, that traditionally is what researchers have been looking for—the answer is "probably not."

These days, though, many of our colleagues who study AFib are increasingly interested not only in the ways in which this arrhythmia ruins people's lives, but also in the ways in which people with AFib can make their lives better. And now that you have a better understanding of what causes AFib, what it does to our hearts, and what it does to the rest of our bodies, you have the tools you need to understand the different treatment, therapy, and lifestyle options that are available to you. Not only that, but you also have the power to truly evaluate these options and figure out which ones are right for you.

And "you" is the operative word here.

If you're going to embark on this journey, you're going to need *a lot* of encouragement. Yes, that encouragement can come from your friends and family. It can certainly come from your doctors. And sure, it can come from this book, too. (Hooray for you! You can do this! We believe in you!) But the strongest inspirations—the ones you're going to need more often than any other—are those you don't have to look to someone else to get.

These inspirations have to come from you.

## MAKING PURPOSE-DRIVEN GOALS

Atrial fibrillation is a shrewd enemy.

It saps you of your strength. It steals your breath. It attacks just about every system of your body. It conspires with other enemies—from inflammation to dementia—to destroy your body, cell by cell and piece by piece. Somehow, it has managed to convince a whole lot of people that it can't be beat. And in some way, it seems, it has even managed to trick us into fighting it with weapons—medications intended not to cure but to make things a little more tolerable on the way to the grave—that often leave people feeling even *more* tired, even to the point of depression, sometimes making submission feel like the only move we have left.

As such, anyone who wants to fight back is going to need to dig deep. And the best weapon for this fight is a purpose.

Does that sound like a bunch of pseudo-psychological mumbo jumbo? It's not. There is scientific evidence—lots of it—demonstrating that being able to define one's life purpose is significantly effective when it comes to fighting numerous diseases.

One study from Rush University Medical Center in Chicago showed that people who could articulate their life's purpose were less likely to suffer from cognitive decline, including Alzheimer's disease.[25] Other studies have shown that having a strong sense of purpose can prevent plaque from building up in our hearts and brains, and can help keep blood clots from forming.[26] Having purpose has also been shown to reduce stress.[27] Other studies have found a correlation between purpose in life and better health outcomes regardless of age, sex, education, or race.[28] Bring all of these effects together, and what results is, on average, an extra four years of life.[29]

Why? Well, aside from the supervillains you see in comic-book movies, it's rare to find anyone who will tell you that the purpose of their life is something *negative*. Even supervillains often frame their nefarious actions in terms of something positive.[30]

There's plenty to be said about the power of positive thinking. But positivity itself probably isn't enough to power clinically significant changes in disease outcomes. So what really accounts for the power of purpose? The effect of purpose on our life goals.

Take Laura, for instance. When she was asked to articulate her life's purpose, she had no problem doing so. Her purpose was to have a meaningful relationship with her two children. Twenty-one and twenty-three at the time of Laura's AFib diagnosis, "they had just gotten over the period of their lives in which I wasn't cool enough to hang out with," Laura recalled. "Now, they seemed to genuinely enjoy being with me again, and I wanted that more than anything else."

From the time they were toddlers until their teens, Laura's kids had spent almost every winter weekend skiing with their mother. Now, after several years that felt like a painful eternity, "they wanted to ski together as a family again," Laura lamented, "but I couldn't."

That's what Laura kept in her mind as she embarked on a journey to send her AFib into remission. Her purpose was to be there for her children. And that purpose drove her decisions as she went to battle against this disease. Whenever she needed to do the things vital to staying on track to fight her arrhythmia, she envisioned the day upon which she would strap on skis with her kids again. When she felt fearful in the days before a medical procedure that would return her heart to rhythm, she remembered the joy that she felt whenever she and her children were gliding quietly through a snow-covered forest.

Finding purpose in life makes us more resilient. Using that purpose to build goals gives us an extra helping of willpower. It's not magic. It's not perfect. But, as we've noted, AFib is a mighty foe, and to fight it we need all the help we can get.

Purpose is powerful. That's why the most important thing that happens *inside* someone when they decide it's time to fight back against AFib has nothing to do with their blood flow, the electrical signals moving through their bodies, or the biochemicals that are supposed to balance all of these things. Rather, it has everything to do with what they *think* about their lives.

So let's do some thinking:

- What is your life's purpose?
- What does the fulfillment of that purpose look like in your mind's eye?
- Could more healthy years of life help you fulfill that purpose even more?
- Could a life without medications give you more energy and vitality to achieve your life's goals?

Rather than relying on memory, write down your answers to these questions and post them somewhere you will see them every day. Even better, put those answers in several places. On your bathroom mirror. On your refrigerator door. On the dashboard of your car. On your desk at work.

Again, this is not just a mental exercise. It is the first step in a research-based treatment regimen. In a test of the AFib Cure, a daily reminder to consider life's purpose was part of a protocol that helped more than 92 percent of the participants adhere to the program and achieve significant positive health effects.[31]

Are you struggling with this? That's okay. A lot of people do—especially those who have been beaten down by the wily foe that is atrial fibrillation. If that's the case for you, a series of conversations with your family members, close friends, coworkers, a faith leader, or a therapist can help you either bring your life's purpose back into clarity or develop a new purpose for the years ahead. If that's not something you're able to do right now, that doesn't mean you should stop here. Still, even if you move ahead without being able to answer these questions, you should return to them again and again, until you can.

Because once you understand what your purpose is, you will be in a much better position to consider the different avenues for fulfilling it.

## FOUR TYPES OF ATRIAL FIBRILLATION

### Paroxysmal
- AFib that starts, then stops, all by itself
- In most cases, limited fibrosis has developed

### Persistent
- Medication or electrical shock needed to return the heart to rhythm
- Depending on the duration of the AFib, fibrosis may be limited to significant

### Long-standing persistent
- No normal rhythm for more than one year
- Fibrosis may be severe

### Permanent
- Many doctors have given up hope of ever restoring normal rhythm
- Fibrosis is likely extensive

Regardless of your type of AFib, improvement in quality of life and longevity are definitely still possible.

## Chapter Three

# ⎯⎯⎯⎯⎯ ⎯ᛉᛚⴼᛉⴼ⎯ THE WELL-WORN PATH ⎯ᛉᛚⴼᛉⴼ⎯ ⎯⎯⎯⎯⎯

### Why a deep understanding of medications and supplements is vital for anyone suffering from AFib

Something was missing. That's all Peri could think about when she was driving home from her doctor's office on the day after her first episode of atrial fibrillation.

"It was such a crazy night," she recalled. "It was just about 3 AM when it started. At first, you know, I thought I was dying. My heart was beating so fast and so hard. And then, suddenly, it stopped on its own."

The doctors in the emergency room sent her away with instructions to follow up with her primary care doctor. "And so I just drove straight to my doctor's office and waited for them to open up," she said. "My doctor was pretty gracious to see me."

While he might indeed have been gracious, he wasn't really much help. "I was expecting some answers, some guidance, some anything," the fifty-two-year-old factory floor supervisor recalled. "But he just said, 'You know, this is going to get worse as you get older, and you already have high blood pressure, so here's a prescription.' And just like that, we were done, and I was standing there with a prescription for some drugs that I was supposed to take for the rest of my life."

It wasn't until she was back in her car that she realized there were so many more questions she wanted to ask. "And I just thought, 'Goodness, this just can't be it. There has to be something else I can do,'" she said.

Peri's instinct was right. But her experience wasn't unusual. For all of the reasons we discussed in chapter two, and more, many doctors are still treating people with AFib as the victims of an inevitable condition that just gets worse over time. In this chapter, we're going to talk about why doctors' first impulse is almost always to prescribe medications—and why drugs can be both important for some patients and unnecessary in the long term for others. We're also going to take a deep dive into the benefits and drawbacks of the most common medications—antiarrhythmics, rate controllers, anticoagulants, and drugs that counter heart failure—which are commonly prescribed both individually and in different combinations as needed. And since we're hearing from an increasing number of AFib patients who are trying to treat their AFib with supplements, or would like to, we'll discuss the pros and cons of some of the most popular non-prescription chemicals out there.

Because many people are paroxysmal when they first experience AFib, diagnoses can be disastrously delayed. Of those who are diagnosed, only some will even be referred to a cardiologist for stress testing. Even fewer will ever make it to a cardiac electrophysiologist. This is tragic because, as you know, with each passing day and each new episode of AFib, it gets harder and harder to correct this condition. If you don't arm yourself with knowledge and advocate for yourself with feisty resolve, chances are quite good that you'll just be prescribed medications to slow your heart and to thin your blood, then be sent on your way as Peri was.

And yet this can't really be called "bad medicine." The doctors who send their patients down this path are certainly not terrible people who are trying to sentence the people they care for to a life of misery. What they're advising their patients to do is backed by decades of research and lots of studies demonstrating that AFib is indeed very common in old age. And those who miss the diagnosis because their patients aren't actively having an arrhythmic episode aren't necessarily bad diagnosticians. After all, the telltale 20 to 30 percent drop-off in cardiac performance that comes with AFib is also indicative of aging, since people tend to be more sedentary as they get older.

Doctors whose first impulse is to prescribe drugs aren't "pushers" or "owned by Big Pharma," as people seem increasingly prone to allege. Their prescriptions are backed by research that supports the idea that AFib sufferers can indeed be made to feel "less bad" when given medications that slow their hearts. Further, by slowing the heart, these drugs may also prevent heart failure. It's also true that blood thinners can prevent stroke. These are treatments that can work.

To a point.

But what many doctors still don't understand is that making AFib more tolerable in the short run, without focusing on long-term goals, can quickly leave patients in an impossible place, for AFib is a race against time. Because AFib begets AFib, doctors have a brief window of time in which their patients' hearts will best respond to treatment and, according to our research, put AFib into remission.[1] Many doctors also don't realize that, for a typical AFib patient, an antiarrhythmic drug offers about a fifty-fifty chance of maintaining normal sinus rhythm for a year. For some patients it could be decades; for others, never.

How long is your window of opportunity? Well, that varies from person to person. If you just have very occasional episodes of AFib that self-correct, that window could be years (sometimes decades for people with familial AFib and otherwise normal hearts). However, if your heart doesn't self-correct, then the window could be just a few months—if it hasn't already closed.

There's another reason many doctors are hesitant to change the way they view this condition. There's simply not as much peer-reviewed research (the sort we generally want doctors to be adhering to when they dole out medical advice) demonstrating that AFib can be put into remission, that patients can get off drugs, and that they can have measurably and mean-ingfully better lives. To be certain, peer-reviewed studies that support these ideas do exist in droves (as the endnotes to this book confirm), but they are stacked up against centuries of prior thought and relative inaction, and have been slow to impact the mainstream medical view.

Change is absolutely afoot. Increasing numbers of physicians and researchers at atrial fibrillation conferences around the world are present-ing on the very sorts of revelations we're discussing in this book. Few of these doctors believe we're anywhere close to an AFib-free world. Most recognize that lifestyle changes are hard, we're a long way away from being able to do anything about the genetic causes of AFib, and it might be even longer before there are enough enlightened EPs for every person in the world with AFib. And yet, in just the past few years, these conferences have gone from pessimistic affairs to optimistic celebrations of what is possible.

Nonetheless, treatment paradigms shift slowly, and that's probably a good thing. We want to be as certain as possible that we're doing the right thing before we advise a patient to "stop doing X and start doing Y."

That's why, if you've been diagnosed with AFib, or know someone who has, you're likely familiar with the sort of advice Peri got: take meds.

In the very short term, after her first AFib episode, that was actually the right advice. The substrate causes that contributed to her AFib, after all, had developed over many years. It was going to take time to address those issues, and the drug she was prescribed was helping her buy some time.

But drugs are a double-edged sword. For one thing, they can come with a lot of side effects.

The good news is that most of those side effects are well known. The drug-creation process from development to FDA approval in the United States can take ten years, a period that ensures drugs have been rigorously tested before they make it into the medicine cabinets of patients across the United States. (Other national and transnational regulatory agencies, such as the European Agency for the Evaluation of Medicinal Products, have similar timelines.) Once drugs are being widely used, the breadth of pos-sible side effects becomes better understood. Since nearly all of the most common AFib drugs gained FDA approval decades ago, anything really bad that they can do has likely been reported.

It's natural that many people get anxious about taking drugs when they look at all of those side effects. That's one of the big reasons why AFib patients are increasingly turning to supplements. But these products exist in a largely unregulated industry—one with a long and sordid history of failing to disclose what is actually in the products being sold.[2]

In fact, what makes use of drugs and supplements complicated is that the biological functions they are designed to affect are simply far too complex and important for that impact not to be felt in systems elsewhere in a user's body. The endless genetic and epigenetic X factors are too vast to account for them all. All of this means that few AFib patients will ever find that drugs or supplements alone are enough to restore the quality of life they truly want.

To be honest, a lot of what we're going to tell you about using AFib drugs and supplements is going to sound like bad news. That's because a lot of it is. But it's important to understand this path, because the other path— the one that we will put before you in the rest of this book—isn't always an easy one. If you choose our path, which for most of the patients we treat offers a drug-free solution, it will be helpful to have a strong understanding of what the other option would have looked like. And that starts with a good understanding of the drugs typically prescribed to AFib patients.

## THE RHYTHM KEEPERS

Wherever you find a medical condition that afflicts millions of new people each year, you will find a medication designed to address that condition. In fact, you'll usually find lots of medications. After all, that's where the money is.

However, in the world of atrial fibrillation treatment, there just aren't many antiarrhythmic medications—drugs specifically designed to keep your heart in rhythm. And, since most of these medications are fraught with side effects, few pharmaceutical companies venture into this space, meaning it's unlikely that many better choices are coming along. As you've learned, these drugs are only about 50 percent effective at holding your heart in rhythm after one year. They also come with the risk of some pretty bad side effects, including cardiac arrest.

You might think that, given all of the people in the world with AFib, drug companies would be spending big on research and development to bring better medications to market. Sadly, this isn't the case. And now that you understand what AFib does to your heart, you have the background to understand why. It simply isn't possible to fix all of those misfiring heart cells with a drug, and any attempt to do so would create huge liability issues for pharmaceutical companies, since a drug developed to "rewire" heart cells could instead "miswire" them, causing an even worse arrhythmia. That's right: a drug specifically given to treat one arrhythmia may end up causing another arrhythmia. This is a condition called proarrhythmia, which can be either atrial in origin—meaning that the drug designed to stop AFib actually causes more AFib or converts your AFib into something else, like atrial flutter—or ventricular, like ventricular tachycardia or ventricular fibrillation—both of which can quickly result in death if not treated immediately.

No drug comes without the chance of side effects—and any drug strong enough to fix the damage done by AFib would likely have a tremendous impact on the rest of your body. How tremendous an impact? Well, have you ever tried to wire a house? It's not easy. There's a reason why great electricians are so expensive. One wrong move and—zap!—that's it. The human body is infinitely more complicated than a house, and far more precious, too. When we mess with the way our cells interact with the electrical signals that are constantly moving through our bodies, it puts us at risk in all sorts of other ways.

Given how severe the symptoms of AFib can be, though, some people would take any risk for a little relief. And before we judge these people, we should make sure we understand that this isn't a behavior that is limited to those with AFib. If you've taken ibuprofen for a headache or back pain, you've accepted immediate relief in exchange for an increased risk of heart attack, bleeding ulcer, heart failure, and kidney failure.

But just as ibuprofen shouldn't be taken willy-nilly, antiarrhythmics should only be used after a careful evaluation of the risks and benefits. Also, AFib treatment guidelines recommend a trial of antiarrhythmics for most patients before moving on to an ablation, the procedure we'll discuss in depth in chapter six.[3] So even though these drugs won't make you live any longer, as we described in our published *Journal of Atrial Fibrillation* article,[4] and even though they're generally effective for a short time, and even though they can come with quite a few negative side effects, there are some perfectly valid reasons to warrant taking an antiarrhythmic.

As such, you should get to know some of the most common kinds of these drugs.

**Amiodarone** is a good place to start this discussion. Belgian scientists first developed amiodarone in the early 1960s as a medication for angina pectoris, the telltale chest pain caused by coronary heart disease.[5] The only problem was that amiodarone had too many significant side effects at the dosage required to treat chest pain.

It wasn't long, though, before it was recognized that amiodarone was also quite effective for AFib. In fact, of all the antiarrhythmics, amiodarone is by far the most potent. While the other antiarrhythmics only get you a fifty-fifty chance of holding normal sinus rhythm for a year, amiodarone could get you many years, sometimes decades.

Also known by the brand name Cordarone, this drug works by rewiring the electrical connections between heart cells. It also *really* slows the heart rate.

Like many antiarrhythmics, amiodarone is relatively cheap. Depending on their insurance, some of our patients have gotten this drug for as little as $4 a month. Because it's so cheap, though, it is probably prescribed more than it should be—especially since, by many accounts, it's the most dangerous of the antiarrhythmics.

Amiodarone has many potential side effects. There's inflammation. There's potential injury to the lungs, thyroid, and liver. There's bluish discoloration of the skin. And, in rare cases, there's damage to the nerves and eyes. In some cases, these situations can be hard or impossible to reverse.

Sometimes, though, physicians don't have much of a choice but to advise the use of medications that have significant side effects. The potential benefits may outweigh the risks—particularly with careful monitoring. But the fact that a medication with such risks is commonly used for atrial fibrillation is a troubling testament to how bad AFib truly is.[6]

While amiodarone does indeed have a lot of scary side effects, it is important to remember that when it is used for just a few months and under careful supervision—as part of a plan to buy some time so that other interventions can work—adverse effects are rare. In general, the nastier side effects only come after years of taking this drug. Nonetheless, amiodarone should generally be limited to use as an end-of-the-line drug—a medication used when no other substitute is likely to work.

**Flecainide** is another popular antiarrhythmic, one that works by blocking the sodium channel electrical connections between heart cells. Also known by the brand name Tambocor, its development came as the result of efforts that began in the 1960s to see what would happen when the electronegative chemical element fluorine was swapped into potential drug molecules for other elements.[7] After nearly two decades of work, the Food and Drug Administration approved it in 1984.[8]

Like amiodarone, flecainide is relatively inexpensive, often costing less than $20 a month. For this and many other reasons, it is the most popular antiarrhythmic used to get patients to and through an ablation procedure, according to our study of 141 of the leading AFib hospitals in the United States.[9] It is also generally well tolerated and it works well enough with relatively few significant side effects.

That doesn't mean there are no side effects, though. The most common adverse reactions include dizziness, tremors, vision problems, and diarrhea. Anxiety and depression are also common among flecainide users. And even though this medication can substantially reduce a patient's risk of another AFib episode, it has long been implicated in a greater risk of proarrhythmia in patients who have a history of heart attacks or heart failure, which is why we don't give this medication to people with abnormal stress tests or heart failure. When it is prescribed, many physicians will periodically administer EKGs to look for significant slowing of the heart's electrical system.

**Sotalol** is another commonly prescribed antiarrhythmic. It was first marketed in the 1970s as a hypertension medication, but was found in the 1980s to also be effective at addressing arrhythmias, and was approved by the Food and Drug Administration in 1992. The reason why sotalol is effective at holding patients in rhythm is that it prevents the stimulation of the nerve receptors responsible for cardiac action and blocks the potassium channel electrical connections between heart cells.

Another relatively inexpensive antiarrhythmic, sotalol is available for as little as $11 a month. But it also has significant proarrhythmic effects—which is why we generally start this medication in the hospital—as well as some other side effects, including fatigue, weight gain, erectile dysfunction, chest pain, slowed heart rate, and dizziness. Sotalol can be used in patients with AFib who otherwise have relatively normal stress tests and no heart failure. And unlike flecainide, it can also be used in patients with coronary artery disease or mild cases of heart failure.

If you are on sotalol, you need your heart rhythm checked regularly. This is because sotalol may lengthen the time it takes for the cells in the ventricles to be electrically stimulated and then recover, a period known as the QT interval. If this interval gets too long, it increases the risk of abnormal ventricular rhythm and cardiac arrest.

You'll also want to get your kidney function regularly checked, because if your kidneys were to falter for any reason, sotalol could build up in your body to unsafe levels, putting you at risk for a life-threatening proarrhythmia.

**Propafenone** was developed in the 1980s as researchers worked to find a new drug option for patients who had severely negative responses to other antiarrhythmics. And, at first, it seemed very promising. Propafenone, the scientists found at the time, was effective at significantly reducing arrhythmias in 70 to 80 percent of test subjects.[10] After widespread use, doctors have continued to find the drug beneficial enough to recommend and prescribe over other antiarrhythmics, even though it also tends to be quite a bit more expensive.

Also known by the brand name Rythmol, propafenone, like flecainide, works by blocking the sodium channel electrical connections between heart cells. But, like all of the antiarrhythmics we've discussed so far, it has some relatively common side effects, with up to 45 percent of patients reporting cardiac issues; up to 20 percent reporting non-cardiac problems; and up to 15 percent experiencing central nervous system effects, including dizziness, fatigue, confusion, and paranoia.[11]

Propafenone is generally used for the same patients as flecainide—those with symptomatic AFib, a normal stress test, and no heart failure. It also works at about the same rate as flecainide. And, like flecainide, the potential for proarrhythmia is definitely a problem.

So why would one be used over the other? We have found over the years that if flecainide isn't tolerated, for one reason or another, propafenone may be a better fit. In this regard, it could be thought of as a backup to flecainide. It can, however, be a medication that requires quite a bit of commitment: the cheaper form of the drug may need to be taken three times a day, which can be a challenge for long-term use.

**Dofetilide**, also known by the brand name Tikosyn, works by blocking the potassium channel electrical connections between heart cells. Of all the antiarrhythmics we could start a patient on, dofetilide may be one of the best tolerated. Unfortunately, along with sotalol, it also comes with a significant risk for proarrhythmia—especially if your EKG and kidney function lab tests aren't checked regularly. Sadly, we have seen cardiac arrests over the years among patients whose doctors prescribed dofetilide and sotalol without closely following their QT intervals and kidney function lab tests.

That's not the main reason why dofetilide is so rarely used, though. Rather, it's because this drug is quite expensive, even in its generic version, and it requires a three-day hospitalization while starting the drug to monitor for the possibility of a life-threatening proarrhythmia.

Despite the risks of dofetilide and sotalol, however, we have seen excellent AFib control on these medications. When they are dosed properly, those effects can last for decades.

**Dronedarone**, more commonly known by the brand name Multaq, is the final antiarrhythmic we'll discuss, and the only one the FDA has approved in recent years. The fact that most of the antiarrhythmics we have discussed were developed decades ago should highlight how challenging it is to make these types of medications safely.

The dronedarone molecule closely resembles amiodarone's, except that it lacks iodine. Long before its approval, we had hoped it would do everything that amiodarone could do but without all the nasty side effects. But while Multaq may indeed be the safest of all antiarrhythmics, it is also the weakest when it comes to keeping the heart in rhythm. This is one reason why researchers have explored combining Multaq with other weak antiarrhythmics, like ranolazine, which is also known as Ranexa. Many EPs feel the Multaq–Ranexa combination's potency nears that of amiodarone, and a trial that explored the combination of these two drugs showed a reduction in AFib episodes compared to dronedarone alone.[12] As of the time of this writing, however, their use in a combination pill has not been approved. An EP physician who does combine these drugs will need to closely follow your QT interval, as together their impact on this interval and your risk of proarrhythmia may be greater.

Multaq cannot be used if you have heart failure as it can increase the risk of death. In addition, if your heart is out of rhythm more often than it is normal, Multaq can do more harm than good. And since Multaq is still a brand-name drug, without a generic version in the United States at the time of writing this book, it is often the most expensive of all the antiarrhythmics.

Amiodarone, flecainide, sotalol, propafenone, dofetilide, and dronedarone aren't the only antiarrhythmics, but they are the most common. No matter what antiarrhythmic you are considering taking, have been advised to take, or are already on, there are some important things to remember:

- If one antiarrhythmic fails to control your AFib, then it is unlikely that any of the other antiarrhythmics will work. The most common exception to this general rule is amiodarone.
- It bears repeating that keeping your heart in rhythm with an antiarrhythmic isn't likely to make you live any longer. What's more, if these drugs are not carefully used and monitored, they can harm your life expectancy.

- Because the *only* purpose for taking an antiarrhythmic is to improve your quality of life by keeping your heart in rhythm, the benefit of the drug must outweigh any possible side effects.
- Most antiarrhythmics have a relatively short window of effectiveness. As noted, these drugs generally give you a fifty-fifty chance of keeping your heart in rhythm for a year. (Amiodarone is the exception, but, as you now know, it can come with quite a few very negative side effects.)

The bottom line: These drugs should be used as stopgap measures to buy you time for other interventions to work. They are simply not a long-term solution for most people.

Peri really should have learned that from her doctor. Instead, she figured it out after a few days of frantic searching on the internet.

"When I really dove into the information that is available about the dangers of antiarrhythmics, I was honestly freaked out," she said. "Over the next few days, I suppose I came to an understanding that all the side effects and risks were better than living with my heart out of rhythm, which is an absolutely terrifying experience, but it felt like being stuck between a bad option and a really bad option."

And those were Peri's concerns after she began investigating antiarrhythmics. She hadn't even gotten around to researching rate-controlling drugs and anticoagulants yet. When she did, she was even more determined to find another way.

| Antiarrhythmics | Amiodarone, flecainide, sotalol, propafenone, dofetilide, and dronedarone | <ul><li>Affects heart's electrical channels with the goal of keeping your heart in rhythm</li><li>May increase risk of a life-threatening ventricular arrhythmia, in addition to the usual nuisance side effects</li></ul> |
| --- | --- | --- |

# THE RATE CONTROLLERS

Of all the drugs that doctors prescribe for AFib, rate controllers are probably the most popular. And yet, in most of the cases we see, these drugs usually don't reduce AFib attacks and seldom prevent them altogether. They also don't always prevent heart failure—because, when it comes to heart failure, rate control alone may not be enough. Many doctors don't even know this yet, but research suggests that just the irregularity alone from AFib is enough to put some hearts into heart failure.[13]

What do rate controllers do, then? They slow your heart down. And sure, when your heart is pounding away at 150 beats per minute, slowing it down is a good thing. But rate controllers slow your heart no matter if it's in an active state of AFib or not. And that can result in bradycardia, a condition in which the heart is beating too slowly and thus not pumping enough oxygen-rich blood to the rest of the body. We've seen countless patients—usually older ones—admitted to our hospitals' emergency rooms with heart rates of under forty-five beats per minute, who are either fainting or coming close to fainting as a result. That's why, if you are on a rate controller, it's vital to invest in a smartwatch or other device for monitoring your heart rate.

Like antiarrhythmics, rate-controlling drugs do serve a purpose. In addition to making AFib feel "less bad," they also help prevent your heart from beating so fast with AFib that it could put you into heart failure. Our hearts simply cannot keep racing twenty-four hours a day, seven days a week, and still function properly.

So how much rate controlling do you need? As long as you aren't having any symptoms, studies suggest an AFib resting heart rate below 110 beats per minute is best.[14] Under the right conditions, rate controllers can help with that. And fortunately, these drugs tend to be available as inexpensive generics. But they're not all the same, so let's look at the three main classes of these medications.

**Beta-blockers** are the most commonly prescribed rate controllers. They are also the only rate controllers that might actually help prevent

AFib episodes, particularly in situations when your body releases a lot of adrenaline, such as when you are stressed out, exercising, or angry. That's because these drugs—which include metoprolol, carvedilol, atenolol, and basically any medication whose generic name ends in "olol"—shield the heart from adrenaline.

This is good when your heart is in AFib. If you're in normal rhythm, though, the adrenaline-shielding property of these drugs can literally put you to sleep. That's why fatigue is one of the top complaints among users of these drugs. In women, beta-blockers are often also associated with weight gain. In men, one of the big problems is erectile dysfunction.

One of the most beneficial effects of beta-blockers is that they often have a calming effect on users, which is good for people with AFib that is triggered by stress or anxiety. These drugs also tend to lower blood pressure, and since most people with AFib have high blood pressure, that's a good thing, too. Beta-blockers also often improve sleep, and since a lack of sleep can be a trigger for AFib, that's also a significant benefit.

So who should use beta-blockers? The main group of patients who can most benefit are those whose AFib is induced by exercise, anger, stress, or heart failure. On the other hand, taking beta-blockers for exercise-induced AFib can also be counterproductive since they can make it hard to get your heart rate up sufficiently to engage in vigorous exercise (which, as you'll learn in chapter five, is a vital component of the interventions nearly everyone needs if they want to put their AFib into remission).

Unlike antiarrhythmics, beta-blockers are quite safe for almost everyone. Indeed, our sickest cardiac patients—those with a history of a major heart attack or heart failure from a low ejection fraction (ejection fraction, or EF, is a measurement of how strong your ventricles are pumping, calculated from an echocardiogram or other heart imaging test)—generally live longer on beta-blockers. If there's a single type of drug that has the best ratio of benefits to drawbacks, it's beta-blockers. But, of course, that doesn't make these drugs right for everyone. That's why there are two other classes of rate controllers.

**Calcium channel blockers** that are used for rate control work by blocking calcium channel electrical connections between heart cells.

Some patients get nervous when they first learn about these drugs. Calcium is vital, after all, for strong bones, among other important functions. But these drugs don't significantly block calcium absorption in your gut, or affect either calcium metabolism or your bone health.

While calcium channel blockers aren't used as frequently as beta-blockers, they can be a good second-line rate-controlling strategy in the event there are intolerable side effects with beta-blockers. Yet these drugs, whose generic versions include diltiazem and verapamil, can have many of the same side effects on the body as beta-blockers. Calcium channel blockers may also cause swelling of the legs, and you should be sure to tell your doctor if you notice your legs getting a little "puffy" with diltiazem or verapamil. Additionally, calcium channel blockers aren't safe for people with heart failure from a low ejection fraction.

**Digoxin**, which is also known by the brand name Lanoxin, is the least-prescribed rate controller. You might recall from chapter two that this drug was derived from the foxglove plant. As the very first AFib medication, it has been used to treat arrhythmias for a very long time. You might also recall that it is falling out of favor among doctors. That's because research has indicated that it might increase users' risk of premature death.[15] Even before this startling concern was revealed, however, this nearly century-old medication was losing market share due to its multiple negative side effects, including loss of appetite, vision problems, fatigue, and confusion. It also has a very narrow margin between a dose that is strong enough to be effective and a dose that is strong enough to be toxic,[16] making precise dosing precarious. And, compared to other rate controllers, its rate-slowing effects are relatively weak.

Despite all of this, however, digoxin is quite inexpensive and can be helpful in a small subset of patients. One possible advantage of this drug, which comes from a class of heart-slowing medications known as cardiac glycosides, is that it doesn't lower blood pressure like beta-blockers or calcium channel blockers. That can be good for people who struggle with low blood pressure.

Beta-blockers, calcium channel blockers, and digoxin all have an appropriate place in the pharmaceutical quiver that doctors use to treat their patients. But given the side effects and other concerns, people often wonder if they really need these drugs, especially if they are also on an antiarrhythmic. If the antiarrhythmic your doctor has prescribed is flecainide or propafenone, the answer is probably yes. This is because the atrial-flutter proarrhythmic effects of flecainide and propafenone are serious enough that most patients need a rate controller to make sure the heart never beats too fast.

However, some antiarrhythmics do have some rate-controlling effects. This is especially the case with amiodarone, sotalol, and Multaq (dronedarone). As a result, if you are combining antiarrhythmics with rate-controlling medications—and especially if you are elderly—you will need to monitor your heart rate very closely, lest it drop so low that you pass out from lack of oxygen to your brain or develop severe low blood pressure.

| **Rate Controllers** | Beta-blockers (like metoprolol), calcium channel blockers (like diltiazem and verapamil), and digoxin | • Primarily slow your heart down, with the slight benefit of keeping your heart in rhythm<br>• Generally safer than antiarrhythmics |
| --- | --- | --- |

## BLOOD THINNERS: KEEPERS OF THE FLOW

Because atrial fibrillation increases stroke risk, doctors are often keen to prescribe an anticoagulant. These medications, also called blood thinners, help prevent clots from forming inside your heart. And the less likely you are to form a blood clot in your left atrial appendage, which can happen when the upper chambers of the heart stop beating during AFib, the less likely it is that a clot will break off, cutting of the blood supply—and thus the oxygen—to the brain or other organs or structures.

For a long time, aspirin was thought to be protective against AFib strokes. It turns out, though, that this cheap and common remedy is actually not all that helpful. While it would be nice to think that lowering the risk of stroke was as easy as "an aspirin a day," a study we did a few years ago demonstrated that aspirin, even in people at lower risk of an AFib stroke, simply doesn't work very well for this purpose. Instead, it puts AFib patients at risk in other ways by increasing their risk of internal bleeding.[17]

Even though it's obviously important to prevent devastating AFib strokes, when you block the body's natural blood-clotting ability, you interfere with a process that is vital to keeping us alive. But, of course, *not* having strokes is vital to life, too—so anticoagulants represent yet another pharmaceutical tradeoff.

Given the considerable risks, many of which we'll detail in the following pages, the guidelines call for "shared decision making" between doctors and patients before these drugs are prescribed.

For those who have had an AFib episode lasting longer than forty-eight hours and requiring a cardioversion, however, the decision is quite simple: everyone in this situation should be on a blood thinner for a minimum of one month. There's nothing magical about this forty-eight-hour rule; it is a rough if conservative estimate of how long it may take for a blood clot to develop in your left atrial appendage. Some research, however, suggests they can form in twenty-four hours, or even as little as six minutes.[18]

For anyone else, the decision to take a blood thinner should be made only after a thorough and thoughtful evaluation of the risks. Before we explain how to conduct that evaluation, though, it's helpful to understand a bit about the history of these drugs.

It all started with an epidemic of cow deaths in the 1920s, when, across the United States and Canada, ranchers were reporting that their cows were bleeding out from minor injuries. It took the work of one of the world's first and most brilliant poison-plant detectives, a North Dakota veterinary pathologist named Lee Roderick, to reveal the culprit: a toxic mold that grew on two invasive, sweet-smelling clovers called *Melilotus alba* and *Melilotus officinalis*.[19]

You might think that the death of so many cows would have prompted humans to stay as far away as possible from the chemical compounds responsible for the carnage. But it was the fatal potential of this chemical that drew scientists to study it, synthesize it, and turn it into a rodenticide. And this chemical might have remained nothing more than a rat poison had researchers not also been on the hunt for chemicals that could keep human patients' blood from clotting *too much*. And while it was quite deadly to some of the very animals we commonly use as model organisms for research, in the right doses in humans this chemical was found to be effective for preventing dangerous clots. That's how the drug known as warfarin was born.

**Warfarin**, which is often sold as Coumadin, was approved for human use in 1954 and has been widely used ever since, backed by decades upon decades of evidence showing that it is quite effective in lowering the stroke risk of AFib patients and treating people with blood clots in other areas of the body.[20] But, as you might expect now that you know its history, warfarin doesn't come without *serious* risks and side effects for humans; also, like the antiarrhythmic digoxin, the effective dosing range is very narrow. Too much and you run the risk of adverse effects. Too little and you might actually *increase* the risk of stroke.[21]

The main risk, though, is exactly what happened to all those ill-fated cows: bleeding. In fact, when a research team of doctors, nurses, and pharmacists looked at the hospital records of nearly 19,000 patients in Great Britain, they found that warfarin was one of the most common causes of adverse drug reactions necessitating hospitalization. As a *singular* drug, the researchers discovered, it caused more hospital visits than all but two other entire *classes* of drugs.[22] And the warfarin patients' symptoms were a veritable house of horrors. They had blood in their stool and urine. They coughed up blood. They had vomit that looked like dirt. They experienced joint pain and swelling. They got bruises even when they could not recall being injured. Sometimes, for no apparent reason, they even bled into their brain—a condition known as a hemorrhagic stroke.

In addition to bleeding, warfarin has many other serious side effects. For example, warfarin works by blocking vitamin K in the body. As you probably know, many of the world's healthiest foods—foods like kale, broccoli, and spinach, among many others—are loaded with vitamin K. Because of this, most people taking warfarin are told to avoid green leafy vegetables. And since not getting enough vitamin K has been associated with coronary artery disease and bone metabolism issues, it should come as no surprise that people taking warfarin may be at more risk of these problems.[23]

Fortunately, there are an increasing number of other choices.

**Apixaban** is one common alternative. Often sold as Eliquis, it appears to be far more effective than aspirin at preventing stroke, which is predictable given our study that failed to show an AFib stroke-prevention benefit of aspirin.[24] It also appears to have a significantly lower rate of internal bleeding than warfarin—about the same risk as aspirin—which is quite reassuring for people who need to take this medication.

**Xarelto**, **Pradaxa**, and **Savaysa** are a few of the other popular alternatives. These may also be safer when compared to warfarin,[25] but, like Eliquis, they are considerably more expensive. While antidotes are available for the newer blood thinners, if you present with a bleeding complication at a small rural hospital, there is no guarantee they will have one of these antidotes on hand (antidotes for warfarin should be readily available at any hospital). Some patients—even those who have what might be described as "good insurance"—can end up paying hundreds of dollars a month for some of these anticoagulants. For a lot of people, that's simply a nonstarter. Fortunately, at the time of writing this book, generics to these new blood thinners were starting to get FDA approval. How long it will take before these generic options make it to the market, however, is yet to be determined.

It's worth noting here that any of the newer blood thinners may offer additional benefits beyond just stroke prevention and a decreased risk of bleeding where it matters most—your brain. For example, our research has shown that long-term cognitive performance is better with one of the newer blood thinners versus with warfarin.[26] This is probably because warfarin is so very difficult to dose properly. Even with all of the frequent blood tests warfarin patients need, it can be next to impossible for many of them to stay in a "safe therapeutic zone," a place in which anticoagulation levels are not too thin and not too thick. The newer blood thinners are far more predictable, and you don't need regular blood tests to make sure you're in the zone. This may help explain why we showed a much lower risk of long-term dementia with the newer blood thinners.

But lower risk doesn't mean "no risk." And the decision to take or decline blood thinners should come only after a thoughtful evaluation of their potential risks and benefits. That evaluation should be informed by a doctor's assessment of your specific annual risk of major bleeding if you do choose to take them, as well as your specific annual risk of stroke if you choose *not* to take them.

And if you do choose to take them, it doesn't have to be for life. The AFib treatment guidelines aggressively promote blood thinners, but these recommendations don't say that everyone with AFib needs to take blood thinners forever.

Who does? That's determined by a clinical prediction rule, specifically designed for patients with atrial fibrillation, known as a CHADS-VASc score.

Calculating your CHADS-VASc used to be easy, but like everything in medicine, these days it's getting more complex. That's not necessarily a bad thing, though, because that complexity brings greater accuracy.

At a glance, though, the score goes like this:

**C**ongestive heart failure: Have you been diagnosed? You get one point.

**H**ypertension: Got that, too? Add another point.

**A**ge: Are you over sixty-five? That's one point. Over seventy-five? That's two.

**D**iabetes: That will buy you yet another point.

**S**troke or transient ischemic attack: Two points.

**Va**scular disease: A blockage in any artery in your body gets you another point.

Sex category: If you're a woman and over sixty-five, or you're a woman under sixty-five and have two other risk factors, you get one more point.[27] (If you are a woman under age sixty-five with no other stroke risk factors, then gender doesn't add anything to your score.)

Add 'em up. If your score is zero, then you are not in need of blood thinners in the long term until your age goes past the sixty-five or seventy-five mark, at which point you "earn" one or two points, respectively. (In the short term, your doctor may recommend these drugs after a cardioversion or ablation procedure.) If your score is 1, then long-term blood thinners are optional until you reach those age-based thresholds. But for scores of 2 or higher, the AFib treatment guidelines recommend lifelong blood thinners.

It's easy to see how people could get stuck on blood thinners under this system. If you've had AFib, just being a woman over the age of sixty-five puts you in the "thinners for life" category, under the recommendations. But the relatively low risk score of 2 is controversial. When we studied tens of thousands of patients, our research showed that the blood thinner warfarin provided limited stroke benefit for people with a CHADS-VASc score of 2, even though AFib treatment guidelines advocate for blood thinners in this group of people.[28]

While the CHADS-VASc scoring system is the "accepted" scoring system for determining who should remain on blood thinners for life, and is used around the world, it certainly isn't optimal.

For one thing, it doesn't apply to special cases, like when AFib is combined with other conditions, such as hyperthyroidism, hypertrophic cardiomyopathy, and mitral stenosis, that increase the risk of stroke. And, as you know, atrial fibrillation isn't a condition that usually "travels alone." Many people with AFib also have one or more of these other conditions.

Another problem: CHADS-VASc totally disregards whether a person has had a successful ablation to eliminate AFib, which our research shows may lower the risk of stroke.[29] It also doesn't account for how much left atrial fibrosis or left atrial enlargement a person has, nor the shape or size of their left atrial appendage, nor whether they have any stroke biomarkers. It doesn't distinguish between people who have their blood pressure or

diabetes well controlled or even reversed, nor does it recognize the importance of a person's metabolic profile, nor whether their AFib is paroxysmal
or persistent. And it doesn't factor how long they have been in AFib—there's
a huge difference between one minute a year and 525,600 minutes a year,
after all.

All of this highlights the need to find new scoring systems, and many
others have been proposed.[30] We've even developed a system that we believe
would overcome many of the shortcomings of the CHADS-VASc system.[31]

But that doesn't mean it's worthless. It's actually pretty decent at offering an estimate of one of the two conflicting risks at play when considering
whether to take a blood thinner: the risk of stroke. For a CHADS-VASc
score of 0, your annual stroke risk is almost 0 percent (every living person
has at least some small risk of stroke). For a score of 1, your annual stroke
risk is approximately 1 percent. For a 2, it is 2 percent, and for a 3 or 4, it
is 3 percent and 4 percent. The risks start shooting upward once you get to
a score of 5. That score gets you an annual stroke risk of 7 percent without
blood thinners—and it only goes up from there.

The other risk is bleeding. Mostly, this is "nuisance bleeding," the sort
that happens after getting a nick while shaving, for instance. Since thinners reduce clotting, they can make it a lot harder to staunch such bleeding. That's annoying, but generally not dangerous. But thinners can also
increase the risk of bleeding into the brain or stomach—and that can be
life-threatening.

What is your risk of dangerous bleeding on a blood thinner? A simple if rough estimate can be taken from a study that was used as support
in the FDA approval process for Eliquis. Patients taking Eliquis had a
2.13 percent annual risk of major bleeding, versus 3.09 percent with warfarin.[32] It's important to note, though, that the median age of patients in
this study was seventy. If you are younger, in good health, and not taking any other medications or supplements that increase your bleeding risk,
then your annual major bleeding risk on Eliquis will be much lower than
2 percent. Of course, if you are over the age of seventy, have other medical
conditions, a bleeding history, or are taking other drugs or supplements that

also cause bleeding, then your annual major bleeding risk while taking this drug will be much higher than 2 percent.

For the other newer blood thinners, your annual risk of major bleeding is probably going to be something close to that of Eliquis rather than the higher bleeding risk observed with warfarin. But just as everyone comes to AFib under different circumstances, not everyone has the same bleeding risk, and lots of factors influence your actual risk.

One of the big factors is other medications. Many of our AFib patients are on a blood thinner—or several—for other conditions. For example, if they have had a heart stent, their interventional cardiologist will want them on an antiplatelet drug, like aspirin or clopidogrel (often sold as Plavix), for the rest of their lives. These drugs can raise the risk of bleeding, and the more drugs you throw into the mix, the higher the risk goes. For instance, as we reported in another study, combining some blood thinners with antiplatelet medications like Plavix, and any of the various NSAIDs like aspirin and ibuprofen, can significantly raise the risk of bleeding.[33]

This factors into a slightly more complicated way to figure your blood thinner bleeding risk—a clinical prediction tool called the HAS-BLED score. This score takes into account:

Hypertension: That's one point.

Abnormal kidney or liver function: One point for each.

Stroke history: Another point.

Bleeding history: Prior major bleeding is one more point.

Labile International Normalized Ratio, also known as an INR: If the results are unstable (labile) or high, that's yet another point.

Elderly: If you're over sixty-five, you get a point.

Drugs used, such as ibuprofen or alcohol: One point for more than eight drinks a week, another point for medications that predispose you to bleeding.

Typically, any score more than 3 is considered "high risk."[34]

Unlike the CHADS-VASc test, which most people can figure out for themselves if they've been diagnosed with or tested for the associated conditions, the HAS-BLED score can't easily be derived without a doctor's help and quite a few tests. But given the gravity of the "thinner or not" decision, it's a worthwhile exercise for many people to undertake with their cardiologist.

Even if you and your doctor decide that blood thinners are best for your AFib, it is no guarantee against an AFib stroke. President Nixon, for instance, had been on warfarin for years when he developed the atrial fibrillation blood clot that dislodged from his heart and traveled to his brain, causing a massive stroke.

It's important to go into these decisions with open eyes. It's also important not to let the risks terrify you into not taking a drug that could help save your life. As is the case with antiarrhythmics, it is absolutely possible for patients to find a safe and effective dose of blood thinners that doesn't result in a life of absolute misery when it comes to side effects.

The important thing to understand is that the risk-versus-benefit balance between stroke and bleeding is *always* quite delicate, and is made all the more precarious if you have to add yet another set of drugs to the mix: heart failure medications.

| Anticoagulants | Warfarin, Eliquis, Xarelto, Pradaxa, and Savaysa | • Thin the blood to significantly decrease the risk of a blood clot stroke<br>• Increase the risk of bleeding |
|---|---|---|

## HEART FAILURE MEDICATIONS

The relationship between atrial fibrillation and heart failure is so deep that researchers writing for the journal *Circulation* once called the two diseases "a dual epidemic," while scientists writing for the *Korean Circulation Journal* called this comorbidity combo punch "a therapeutic challenge of our times."[35] Danish health scientists have found that nearly 10 percent of patients with heart failure have or will develop atrial fibrillation within three and a half years.[36]

Now, heart failure doesn't mean your heart has stopped working; after all, if that were the case, there would be no need for medication. Rather, the hearts of people who suffer from this condition have ventricles that can no longer contract as vigorously or fill as efficiently as they should. And, as is the case when it comes to atrial fibrillation, if this condition is left untreated it will likely get worse over time. So, all too often, heart failure can eventually lead to hearts that indeed stop working.

Even a few days of a heart beating in active AFib may be enough to degenerate into heart failure. If that heart failure is entirely due to AFib, then a few months of normal sinus rhythm is usually enough time to put the heart failure into remission. Either way, though, if you have been diagnosed with the dual epidemic of AFib and heart failure with a low ejection fraction, you can expect your doctor will want you to take at least a few more drugs, including angiotensin-converting enzyme (ACE) inhibitors, which dilate blood vessels and thus reduce blood pressure; angiotensin II receptor blockers (ARBs), which help relax your veins and arteries for the same purpose; angiotensin-receptor neprilysin inhibitors (ARNIs), a combination of two blood pressure–lowering peptides that reduce blood volume; beta-blockers, which reduce heart rate and pumping force; and diuretics, to get rid of the extra fluid you retain from heart failure—among other possible drugs.

| Heart Failure with Low Ejection Fraction Medications | Beta-blockers, ACE inhibitors, ARBs, diuretics, and neprilysin inhibitors | • Prescribed only if you have heart failure in addition to AFib |
| --- | --- | --- |

Suffice it to say there is a veritable sea of drugs out there, each with potential benefits. They don't all work the same way or with the same effectiveness in all people. And most come with side effects and risks that make taking them for the rest of one's life a rather unpleasant thought.

Small wonder that so many people want to know if there are any supplement alternatives. And yes, there are.

## THE SUPPLEMENT STORY

Does this long discussion on medications, medications, and more medications leave you feeling a bit hopeless? If you're anything like the patients we see every day, you probably feel either a bit lost in the haze or angry that your doctor wasn't more clear with you about the numerous hazards related to AFib drugs before they jetted off to write a prescription. It is for these reasons that many of our patients have gone looking for another path—and one of the first things they discover is the Wild West world of supplements.

Supplements include vitamins, minerals, herbs, and chemicals that can play an important role in a person's health, but have not gone through the rigorous testing of pharmaceuticals. There are no FDA-approved AFib supplements. In fact, no one is even regulating the supplement industry itself, so it can be difficult to know if you are even getting the supplement you desire, in the amount you need, and free of any toxic contaminants. So, if you choose to take supplements, you absolutely must know that you do so at your own risk—and we cannot stress enough how important it is to first discuss this choice with a cardiologist.

Some might argue that because supplements aren't regulated, doctors shouldn't even talk about them. That's silly. Whatever the concerns, people with AFib are increasingly turning to these substances for help—and there is good evidence that some supplements may indeed be effective.

**Magnesium** is a good place to start, because if ever there was a supplement that even the most traditional of all traditional doctors could accept, it would have to be this essential mineral, which is responsible for hundreds of biochemical reactions in the human body. Nonetheless, the plant-light diet of most Americans means millions upon millions of people are magnesium deficient. Prominent cardiologists have even called magnesium deficiency a principal driver of cardiovascular disease and a public health crisis.[37]

Low magnesium levels have long been observed in AFib patients.[38] Magnesium works its magic by calming the cell-to-cell electrical channels in the heart.[39] It has even been shown to help treat AFib in many studies, and it can make some antiarrhythmics like sotalol or dofetilide much safer.[40] Magnesium can also calm palpitations from premature atrial or ventricular contractions, known as PACs and PVCs.

We have some patients who swear magnesium is the secret to treating their AFib. If that's true—and some research suggests it may indeed be[41]—it might partly be because it is quite effective at also helping people sleep—and deep, restful, restorative sleep is absolutely vital for anyone who wants to put their AFib into remission.[42]

So long as your kidneys are healthy and you don't take more than the recommended dosage, magnesium is remarkably safe. The most common side effect is loose stools, which can usually be resolved by simply taking a lower dose or switching to a different form of magnesium.

Perhaps the best news when it comes to magnesium is that most people don't need to supplement for it. Unless you are taking a stomach-acid-blocking medicine, or have other gut absorption issues, you can pack your diet full of magnesium just by eating nuts, seeds, and greens—the more greens the better, in fact. If you do need extra supplementation, and you are concerned about the purity of supplements, your doctor can prescribe a prescription version of magnesium.

**Potassium** is another supplement that some of our patients believe has made a world of difference in their AFib treatment. As with magnesium, potassium deficiency has also clearly been linked to atrial fibrillation.[43] However, the big difference is that while magnesium supplementation is safe for almost everyone, it can be trickier to safely supplement with potassium because, in people with weak kidneys, potassium levels can quickly build up, increasing the risk of cardiac arrest. (Dr. Jack Kevorkian's approach to physician-assisted suicide was potassium overdose.) For this reason, supplemental potassium tablets are very low dose.

But if your kidneys are strong, your heart will thank you for eating spinach, tomatoes, asparagus, bananas, broccoli, oranges, and other potassium-rich foods. If you have a more severe case of potassium deficiency, it can be beneficial to work with a doctor to get a prescription-strength potassium supplement to help keep your heart in sinus rhythm.

**Nattokinase**, an enzyme extracted from a popular Japanese health food called natto, is one of the many "natural blood thinners" that some AFib patients take in hopes of avoiding the prospect of being on a pharmaceutical blood thinner for the rest of their lives.

Here's the problem: while studies do indeed show that nattokinase can prevent some blood clots, it has never been shown to prevent atrial fibrillation clots.[44] And, like other weak blood thinners such as aspirin, we suspect that nattokinase isn't strong enough to prevent AFib strokes. That probably explains why, anecdotally speaking, we've seen strokes in patients who've opted for nattokinase over prescription-strength blood thinners.

That doesn't mean nattokinase can't help at all. If you use the tactics described in this book, have a low CHADS-VASc score, and are no longer experiencing AFib attacks, nattokinase could possibly offer just a bit of extra assurance, as can other herbal blood thinners like turmeric, garlic, cayenne peppers, fish oil, cinnamon, and gingko. However, none of these other natural blood thinners have ever been shown in clinical settings to prevent AFib strokes. And it's very important to know that, as we described in a study for the journal *Cardiology* in 2010, combining these natural blood thinners with prescription-strength blood thinners could send your bleeding risk sky-high.[45]

**Vitamin D** has been shown in some studies to be associated with atrial fibrillation,[46] but correcting vitamin D deficiencies with a supplement hasn't yet been shown to prevent AFib. Nonetheless, guided vitamin D supplementation, under the direction of a doctor to keep your vitamin D levels in the normal range, could be helpful—and since most people living far from the equator have a vitamin D deficiency, it can be beneficial in several ways.

It's important, however, not to overdo it. Our research has demonstrated that taking *too much* vitamin D could actually be a risk factor for developing AFib.[47]

**Fish oil** *should* work wonders for AFib. After all, it has been clearly shown to change the heart's electrical properties through its antioxidant, anti-inflammatory, and anticlotting effects. Yet when fish oil has been studied in numerous different situations for AFib, the results have been confusing. A number of studies say it helps. Others suggest it has no effect or might even make things worse.[48] What mixed results like these often mean is that there really is no significant difference or that an intervention has different effects on different people, based on factors that are yet unclear.

So, what should you do when it comes to fish oil? If your cardiologist has recommended fish oil for another condition, such as high triglycerides, and it feels as if it is helping with your AFib, too, then carry on. But if you're not confident that it's working—and certainly if you feel it might be adversely impacting your AFib or your bleeding risk—you shouldn't just keep taking it. Rather, it's time to renew the discussion with your doctor about whether the benefits for one condition outweigh the potential risks for another.

**Coenzyme Q10**, or CoQ10, is another very popular cardiac supplement. CoQ10 is a naturally occurring enzyme in our bodies that protects cells from oxidative stress—especially the mitochondria, which are the energy storehouses of our cells.

Some studies have suggested CoQ10 might improve heart function in patients with heart failure and might be protective against some of the side effects that often come with statin use.[49] It also appears to be quite safe and is widely available as a supplement.[50] Further, early studies have shown a possible beneficial effect of CoQ10 for people suffering from both heart failure and AFib.[51] Like all supplements, however, it should be taken under the direction of a doctor.

**L-carnitine** is another popular AFib supplement among our patients, but it is difficult to assess this supplement as there are quite a few conflicting study results. Some studies have shown that L-carnitine may help with both AFib[52] and ventricular arrhythmias.[53] But we also know that L-carnitine may cause your gut microbiome to start producing potentially toxic levels of the molecule trimethylamine N-oxide, or TMAO,[54] which has been linked to heart attacks, AFib, and even death.[55] Thus, the bottom line is that we desperately need more studies on this supplement, for while L-carnitine might help your AFib, it could just as easily increase your risk of a heart attack or death. Until we know with greater certainty, it's advisable to avoid this supplement unless under the direction of your cardiologist.

**Vitamin K$_2$** hasn't been shown to do anything for AFib, but many of our patients like this supplement because of some early studies showing it may help prevent both osteoporosis and coronary artery disease.[56] It also appears to have a rather favorable "side effect profile," meaning it's unlikely to make you feel miserable.

We always advise our patients that healthy food is the best medicine, and this is advice that can be followed with K$_2$. While your body will convert some of the K$_1$ from broccoli, kale, spinach, and other greens to K$_2$, you can also eat K$_2$ directly. For example, K$_2$ is quite prevalent in natto, which is made from fermented soybeans and is available at most Asian grocery stores in the United States. In addition to being a probiotic, packed with nattokinase and more vitamin K$_2$ than any other food on this planet, studies suggest natto may be one reason why the Japanese have such low rates of cardiovascular disease and exceptional longevity.[57]

**Hawthorn**, or, more specifically, the extracts from the flowers, leaves, and berries of the hawthorn plant, have been used for centuries to treat various cardiovascular conditions. But while some studies have shown hawthorn might be successful in treating heart failure,[58] and it has been shown to change the heart's potassium channels,[59] there are no studies showing whether these electrical changes make AFib better or worse. We do know from antiarrhythmic drug studies, however, that whenever you change the heart's potassium channels, there is a chance of causing cardiac arrest. Thus, until research shows if hawthorn is good or bad for AFib patients, it would probably be best to leave this one alone.

**CBD oil** will fix just about anything that ails you—or so it might seem these days, as this chemical compound, derived from the cannabis plant (also known as marijuana), is showing up just about everywhere.

You can't get "high" from CBD oil; that effect comes from a different chemical in the plant, tetrahydrocannabinol, or THC. But that doesn't mean it has no effect. Indeed, many of your friends may swear by CBD oil for treating their chronic pain, anxiety, depression, cancer, acne, neurological conditions, high blood pressure, or diabetes. There is some clinical evidence that supports some of these anecdotal points of view, but, to date, there are no studies looking at whether or not it helps AFib.

Given the enormous popularity of CBD oil, it is probably just a matter of time before a researcher somewhere in the world starts studying CBD oil for the treatment of AFib. In the meantime, though, a wait-and-see approach is advised, especially given reports of liver damage from CBD oil.[60]

| Supplement | Key Points |
| --- | --- |
| **Magnesium** | May help with AFib, palpitations, sleep, and anxiety. Minimal risk. |
| **Potassium** | May help with AFib and palpitations. Very narrow therapeutic window. Significant risk if potassium levels get too high. |
| **Nattokinase** | Most popular "natural" blood thinner. Never studied with AFib. Likely not potent enough to prevent AFib strokes. Significant bleeding risk if combined with prescription-strength blood thinners. |
| **Vitamin D** | May help with AFib if deficient in this vitamin. Take under your physician's direction to make sure vitamin D levels are in the normal range. Over-supplementing with vitamin D may worsen AFib. |
| **Fish oil** | Recent studies question benefit for AFib. Has some blood-thinning effects. Good for high triglycerides. Minimal risk if taken as directed. |
| **CoQ10** | Very popular heart supplement. May help with heart failure, and those on cholesterol-lowering statins. Minimal risk if taken as directed. |
| **L-carnitine** | May help AFib. May worsen AFib and heart arterial blockages through TMAO production. Probably best to avoid. |
| **Vitamin K$_2$** | May help prevent calcification of arteries (especially in heart) and promote bone health. Avoid if taking warfarin. Minimal risk if taken as directed. |

| Supplement | Key Points |
|---|---|
| Hawthorn | May have some benefit in heart failure. Changes potassium channels of the heart with unknown effects. Probably best to avoid until more research is available. |
| CBD oil | Not studied for AFib but a very popular supplement with our patients. May help with diabetes and hypertension. Reports of liver damage. Probably best to avoid until more research is available. |

## DRUGS AND SUPPLEMENTS: THE BOTTOM LINE

Whether you choose to treat your AFib with meds, supplements, or a combination of both, it's important to remember that, either way, you are putting chemicals into your body.

Sometimes, sure, there is simply no other choice: your body needs these substances to survive. Most atrial fibrillation patients will need some drugs, and possibly a few supplements, at least temporarily, until the underlying atrial fibrillation causes can be addressed and the disease put into remission. But many patients succumb to the idea that they are hooked on antiarrhythmics, blood thinners, and heart failure meds for the rest of their lives.

It's easy to get complacent after starting on AFib meds. Symptoms are alleviated. Side effects are limited. As such, it starts to feel like things are getting better. But medications and supplements that seem to be working right now won't likely have the same effect a few years down the road. A lack of side effects now doesn't mean there won't be side effects in the future.

You cannot solve all of the problems from AFib with a pill. Eventually it may catch up with you again. If you're okay with that, then there is nothing left to do. But if you're reading this book, you're probably not okay with that. And you shouldn't be.

Peri came to understand this very early into her AFib journey—and she didn't like it at all. That's good, because it was a strong indication that she would be motivated to get off the drugs as soon as possible.

And that's just what she did. But she absolutely couldn't do that without taking a few other steps first.

The rest of this book describes the process Peri and many other people have taken to not just put AFib drugs in the past, but to put AFib itself in the past. And, since everything needs a catchy acronym these days, we call it "BLAST," which stands for:

**B**iomarker Monitoring: It's hard, if not impossible, to manage things that we do not measure. That's why biomarker monitoring is so important. This is the process of watching a variety of substances that exist in your body that are known to be indicators of increased AFib risk.

**L**ifestyle Optimization: You can't control your genes. You also can't change the past. But there are a lot of steps you can take to exert influence over the areas of your life that impact your AFib and ensure that your health gets better over time.

**A**blation: Not everyone with AFib, and certainly not everyone at risk of AFib, will need to have an ablation procedure to fix faulty electrical pathways in their hearts. However, everyone with AFib should understand what happens in an ablation procedure, and what the various options for getting an ablation are.

**S**topping Unnecessary Drugs: Many people who are on AFib medications think they are stuck with those drugs for the rest of their lives. This simply isn't true. Most determined patients can significantly reduce, and sometimes altogether eliminate, the medications they have been prescribed for AFib.

**T**racking: Putting AFib into remission—and keeping it there—is a lifelong endeavor. It doesn't have to be hard, but the patients who are most successful are those who dedicate themselves to measuring their biomarkers periodically, monitoring their lifestyle-optimization strategies, keeping a close eye on their medication intake, and noting any incidence of arrhythmia.

You can take *some* of these steps out of order. If you've already had an ablation, for instance, that doesn't mean you can't start monitoring your biomarkers. But the decision to reduce or eliminate medications is one you should absolutely make in consultation with your physician after the other steps begin to affect your health. If you're on AFib medications right now and you quit "cold turkey," you're potentially putting your life at risk. Quickly ending a drug that your body, and in particular your heart, is accustomed to having is not going to help you cure your AFib; it could very well be suicide.

But if you're determined to get there, know this: most people who follow this process can indeed significantly reduce the need for AFib drugs and supplements, and many have been able to throw all of their medications in the trash.

The BLAST approach really does work—and we have thousands upon thousands of patients who are living proof of this.

## Chapter Four

# BIOMARKER MONITORING

## How to understand what your body is telling you

Theresa had spent more than thirty years of her nursing career caring for heart patients in the thoracic intensive care unit of a large hospital. So, when she had her first episode of atrial fibrillation just six months after retiring, she couldn't help but laugh a little at the irony.

That is, *eventually* she laughed. First she was scared. Really scared.

Theresa and her family were gathered to celebrate her husband's birthday when she began feeling unwell. Once she got home, she found a small finger oximeter (the medicine cabinets of nurses and doctors have all kinds of cool toys) that measures oxygen saturation in the blood and the pulse rate.

Her heart was beating irregularly—and at 165 beats per minute.

That was her first episode of atrial fibrillation. It would not be her last.

Theresa's AFib episodes came and went every few months after that. Slowly but surely, they became more frequent and more severe. And then, one day while rushing to catch a flight at the airport, the need to get help became terrifyingly clear.

"It was a long walk to the gate in the airport," she recalled. "By the time I arrived, I was having difficulty breathing."

She was sweating, shaking, nauseated, and dizzy. Her temples were throbbing. Her heart rate was 180. Then 200. Then 220.

Then 240.

"This is it," she remembers thinking. "I'm going to die. My heart can't keep going this fast much longer."

Theresa was definitely in a bad situation—a dangerously bad situation—but she survived, and got the "come to God" moment she needed to take the big steps necessary to save her own life. Indeed, as of this writing, she is still going strong. Stronger than ever, in fact—because she has put her AFib into almost complete remission!

To be able to say that, Theresa had to make *a lot* of life changes. But one of the first, and most important, is that she became a student of her personal biomarkers.

In this chapter, we'll discuss the B in BLAST—biomarker optimization—and introduce you to the ten biomarkers most important for AFib patients to watch. We'll discuss the research that has connected these biomarkers to atrial fibrillation, and talk about ways to optimize each one, to maximize your chance of putting AFib into remission, or to stop it before it does to you what it was doing to Theresa.

## THE BIOMARKER REVOLUTION

Published in 1990 by Oxford University Press, *Biological Markers in Epidemiology* was one of the first and most comprehensive attempts to explain what was then a cutting-edge field of science. In it, editors Barbara Hulka, Timothy Wilcosky, and Jack Griffith explained how scientists had identified ways to "see" a disease long before it was more traditionally diagnosable, and to monitor its progression with relatively easy tests, rather than invasive procedures. But alas, they warned, lest anyone get too excited at the paradigm-shifting potential, "considerable groundwork is needed to relate biomarkers in tissues readily available for human monitoring."[1]

Ah, what a difference a few decades makes. Today, researchers have identified thousands of biomarkers. While the term *biomarker* is most often used to describe a protein or chemical in our body that we can measure from the blood, it can also be applied to *any* indicator of health that can be measured over time to track biological processes. These markers can be clues to the presence, status, or extent of a disease, and they can also provide evidence of the extent to which a treatment or therapy is working.[2]

That's not just important for people who want to keep their AFib at bay—it's essential. That's because most medical conditions aren't nearly as binary as many of us have come to think. Between "being well" and "having AFib" are millions upon millions of tiny steps that are not perceivable by patients, nor by the traditional methods doctors use to diagnose this condition. These processes used to be invisible to us. Now, through the use of biomarkers, we can monitor these steps.

As you might suspect, that's going to be quite important when we get to the tracking part of the BLAST process. But for now, it will immediately help you prioritize what lifestyle optimization strategies you need to adopt, determine whether and when to pursue an ablation, and know which drugs are necessary and which can be curtailed.

You've probably had some of your biomarkers checked quite a few times—even if you didn't realize it. One commonly known biomarker is prostate-specific antigen, or PSA, which is frequently used to monitor and assess the status of patients with or at risk of prostate cancer. But every time you've had your body temperature taken, slipped your arm into a blood pressure monitor, or had blood drawn for a cholesterol check, you've engaged in the process of assessing your biomarkers to monitor your health. (Want to know what you've already had done? Most US medical providers now have a patient portal where you can log on and view all of your lab results in comparison to the normal ranges of various biomarkers.)

These days, the options for biomarker testing are virtually endless. The global market for diagnostic tools that measure biomarkers is in the tens of billions of dollars, and growing fast,[3] and you could spend a very large fortune trying to get all of your markers tested. When it comes to AFib, however, there are ten simple blood tests that any doctor can easily order—and some you can do yourself at home—that you should consider getting on a semiregular basis. In the United States, many if not all of these tests are covered by insurance companies. In nations with more significantly socialized systems, many of these tests are available for free with a doctor's order. No matter where you are, though, it's a good idea to check into what is covered to make sure you don't get any surprise bills and, of course, to consult regularly with your doctor about the purpose of the tests and what they are telling you about your condition.

Do you need to get *all* of these checked on a regular basis? Almost assuredly not. But it's a good idea to get each one done at some point, and to keep an eye on the ones that are most related to the AFib symptoms that you are experiencing or concerned about. A doctor can help you with those decisions—but you can help your doctor a lot if you're up to speed on what these tests are, what they mean, and how they are measured.

## Highly Sensitive C-Reactive Protein

Back in the mid-2000s, we conducted a study of more than 2,300 patients between the ages of fifty-two and seventy-six in search of biomarkers that might help us predict and prevent atrial fibrillation. When we published our results in 2009, many people were stunned. We had demonstrated that a blood biomarker known as C-reactive protein, or CRP, was a powerful predictor of who would get AFib.[4]

The reason why this came as such a surprise was that CRP isn't commonly associated with the heart. Rather, it's produced in the liver, and it's most commonly used as a blood test marker for inflammation.

What does inflammation have to do with a condition most commonly associated with the abnormal firing of electrical impulses in the heart? Well, as it turns out, quite a bit. While the precise mechanistic links aren't yet fully known, researchers believe that atrial fibrillation could be both a cause and a result of inflammation[5]—a very horrible example of a "vicious cycle" in which heart scarring causes inflammation (in part because of the migration of immune cells toward injured tissue) and inflammation causes even *more* heart scarring.

The good news—if there can be any good news when it comes to the dangerous combination of inflammation and AFib—is that because of this relationship, CRP can be a tremendously useful biomarker. And yet, of all the blood tests doctors can order for atrial fibrillation, CRP is probably the most commonly overlooked. That's too bad, because at around $30 over the counter (and often cheaper with a prescription and some insurance plans), this is a simple and relatively inexpensive test that can tell us a lot about our overall risk.

If you've already had your CRP tested, you might know that there are two different CRP tests. The first is for the standard CRP, which is best for detecting inflammation related to autoimmune diseases. The second is for highly sensitive CRP (hs-CRP), which is best for detecting inflammation of the heart. The results from these tests correlate quite well—if the CRP is high, the hs-CRP will probably be high as well; likewise, a low CRP usually translates to a low hs-CRP. That doesn't mean the tests are interchangeable for the purpose of tracking your progress—getting CRP tested in January and hs-CRP tested in July won't tell you much about how you're doing. But if your doctor or insurer prefers one over the other, for whatever reason, you're not missing out.

Both tests are measured in milligrams per liter (mg/L). Doctors who treat AFib patients and who are attuned to the importance of this bio-marker often see some very high CRPs (anything above 3 mg/L), while a very healthy CRP is nearly undetectable. The magic number, though, is 1: if your CRP is higher than 1 mg/L, then you have to work on decreasing your risk.

If your CRP comes back sky-high, though, please don't panic. By itself, all this number tells you is that there is an "inflammation fire" burning somewhere in your body and that your immune system is working overtime to put it out. That could be a result of AFib, but it could also be the result of a simple viral infection, an intense bit of exercise, an undiagnosed autoimmune disease, cancer, bad genetics, or, all too often, lifestyle and eating choices that have led to an unhealthy chronic activation of your immune system.

The single best thing you can do to lower your CRP is to get your waist size down. Why? Because waist size tracks quite closely to visceral fat,[6] which is every kind of fat stored within the torso—including in the pericardium, a thin, membranous sac holding the heart. Sometimes, the pericardial fat layer surrounding the heart can be more than an inch thick. This fat releases cytokines, which can cause particularly intense inflammation. Everyone's body is different, but research indicates that to keep visceral fat at bay, men want to get their waist size below thirty-five inches, while women should shoot for less than thirty-two inches.[7]

Cutting inches off your waist isn't the only way to address a high CRP. The tips and tactics we'll discuss in later chapters, like following the anti-inflammatory AFib diet, daily exercise, and optimizing your sleep and stress levels, will also help you get your CRP down—and keep it there.

The key to making any biomarker worthwhile is regularity. Getting your hs-CRP checked just once, after all, gives you little more than a snapshot of inflammation on a single day. If your hs-CRP is above 1, you should have it checked periodically to track your progress and to make sure you can get it below 1. Simple and relatively inexpensive home kits are even available online without the need of a doctor's prescription. Once your hs-CRP has been optimized and is steadily below 1, you should recheck it every few years, or sooner if something has changed in your life that is likely affecting your health.

## Hemoglobin A1C

Most people seem to know that high blood sugar can be a big problem for people with diabetes. What many don't know is that glucose—the simple sugar that serves as one of our bodies' most common sources of energy—is an important biomarker for many other medical conditions, including atrial fibrillation. That's in part because people with diabetes have about a 50 percent increased risk of AFib,[8] and the longer you have diabetes, or the higher your blood glucose tends to run, the more likely AFib becomes.[9] But high blood glucose may damage the electrical system of the heart long before you're ever diagnosed with diabetes, and even if you never become diabetic at all.

The mechanistic causes of this association aren't entirely clear, but some researchers have suggested that it's not the blood glucose levels so much as the *fluctuations* of those levels that upregulates the expression of a gene called *TXNIP*. That gene, in turn, orders up increased levels of reactive molecules that can cause cells to die—an evolutionary response, perhaps, to the body's need to ward off the growth and spread of harmful microbes.[10] In a manner of thinking, our bodies treat the waxing and waning of glucose as an invasion, pulling out all the stops—including the sacrifice of some healthy cells—to fight it. And when a heart cell dies, it leaves behind fibrosis, which may then disrupt the heart's normal electrical conduction.

Fibrosis isn't the only consequence of an elevated glucose level. Studies show that glucose fluctuations might also stoke inflammation in the heart—contributing to the vicious cycle we discussed above.[11] In addition, glucose intolerance and insulin resistance have been shown to cause heart enlargement and abnormal thickening.[12] And, just as diabetes can destroy the nerves in your hands and feet, it can also damage the nerves in your heart, again leading to atrial fibrillation.[13]

Developing a basic understanding of these associations is important for taking ownership of the treatments and therapies we use to move these biomarkers in safer directions, but it's important to remember that *however* this happens, it happens. And that's why people at risk of atrial fibrillation, or who have been diagnosed with AFib, should get regularly tested for hemoglobin A1C, which measures how much glucose in your blood has been sticking to your red blood cells over the past few months, and which is reported as a percentage.

Sugar coating is all well and fine when it comes to gumdrops and chocolate donuts, but it's not good for your red blood cells. So, in general, the lower your average A1C percentage, the better. Indeed, one study demonstrated an astoundingly linear correlation between A1C and the risk of an atrial fibrillation stroke.[14]

An A1C reading over 6.5 percent indicates diabetes, and over 5.7 percent is considered prediabetes. So, to keep AFib at bay, we urge our patients to shoot for an A1C that is consistently less than 5.7.

Not there yet? It's time to get to work. Perhaps not surprisingly, the foods we eat have a tremendous impact on our A1C. You're probably already well aware that any added sugars should be reserved for exceptionally rare occasions, if not eliminated from our diets entirely. Perhaps you're also savvy to the fact that even 100 percent fruit juice, which many people consider to be a healthy part of a balanced diet, can result in a blood-sugar spike—the very sort of fluctuation that research suggests might cause our bodies to assume we're under attack. What many people are also coming to realize is that any processed carbohydrates, like those found in flour, are broken down by our bodies into sugar—and this can actually happen just as quickly as it would after we consume a piece of candy from the grocery checkout aisle. Even so-called "healthy" whole wheat bread, as we noted earlier, can spike your blood glucose levels higher than a candy bar.

Late-night eating can also be tremendously detrimental to our A1C levels. A body at rest simply can't process sugars as effectively as a body in motion, which should also be a big clue that staying in motion is a key factor for keeping blood sugar at bay (more on that in chapter five). Your last meal of the day should come at least three hours before you head to bed, and it's absolutely vital to spend some of that in-between time getting some physical activity—and there are plenty of fun ways to do that.[15]

Whichever diet or eating approach you choose to combat your A1C levels, you should combine it with a healthy dose of exercise that ultimately lowers your weight to normal levels if you want to move the needle on your A1C.

If you can't normalize your A1C by cutting all added sugars and processed carbohydrates (like flour), getting exercise, and losing weight, you'll want to see a diabetes specialist, like an endocrinologist, to explore medications that might help get your A1C below 5.7.

While some will argue that there are better ways than A1C to test for diabetes and prediabetes, the hemoglobin A1C test is a very good start because it is readily available at any doctor's office, is usually covered by US health insurance, gives you a running three-month average of your glucose levels, and has been extensively studied for decades.

Also, because diabetes is such a common condition, A1C home-testing kits are easy to find and relatively inexpensive. You can get a highly accurate, reusable A1C tester for about $60 over the counter. Many people who have successfully fought their AFib have found that it was valuable to use it once every few months until their A1C was reliably below 5.7 every time. After that, testing every year or so might be a good idea, even if you've had a procedure that has successfully treated your atrial fibrillation, because research shows that insulin resistance is an important predictor of AFib recurrence—and while insulin resistance itself isn't usually a routine test, A1C is a very reasonable surrogate.[16]

## Thyroid Panel

It's well known that the forty-first president of the United States, George Herbert Walker Bush, lived well into his nineties—and that he remained in generally good health until the very end. In fact, the onetime pilot, who became one of the US military's youngest aviators after enlisting in the Navy after the December 7, 1941, attack on Pearl Harbor, still had his head in the clouds at an age when many people have long since been underground—he celebrated his eightieth, eighty-fifth, and ninetieth birthdays by skydiving.

But Bush, who was in his mid-sixties when he became president, couldn't escape all of the health woes that come with age. He was diagnosed with atrial fibrillation while serving as the nation's chief executive.

Now, that makes sense, right? Being president is exceptionally stressful. Just look at the before-and-after pictures of US presidents; what a difference a stint in the White House makes in terms of wrinkles and gray hair! And we've known for more than half a century that psychological stress can be a trigger for AFib.[17] Yet Bush's AFib does not appear to have been a consequence of stress alone. Rather, it was initially the result of an overactive thyroid.

As we discussed in chapter one, hyperthyroidism occurs when the thyroid gland, an endocrine gland in our necks that produces hormones necessary for the cells in our bodies to function, starts to overproduce thyroid hormone. In normal circumstances this hormone helps with metabolism—a good thing—but when it is hyperactive or you have been prescribed too much thyroid hormone, it acts as a very potent stimulant. Over time, this can cause unintentional weight loss, tremors, and anxiety, among other serious problems. It can also cause rapid or irregular heartbeats and palpitations. Sound familiar? Indeed, hyperthyroidism and atrial fibrillation go hand in hand. And not only does thyroid hormone trigger AFib; it also changes your blood chemistry such that your body more easily forms blood clots,[18] making AFib and hyperthyroidism a one-two combo punch that often leads to stroke.

An underactive thyroid can also lead to atrial fibrillation.[19] To make matters worse, even if you feel great and are having no symptoms, just a minor abnormality in any of your thyroid hormones may put you at risk for atrial fibrillation.[20]

That's the bad news. The good news is that once an abnormality in your thyroid hormone is diagnosed, it can usually be corrected quite easily. And the first step in that process is getting to know your thyroid panel, which usually includes tests for thyroid-stimulating hormone, thyroxine, and triiodothyronine (known as TSH, free $T_4$, and free $T_3$, respectively). Your goal is simply to work to make sure your numbers are all well within normal ranges.

Keeping these levels as close to the center of the normal range as possible is important. Our research in nearly 175,000 people has shown that, when it comes to free $T_4$, even levels that are ever so slightly on the high side of "normal" are associated with atrial fibrillation.[21]

As with the other biomarkers, you can always do more advanced thyroid testing. However, if you want to do the testing through your physician and increase the chances of insurance covering the costs, then knowing your

TSH, $T_4$, and $T_3$ levels are usually enough to give you the data you need to minimize your AFib and stroke risk. If you are a do-it-yourself sort of person, home tests are also available for about $100.

Because hyperthyroidism can be a harbinger of atrial fibrillation, it's not uncommon for newly diagnosed AFib patients to have already been prescribed a thyroid hormone. If that's your situation, you absolutely need to get your thyroid panel done again. As our research has shown, high doses of thyroid hormones can raise the risk of atrial fibrillation.[22]

Another often overlooked problem that can lead to thyroid abnormalities and higher AFib risk is iodine deficiency. While iodine deficiency was once only seen in developing countries, it is making a comeback in more economically advanced places, as well.[23] The reason is simple: most of the salt in processed foods isn't iodized. So, if you don't eat much dairy, seafood, seaweed, or strawberries, you don't use iodized salt in your home salt shaker, or you don't take a multivitamin that includes iodine, you may be at risk.

The bottom line for thyroid abnormalities is that if any of your thyroid numbers are off, it would be best that you advocate for yourself and at least consult an endocrinologist.

## Comprehensive Metabolic Panel

By now, you understand that atrial fibrillation isn't a disease of the heart; it is a disease of the body that specifically attacks the heart. With that in mind, might a test that offers a broad overview of many body functions be useful? Absolutely. That's why, if you have been diagnosed with AFib, your regular doctor or the emergency room doctor who treated your AFib attack has probably already ordered a comprehensive metabolic panel, or CMP.

Many people have this battery of blood tests done as part of their annual physical. Most Americans, however, don't get an annual physical, and many doctors believe that physicals are an unnecessary and even counterproductive way of going about healthcare.[24] And even people with AFib often go longer between doctor visits than they probably should. But the

CMP offers a lot of information on a lot of different biomarkers. It is relatively inexpensive, too, at about $30, with insurance typically picking up most of the tab.

This test varies from lab to lab, but in general it measures blood sugar and electrolyte levels, and your kidney and liver function. We've already discussed the importance of knowing your blood sugar levels, so let's focus on those other areas.[25]

**Electrolytes** like sodium, potassium, magnesium, calcium, and chloride are important for conducting electrical impulses through the body—and if you think about that role, it's clear why they are of vital importance for people with AFib. Indeed, the depletion of electrolytes is a clearly established risk factor for atrial fibrillation, and electrolyte optimization is critical to maintaining normal sinus rhythm. The reason why electrolytes are so critical to keeping your heart in rhythm is that the electrical channels in each heart cell depend on the right balance of electrolytes to do their job.

Are you low? That's not good when it comes to AFib. But this is usually an easy fix.

Of your electrolytes, the most important ones to prevent atrial fibrillation are potassium and magnesium. These two electrolytes are not only important in preventing atrial fibrillation; they are also critical to monitor if you have been prescribed an antiarrhythmic medication.

For potassium, the goal is to keep your levels as close to 4 millimoles per liter (mmol/L) as possible. Based on the studies available, this is where the heart functions best with regard to atrial fibrillation risk.[26]

For magnesium, you want your number to be at least 2 milligrams per deciliter (mg/dL). In fact, keeping your serum magnesium level above that number cuts your atrial fibrillation risk by about 50 percent[27] and helps with other biomarkers like CRP[28] and blood pressure[29] as well. Magnesium can be tricky, though, because only a tiny fraction is ever in your bloodstream; the rest is inside your cells. Because of this, blood testing misses up to 99 percent of the magnesium in your body.

The two most common reasons why we see people with low electrolyte levels are either they are eating an electrolyte-depleted diet or they are taking a diuretic medication (used for high blood pressure, fluid retention from heart failure, or other causes). You don't have to rob Peter to pay Paul, though, when it comes to taking diuretics—because faithful adherence to the holistic approaches for beating atrial fibrillation discussed in this book may completely eliminate most people's need for diuretics. In fact, simply increasing your intake of foods with electrolytes in them—from spinach to bananas, from butternut squash to avocados—can make a world of difference. In some cases, potassium or magnesium supplementation, as discussed in chapter three, may be required. Some people think they may be able to do this with sports drinks like Gatorade and Powerade. While those drinks might possibly raise your electrolytes, they can also raise your blood sugar, and even the artificially sweetened drinks can bring more risk than benefit. However, if your potassium is on the low end of normal (3.5–3.9 mmol/L), then simply boosting your intake of fruits and vegetables should help correct any deficiency. As long as you have healthy kidneys, it is almost impossible to get too much potassium by eating a healthy diet.

Because the vast majority of Americans suffer from magnesium deficiency, many of our patients have found relief from their atrial fibrillation by eating a diet high in magnesium or by taking a magnesium supplement. But unless you undergo advanced magnesium testing, like the RBC Magnesium Test, which is probably not available through your doctor's office and definitely not covered by insurance, you'll never really know just how depleted of magnesium your body is. It is for this reason that it may take six or more months of magnesium supplementation before you see any beneficial effect. And, if you are on one of the commonly prescribed or over-the-counter proton-pump inhibitors used to reduce stomach acid (omeprazole, lansoprazole, esomeprazole, and pantoprazole, sold under the brand names Prilosec, Prevacid, Nexium, and Protonix, respectively), it may take even more time, since these drugs block the absorption of magnesium in the gut.

**Kidney and liver function** deficits are also associated with atrial fibrillation, although researchers aren't yet sure whether the kidneys and liver cause AFib, if it's the other way around, or if it's another vicious cycle. Whatever the case, poor kidney[30] or liver function[31] significantly increases your risk. So, if the goal is to beat atrial fibrillation, or just enjoy great health, then both kidney and liver function need to be optimized—and the CMP can be a big help in that regard.

Having normal kidney and liver function is also critical to minimizing the risk of any medications your doctor may have prescribed. For example, poor kidney and liver function significantly increase both your bleeding risk and your odds of a life-threatening ventricular arrhythmia if an antiarrhythmic is prescribed. If either of these organs isn't functioning properly, be sure to advocate for yourself to quickly see a nephrologist for your kidneys or a hepatologist for your liver. If you live in a rural area, it is well worth the trip to see a specialist in a nearby city.

Depending on your medical history, you may want to have this test done one or more times annually.

## Lipid Panel

Like the CMP, a lipid panel is another blood test that doctors frequently order—usually in the hopes of heading off atherosclerosis and a future heart attack. Also, as is the case with the CMP, lipid panels are used far less frequently than they could or should be, given this test's potential to tell us so much information about our AFib risk.

Also known as a coronary risk panel, a lipid panel—typically about $50 and usually covered by insurance—generally includes total cholesterol, high-density lipoprotein cholesterol, low-density lipoprotein cholesterol, and triglycerides. It is usually done after about twelve hours of water-only fasting. As with most of the biomarkers we discuss in this chapter, more involved lipid testing is certainly available, but the basic forms, which are generally covered by US insurance plans, suffice in most AFib cases.

When it comes to atrial fibrillation, two of the numbers in the lipid panel are most important. The first is your triglycerides, which are chemicals made by the body from sugar and carbohydrates, stored in fat cells, and released for energy at a later time. Your triglyceride goal is to get your number at least below 150 mg/dL (even lower is better), which decreases your atrial fibrillation risk by 60 percent when compared to people with higher triglyceride numbers.[32]

If your triglycerides are above 150, though, don't panic. Unless you have been diagnosed with a form of familial hyperlipidemia or related genetic abnormality, which is very rare, your high numbers are likely reversible by following the lifestyle practices advocated in this book. Those who do can often get this biomarker into the safe zone in a matter of weeks or months.

The second biomarker to focus on in the lipid panel is your LDL. This is often called "bad cholesterol," and for good reason: a high LDL dramatically increases your risk of a heart attack and doubles your risk of an atrial fibrillation stroke.[33]

So, what number should you shoot for with your LDL? While lower is definitely better when it comes to LDL, at minimum it should be below 100 mg/dL. If you have already had a heart attack or stent placed, however, your LDL target is going to be much lower.

As with the triglycerides number, individuals who consistently follow the path laid out in this book very commonly can get their LDL number below 100 without the need for drugs. Indeed, eating a mostly plant-based diet, exercising every day, and consuming exceedingly high amounts of fiber from unprocessed real foods is all most of our patients need to get their LDL well into the safe zone without medications.


## Vitamin D

Want to know something that will make you feel a little more connected to the cosmos? The building blocks of life on Earth, the atomic matter most frequently found inside of you and every living thing around you—carbon, hydrogen, nitrogen, oxygen, phosphorus, and sulfur—are also the most abundant elements in our galaxy. *Homo sapiens* and the Milky Way galaxy are composed of about 97 percent of the same kinds of atoms, according to astronomers who catalogued more than 150,000 stars for the Sloan Digital Sky Survey.[34]

We are stardust, indeed.

Is it any wonder, then, that one of the most important things we can do for our health is to get outside and soak up some sunshine? And is it any wonder that when we don't get enough vitamin D—a hormone that is created when ultraviolet radiation penetrates our skin—our health can suffer? A low vitamin D level is associated with many chronic medical conditions, and atrial fibrillation is no exception. Vitamin D deficiency can increase the risk of AFib by 31 percent[35]—perhaps because of increased inflammation through vitamin D receptors on cardiac cells, altered calcium metabolism, and fluid balance.[36] That is no small consideration, especially if you are already at risk.

Fortunately, vitamin D testing is cheap and is usually covered by insurance. Even more fortunately, of all the biomarkers to optimize, vitamin D is the easiest to correct for most people. Supplements work for people who don't eat much fish, mushrooms, or dairy, or who might not be able to get much sun time for a few days for whatever reason, but walking out the door is still truly the best medicine. Just getting outside for an extra ten to fifteen minutes a day—a little longer on overcast days—can make a world of difference in levels of vitamin D. Of course, when it comes to sun exposure, a little goes a long way, and you should consult with your doctor to see what dose of sunshine is best for you given your skin color, how far you live from the equator, the time of the year, and whether you live at sea level or at a higher elevation.

So, how high does your vitamin D level need to be? While there is some debate as to whether you want to target 20 or 30 nanograms per deciliter (ng/dL), it is certain that anything below 20 ng/dL is too low. We tend to agree with most integrative doctors and naturopaths in that the 50- to 70-ng/dL range is a very good goal.

Why test at all? Why not just skip the sun and take a high dose of a vitamin D supplement each day? Because, just as with natural sun exposure, there can be too much of a good thing. Indeed, our research suggests that too much vitamin D from supplements (anything over 100 ng/dL) may increase your atrial fibrillation risk two-and-a-half-fold.[37]

## Anemia, Including Red Blood Cell Size

For about a half a century, we've known that anemia, a lack of red blood cells, can be a serious risk factor for atrial fibrillation—and can indicate a potentially more dangerous case.[38]

As with many of the other atrial fibrillation biomarkers we have discussed, doctors commonly test for anemia. But as is the case for many of those tests, most people don't test as frequently as they could or should to ensure they are optimizing all of the most important markers.

Anemia is generally the result of one of two things. Either you are losing blood somewhere in your body, or your bone marrow can't make enough red blood cells. In both cases, the result is that your heart may not be getting enough oxygen, and that stress—like any stress on the heart—increases the likelihood of atrial fibrillation.

Anemia itself is fairly common. That doesn't mean it should be ignored, especially by people with atrial fibrillation, and even less so by AFib patients who are also on blood thinners, which can cause anemia without any visible signs of blood loss. And anemia doesn't just increase your atrial fibrillation risk; it also indicates an increased risk of heart attack, stroke, and all-cause mortality.[39] That's why, if you have been diagnosed with both atrial fibrillation and anemia, you should be working closely with your doctor to correct the underlying cause of anemia and minimize the risk of anything else bad happening.

An anemia test measures the amount of hemoglobin in grams per deciliter (g/dL) of blood. For men, the normal range is 13.5 to 17.5 g/dL. For women, it's 12 to 15.5 g/dL. Generally speaking, you want to be as close to the center of these ranges as possible.

In addition to this number, you also need to know the type of anemia you have, which is based on size and characteristics of the red blood cells. For example, if you are vitamin $B_{12}$ or folate deficient, the resulting type of anemia is macrocytic, meaning the few red blood cells you have for carrying oxygen are too big. In contrast, other medical challenges such as blood loss and iron deficiency can lead to microcytic anemia, in which the few red blood cells you have are too small. Both of these conditions can increase the risk of atrial fibrillation, but, as our recent research demonstrates, the treatments are often different.[40]

Macrocytic anemia can usually be corrected easily with healthy food choices: simply boost your fish and vegetable intake. Supplements may be necessary in some cases. You will also want to make sure you aren't on any medications, like the commonly prescribed proton-pump inhibitors for acid reflux, that may be blocking your absorption of key nutrients.

Since microcytic anemia is usually due to iron deficiency, in most cases the solution is to simply eat more iron-rich foods, such as spinach, tofu, broccoli, wild or organic meat, and dark chocolate. You can also eat foods that aren't necessarily iron-rich themselves but that are good at helping your body absorb iron, as fruits with lots of vitamin C are.

Having too many red blood cells can also adversely impact normal sinus rhythm.[41] This can occur from the body trying to compensate for a lung problem or genetic abnormality, like hemochromatosis, by making too many red blood cells. This is uncommon but nonetheless something to keep an eye on when you're monitoring your biomarkers.

## Homocysteine

You probably know that protein is one of the essential "building blocks of life" and that our bodies can't make protein without amino acids. You might also know that too many amino acids in your system can be a sign that you suffer from the "omnivore's dilemma," in that there is too much meat in the world and not enough time to eat it all. All of this, of course, means it's important to know the state of your aminos. And yet a simple blood test for one of the most potentially dangerous aminos, homocysteine, is rarely done.

That's unfortunate, because the presence of too much homocysteine in our blood has been associated with stroke, heart attack, dementia, and—no surprise at this point—atrial fibrillation. As with many of the other bio-markers we've discussed, the exact mechanism whereby homocysteine may trigger AFib isn't entirely clear, but research suggests that too much of this amino acid may be damaging to collagen, which provides structure and plasticity to our hearts. These are, of course, important traits for a muscle that never stops moving, and the result can be cardiac scarring and atrial enlargement.[42] In addition, high levels of homocysteine have been shown to damage or even kill the cells that line the insides of arteries and the heart.[43]

The healthy range for homocysteine is less than 10 micromoles per liter (μmol/L). Anything higher than that should make you want to spring into corrective action.

Hacking this biomarker isn't hard. Lowering your consumption of land animals can be a big help, so long as you are still getting enough vitamin $B_{12}$, which is found in animal protein; folate from green leafy vegetables and beans; and vitamin $B_6$ from sweet potatoes, sunflower seeds, spinach, and bananas. Some people also think there's a simpler hack—taking $B_{12}$, $B_6$, and folic acid supplements. While you can indeed lower homocysteine levels with vitamin supplementation, three studies of patients with preexisting heart conditions all failed to find any clinical benefit from such supplements.[44]

## BNP

This brings us to the biomarkers with arguably the most intimidating names, B-type natriuretic peptide and N-terminal-pro-BNP (NT-pro-BNP). Everybody just calls these "BNP" for short, and the medical literature suggests there really isn't much difference between the two.[45] After all, both measure the physical stress your heart is experiencing—and if you've been diagnosed with atrial fibrillation or have reason to be worried about it, that's a rather important metric. That's why, if you've been in the hospital and have had any fluid retention problems, you've likely had a BNP test already.

BNP measures the degree of heart failure you have. If your heart is pumping against high pressures, your body is retaining fluid, and the heart chambers begin to stretch and strain under the stress, your BNP will probably be high. For individuals under the age of seventy, a "high BNP" is anything above 100 picograms per milliliter (pg/mL) for BNP, or anything above 125 pg/mL for NT-pro-BNP.

Anything above those numbers is a danger sign for anyone, especially someone with atrial fibrillation, as it is associated with heart failure, stroke, and premature death. Indeed, one of the biomarker-based AFib stroke-risk predictor models uses BNP (along with troponin, which we will discuss in the next section) to determine how high your AFib stroke risk is.[46] All of that is to say that it is incredibly important to keep this biomarker in the normal zone. If your BNP is up, you definitely need to see a cardiologist as soon as possible, as your life may be in danger, and you likely will need medications until you can lower your BNP in more natural ways.

## High-Sensitivity Troponin

The last test that can be a good biomarker for individuals with or at risk of atrial fibrillation is for high-sensitivity troponin, or hs-Tn. If you have ever been to the emergency room for an AFib attack, then you've probably been given this biomarker blood test already. In general, the normal range for troponin is below 0.4 ng/mL.

Since troponin is a heart muscle protein that signifies active heart muscle damage, having *any* troponin elevation in your bloodstream is a bad sign—a really bad sign. Indeed, elevated troponin in someone with atrial fibrillation predicts a much higher risk of heart attack, heart failure, stroke, or premature death.[47] That's why, as with an elevated BNP, anyone with atrial fibrillation and an elevated troponin level must be under the very close care of a cardiologist. In fact, we can't emphasize that enough: an elevated BNP or troponin level is a potential disaster. Dishearteningly, people with elevated troponin levels may also have a harder time trying to get their atrial fibrillation under control.[48]

That doesn't mean all hope is lost. Not at all. With prompt and aggressive therapy, including lifestyle optimization, both BNP and troponin generally go down over time. But while all the biomarkers we've discussed should be met with immediate action if they are too high or too low, these simply cannot be ignored for another minute.

## More Advanced Testing

So far, we've discussed the ten most important atrial fibrillation blood tests that your doctor can easily order for you that also probably will be covered by insurance—or that, in the right circumstances, you can even do for yourself at home with tests available from respected, certified labs. But, as you might imagine, these ten tests are just the tip of the iceberg.

Biomarkers are available for chronic infections, food sensitivities, micronutrient deficiencies, hormonal imbalances, heavy metals, autoimmune diseases, and vitamin deficiencies, all of which have been associated with atrial fibrillation in published studies. Atrial fibrillation affects millions of people and, in many ways, its biological signatures and symptoms are like a thumbprint—everyone's situation is absolutely unique. To get beyond the ten tests we've discussed, then, often requires consultation with a functional medicine physician, naturopathic doctor, or other nontraditional healthcare provider.

However, to do all this advanced testing could easily set you back thousands of dollars, as insurance likely won't cover the costs. So, unless there is something unique about your case, you can likely drive your atrial fibrillation into remission without testing beyond the ten biomarkers discussed in this chapter. In most cases—probably yours as well—some combination of these ten tests will be right for you and your doctor as you monitor your fight to put AFib into remission and keep it there.

## Keeping Track

As evidence of someone who has truly become a master of her biomarkers, Theresa can rattle off her numbers like a baseball fanatic listing the statistics of the players on her favorite team.

"My A1C was 6.5; I got that down to 5.8," she said. "My total cholesterol is down to 141. My LDL is 74. My triglycerides are down from 127 to 96. My CRP is only 0.1 and my vitamin D is at least in the normal range at 39. My homocysteine is normal at 9."

And, most importantly, her episodes of atrial fibrillation have disappeared almost entirely.

That doesn't mean she is done, though. Theresa has become a dedicated biotracker. When any of her numbers move, she pays close attention, and when those numbers keep moving in a direction that concerns her, she takes action. (We'll discuss this in further detail in chapter eight.)

And yes, she'll be doing this for the rest of her life.

But it's likely to be a very long and very healthy life.

## TEN KEY BIOMARKERS FOR AFIB

| Biomarker | Test with AFib Diagnosis? | Further Testing? |
|---|---|---|
| 1. CRP (C-reactive protein) | Yes | Recheck in three months if higher than 1 mg/L and committed to lifestyle changes, periodically thereafter depending on results |
| 2. Hemoglobin A1C | Yes | Recheck in three months if above 5.7%, periodically thereafter depending on results |
| 3. Thyroid hormones | Yes | Recheck if abnormal, check at least annually if on long-term therapy, periodically thereafter depending on results |
| 4. CMP (comprehensive metabolic panel) | Yes | Recheck soon depending on abnormality, most primary care physicians check annually |

| 5. Lipid panel | Yes | Recheck in three months if abnormal and committed to lifestyle changes, periodically thereafter depending on results |
|---|---|---|
| 6. Vitamin D | Yes | Recheck in three months if below 50 ng/mL or above 100 ng/mL, periodically thereafter depending on results |
| 7. CBC (complete blood count for anemia) | Yes | Recheck soon if anemic (below 13.5 g/dL for men or below 12 g/dL for women, timing based on findings); most primary care physicians check annually |
| 8. Homocysteine | Yes | Recheck in three months if above 10 µmol/L and committed to lifestyle changes, periodically thereafter depending on results |
| 9. BNP | Yes | Recheck soon with slightest elevation (timing based on findings), periodically thereafter depending on results |
| 10. HS-troponin | Yes | Recheck soon with slightest elevation (timing based on findings), periodically thereafter depending on results |

## Chapter Five

# LIFESTYLE OPTIMIZATION

### Why setting up a better life for confronting AFib is easier than you think

Remember back in chapter one when you did an assessment of the factors that put people at greater risk for atrial fibrillation? Now we're going to put that information to work. If you struggle to sleep, for instance, you'll want to pay close attention to the section on sleep. If there's a lot of unhealthy stress in your life, the section on stress is specifically for you.

But you'll also recall that atrial fibrillation rarely comes from just one source. A struggle in one area of health often exacerbates initially smaller struggles in others, and our bodies—like any machine—are harder to get back into working order once something's gone wrong. So if you've already been diagnosed with AFib, *all* of the steps in this chapter are especially important.

That means addressing the factors keeping you from getting healthy and restorative sleep, identifying ways to reduce negative stress, taking the vital steps you need to lose weight, and ending terribly unhealthy habits like smoking. This chapter offers strategies for making all of these goals a reality.

You can take one at a time—and generally in whatever order best addresses the causes of your arrhythmia—in the short term. In the medium to long term, however, patients who address every one of these issues are the ones who are most likely to put their AFib into remission and keep it there. And while lifestyle optimization alone may not be enough to put your AFib into remission, it can make antiarrhythmic medications or ablation far more effective than they otherwise would have been.

That's the idea behind lifestyle optimization: not only addressing each of these areas of your life, but doing so in a way that ensures your health gets better and better over time. And that's important, because, as you'll remember, unaddressed atrial fibrillation tends to get worse and worse.

As optimization isn't a one-time thing, these are principles you should come back to again and again. What you're willing and able to do right now to improve your health will set you up for future successes. But, as is the case in any long journey, it's only once you reach your current goals that those new horizons can truly be seen.

## GET BETTER SLEEP

At first, Paula was reluctant to talk to her doctor about the causes of her AFib.

You might recall from chapter one that she didn't initially understand the reason why an honest assessment of the most likely causes of her AFib was so important. Once Paula understood the purpose for that part of the process, though, it didn't take long for her to identify two very likely culprits: sleep and weight.

She knew she needed to address both of those factors and, since she'd fought a lifelong battle to keep her weight down, she figured sleep would be the easier thing to attack. Besides that, she learned, doing so might make it easier to take on the weight issue. Studies show better sleep can result in a reduction of up to 522 calories from a person's daily food intake compared to sleep-deprived people.[1]

People who are chronically sleep deprived not only eat more, but also tend to eat late at night, and late-night food choices tend to be unhealthy and promote weight gain.

"Before, I really hadn't thought much about how important sleep is," she recalled. "So once I understood some of the science, and especially when I read about the studies that show such a strong connection between AFib and the quality of our sleep, I honestly figured that it was just a matter of making more time for sleep."

Easy, right? That's what Paula thought, too.

"But, oh boy, was I ever wrong," she told us. "It turns out that good sleep is something you really have to work at."

Paula might have been wrong about how easy it is to get more sleep, but she wasn't wrong about the importance of making time. The amount of time you dedicate to sleep is exceptionally important when it comes to general health and, more specifically, for keeping your heart in rhythm.

That's why we've made it the first principle in this chapter. For unless you are getting healthy and restorative sleep, everything else in this chapter will be much, much harder.

Everyone's needs are different, but there is almost no one in the world who cannot benefit from getting at least seven hours each night. And, to be clear, that's seven hours of *quality* sleep, free from sleep apnea and other disruptions—not just lying in bed for seven hours.

It's also true that simply *planning* to get more sleep is only the first step. Let's start there.

## Schedule Your Sleep

Take a look at your calendar. If you're like most people, there are blocks of time set aside for work, vacations, dinner with friends and family, visits from family members, and a whole bunch of other things. But does your calendar specifically include a daily block of at least seven hours *completely* dedicated to sleep so that your risk of AFib isn't higher?[2]

For most folks, the hours dedicated to sleep are implied, not blocked out on a schedule.

If irregular or insufficient sleep is a factor in your AFib risk, you absolutely need to join the 10 percent of Americans who actively prioritize their sleep.[3] Indeed, studies show that just one night of bad sleep can increase your risk of an AFib attack the next day by more than threefold![4] And the best way to do this is to actually put it on your calendar. Just as you do everything you can to avoid being late to work, you should do everything you can to avoid being late to bed. This is a simple and powerful step; studies show that the mere act of setting a bedtime and sticking to it results in an entire additional hour of sleep each night.[5]

And remember, seven hours is the target for actual sleep—not for time in bed. If it takes you thirty minutes to fall asleep and you typically have a middle-of-the-night awakening to use the bathroom, get a drink of water, check the locks on the doors, or whatever, then you should probably schedule at least eight hours.

At the same time, you also should schedule the time you'll get up in the morning—and rise no later than that time. This can be a tall order in a world in which more people than ever before are working remotely, with flexible hours and start-of-the-day times that are all too often aspirational rather than required. That can make it seem like hitting the snooze button is a harmless choice. But, contrary to popular belief, getting a few extra minutes of sleep in this way doesn't actually result in *restorative* sleep. In fact, waking, dozing off again, and abruptly waking again can result in sleep inertia—a period of up to four hours of lowered functionality.[6]

This doesn't mean you should stay in bed if you wake prematurely and feel rested. If you wake up and are ready to go, there's no reason not to greet the day. Conversely, if you *need* an alarm clock to wake up in the morning, then you likely didn't get enough sleep the night before. Our bodies have evolved to wake once we've gotten the amount of sleep we need. So once you've figured out how much sleep your body truly needs, you can set your bedtime accordingly.

Alarm clocks should be like insurance policies; they are there to put our minds at ease just in case we oversleep but it's best when they are never needed. Our bodies function best when we are able to wake up naturally, and that is most likely to happen when we schedule our bedtime and stead-fastly adhere to that schedule.

That's the first step Paula took, and it finally dismantled her notion that simply resolving to get more sleep was going to make it easy to do so. "It wasn't easy to get out of the habit of pushing back my bedtime so that I could get other things done," she said. "Every day it seemed like there was something that I needed to get done, and I kept telling myself that just a few minutes wouldn't hurt."

Once she truly committed to getting to bed by 10 PM, even when it meant leaving some things undone, "it was sort of like magic," she said. "It made every other step I needed to take so much easier, because I woke up with the energy I needed to fight the other battles."

## Lights Out

Even if you keep a perfect schedule, it's usually not enough to just show up for work. If you are a police officer on patrol, for instance, you can't do what you do without your badge, your uniform, your handcuffs, and your body camera, among other trappings of the job.

Sleep is the same way. Scheduling a bedtime is important, but once you get to bed, everything needs to be in order so that you can do what you're supposed to be doing there. This includes maintaining a clean, quiet, and cool room with plenty of fresh air. It also means remembering the most important purpose for your bed: sleep. Everything else can be done some-where else, and most things should be done somewhere else.

To be very clear on this point: our beds are not the right place for eat-ing. They're not the right place for working. And they're absolutely not the right place for "screen time" of any sort. While exposure to any kind of light can reduce the production of melatonin, a hormone that helps the body regulate its sleep-wake cycle,[7] blue light—the part of the spectrum commonly emitted by televisions and computer screens—does so with even greater effect.[8] As a result, just having an electronic device in the bed-room can result in an hour less of sleep each night.[9] Put another way, by doing nothing more than removing the television from their bedrooms and committing to not bringing mobile phones and laptop computers into that sacred space, the average American could reset the clock, so to speak, from the just under seven hours they currently get to the just under eight hours Americans averaged in 1942.[10]

If you absolutely must use an electronic device as bedtime approaches, don't do it in the bedroom, and make sure the blue-light-filtering feature is on. Most televisions don't have this option built in, so if you are going to watch a television program after dinner, do so while wearing amber glasses, which are designed to filter blue light.[11] If that just seems too silly to do, consider that whatever television program you're watching might not actually be of great importance to your life; if it was, you'd be willing to trade a little pride to watch it. Meanwhile, begin dimming the lights in your home a few hours before your scheduled bedtime. When it's time to sleep, turn the lights in your bedroom completely off.

## Control the Chemicals

Most people are already aware that caffeine can impact sleep, but they tend to underestimate its effects. Caffeine isn't just a mild stimulant; it's a very powerful drug that can stay in your body for more than a day. For many people, the majority of the effects of this drug are gone in about five hours, but about 50 percent of people have a variant of a gene known as *CYP1A2* that lowers the amount of a certain liver enzyme to a point where their bodies metabolize caffeine more slowly.[12] From one person to the next, in fact, there can be as much as a fortyfold difference in the rate they metabolize caffeine.[13] (These vast genetic differences may help explain why some studies suggest that caffeine can be quite safe while others suggest that it may be dangerous for your heart.)

In most people—even those who are slow metabolizers—it's generally safe to consume up to 100 milligrams of caffeine per day without adversely impacting sleep.[14] But that's not much caffeine; it's the equivalent of one cup of coffee, two cups of tea, three servings of soda pop, or four ounces of chocolate. Start combining those sources, and you'll quickly blow past the limit at which most caffeine consumers can escape significant impact on their sleep. Also, it should probably go without saying that so-called energy drinks, which are packed with lots of caffeine and other stimulants, will put you past the limit faster than you can say the words "Red Bull." For most people, a "caffeine curfew" that comes six hours before bedtime is a good rule. But the best chance of ensuring caffeine doesn't impact your sleep whatsoever is to not use it at all.

Alcohol is the other most common chemical sleep disrupter for many.

If this doesn't immediately make sense to you, you're not alone. Alcohol, after all, is a central nervous system depressant, with an oppositional effect to caffeine. And yes, it's true that a drink before bed can help some people fall asleep more quickly,[15] but that initial benefit is offset by a reduction in the quality of sleep they get. Research shows that people who drink alcohol before bed get less REM sleep,[16] the sort of sleep characterized by rapid eye movement, dreaming, and bodily movement, and which offers the biggest benefits in terms of health and restfulness. REM is also key to keeping our hearts in rhythm. One study, for instance, showed that people who have less REM sleep have higher rates of AFib, with the risk increasing as REM decreases.[17]

A single glass of wine or beer during a dinner that comes several hours before bedtime is unlikely to be detrimental to most people's sleep. But, as is the case with caffeine, there are a lot of factors at play. Biological sex, race, weight, medications, experience with drinking, microbiome composition, and myriad genetic factors can impact how alcohol is metabolized in the body. And, since the hard truth is that there really is no level of alcohol consumption that improves our overall health,[18] and even minimal alcohol consumption results in worse outcomes for people with AFib,[19] the best possible amount of alcohol is none at all.

Not yet convinced that you need to pay close attention to the role these substances are playing in your life? You'd do well to remember that, in addition to the sleep-disrupting properties of alcohol and caffeine, these two chemicals are also the number one and two self-reported AFib triggers, as we noted in chapter one. Accentuating that point, a study published in the *New England Journal of Medicine* showed a significant reduction in arrhythmia recurrences among a study group that abstained from alcohol. If your goal is to beat AFib and you drink, it's time to quit.[20]

## Take a Warm Bath

People often turn to alcohol to unwind from a stressful day and relax. But there are other ways to promote relaxation that can profoundly benefit your sleep quality and duration. Taking a scheduled warm bath or shower at a temperature of 104 degrees can improve the time it takes you to get to sleep, your sleep quality and total sleep time, and how often you wake during the night.

Are you the type who needs a shower to get moving in the morning? Fair enough. Keep that habit, but build in an evening bath as well. This simple lifestyle change can be done with little disruption to your daily routine, after all, and with a pretty significant payoff. In studies that have shown a significant benefit on sleep, the bath or shower can be as short as ten minutes.[21]

## Treat Sleep Apnea

Even if you perfectly schedule your sleep, and you always ensure your bed is a place that is reserved only for what it's meant for, and you consistently turn the lights down when you should, and you refuse to consume chemicals that can impact your sleep, you might *still* have trouble getting truly healthy sleep if you are one of the hundreds of millions of people across the globe who suffer from sleep apnea.

Many people don't realize they have the symptoms of sleep apnea, but their partners usually do—although they usually don't realize what those symptoms mean. People suffering from sleep apnea often snore like a bear, stop breathing, and then gasp for air.

Yet in others, the symptoms of sleep apnea may be much more subtle. In these people the center of the brain that initiates a breath becomes dysfunctional. For people with this type of central sleep apnea, sleep is very quiet, seemingly deep and restful; unless you're paying close attention, you might not even notice long periods of missing breaths. In all forms of sleep apnea, however, these periods of breathlessness cause blood oxygen levels to plummet, increasing the risk of high blood pressure, coronary artery disease, heart failure, and atrial fibrillation.

If you're not sure if you have the symptoms of sleep apnea, you should take an inventory of your symptoms.

First, do you snore? If you have a partner with whom you sleep, it's time for an honest chat. If you don't have a partner, invite a family member or trusted friend for a sleepover, just like in grade school. (Pillow fights are optional, but fun.) Remember, however, that sleep apnea is much more complex than the obstruction in breathing that we may hear, so it is critical to keep assessing even if your partner, friend, or family member tells you that you enjoyed a silent night.

Second, do you experience excessive fatigue during the day and need to take a nap? That's a sign that, no matter how you think you slept, you didn't get the sleep you actually needed.

Third, are you overweight? Just a few added pounds can harm sleep quality, according to researchers from the Johns Hopkins University School of Medicine, while weight loss, and especially a loss of belly fat, can improve sleep.[22]

Fourth, do you have high blood pressure? Obstructive sleep apnea produces surges in blood pressure that can persist into the next day, long after breathing has normalized.[23]

Fifth, do you have a large neck? "Large" in this case means sixteen inches in circumference for women and seventeen inches for men. In many cases, this is a sign of excess fat, which can put pressure on a person's breathing tube.

Finally, are you a guy? Studies show that sleep apnea is more common in men than in women, even accounting for the fact that many researchers believe it is underreported and underdiagnosed in women.[24]

Did you answer "yes" to five or all of those six questions? If so, you are at high risk of sleep apnea. If you answered "yes" to three or four of these questions, you are at some risk, and should absolutely engage your doctor in a conversation about a potential diagnosis, which may require an overnight sleep study, also known as polysomnography. A sleep study is not nearly as fun as a sleepover (and there are definitely no pillow fights allowed), but it can offer the observational and biological data your doctor will need to prescribe a continuous positive airway pressure machine. CPAP machines can feel cumbersome at first, but have been shown to improve sleep quality and reduce the risk of atrial fibrillation.[25]

If you're claustrophobic, or simply cannot sleep with a mask on, there are other options, including dental devices and even a simple T-shirt, called a "stop snoring shirt," with a pocket on the back for a tennis ball or pair of rolled-up socks. The idea is that the lump will keep you from sleeping on your back and, for many people, that's all it takes to promote side sleeping, which typically prevents snoring and sleep apnea. These methods aren't as effective as a CPAP, but both are relatively inexpensive and worth a shot.

---

## TRY THESE THREE EASY, DRUG-FREE SLEEP AIDS

Even if you've scheduled your sleep, controlled your caffeine and alcohol intake, turned the lights out when you should, taken a warm bath before bed, and, if needed, gotten treatment for your sleep apnea, slumber can be an elusive friend. And that can make pharmaceutical sleep aids and supplements very alluring.

Resist! Sleep drugs and supplements should be used only under a doctor's supervision, and only as a last resort. If supplements must be tried, studies show magnesium may not only help your AFib but your sleep as well.[26] Likewise, melatonin is generally quite safe and may help with sleep.

Other than magnesium and melatonin, though, there are a lot of other ways to make sleep easier and better without altering your body's chemistry.

There is no infallible plan for getting the rest you need, but if you've taken the other steps in this chapter and are still having trouble, there are three more things you can try that have worked in our own lives and in those of our patients. Neglect one of these and you may be in for a night of bad sleep. Do all three in addition to taking those other steps toward better sleep, and you'll almost certainly rest like a baby.

First, you've got to work out. We'll talk about all of the other ways in which exercise is an anti-AFib force multiplier later in this chapter, but one of the most important ways exercise helps is that it promotes sleep. In fact, research demonstrates that exercise is especially good at helping you fall asleep quickly and then stay asleep throughout the night.[27] We've found that outdoor exercise is especially beneficial—and the National Sleep Foundation has noted that when you exercise outside, you're exposed to natural light, which is vital to a strong sleep-wake cycle.[28]

Second, unless you are feeling dehydrated, avoid drinking anything after dinner, and make sure to head to the restroom as your last stop before you go to bed. One of the main reasons people get up at night is to use the bathroom and, once up, those who have trouble sleeping in general are more likely to stay up. If you've fully hydrated throughout the day, a few hours without water before sleeping probably won't hurt you. If you do have to use the restroom, it should be a direct to-and-from trip. Don't take a lap around the house to make sure everything is shipshape. Don't get another drink of water (which will begin a vicious cycle). And finally, do not go to the kitchen—especially not to open the refrigerator to get a blast of light that will signal your brain to start waking up.

Third, read something that relaxes you. One of the main reasons why people struggle to fall asleep and stay asleep is because they are occupied with worries about work and family (and increasingly, as we've heard from our patients, politics). But just as it's hard to get an "ear worm" out of your head without another song to replace it, it's easy to get stuck on a thought if there's not something else taking its place. And if we're not otherwise occupied, it's easier to succumb to the urge to surf the internet or check social media—subjecting ourselves to light at a time in which our surroundings should be going dark. While there haven't been many studies on the association of reading and sleep, researchers have known for many decades that just a few minutes of reading can have a beneficial effect on stress.[29] Researchers *have* found, however—and it should really go without saying—that whatever positive effects reading has on sleep are diminished if we're reading from a backlit phone, laptop, or tablet screen.[30] The traditional page or a non-backlit e-reader is the way to go.

Do those three things, in addition to the other guidance we've offered so far, and you're far more likely to get a great night of sleep—one that is at least seven hours long, restful, dream-filled, and quiet. Each night of sleep like that is a tremendously important step toward taking the other steps you need to beat back your AFib, including the other thing that Paula had identified as a likely risk factor for her AFib.

## GET YOUR WEIGHT DOWN

There is absolutely no universal cause for atrial fibrillation. But if there's one characteristic that people with AFib share more than any other, it is that they are overweight. Indeed, outside of the twenty- or thirty-year-olds who come to us with familial AFib, and the endurance athletes who have been shown to be more likely to get AFib as a consequence of their sport, it is quite rare for us to see a patient at a healthy weight with atrial fibrillation.

Weight itself isn't the problem, per se. Rather, it's a strong indicator. It tells us that the balance between constructive metabolism (which occurs when we consume food) and destructive metabolism (which happens when our bodies break down and use the substances in food) may be out of sync. It also tells us that we may be carrying around more fat than we should, including around our hearts, where it often releases dangerous cytokines and makes it harder for the muscle at the center of our circulatory system—which never gets a rest to begin with—to do its vital job.

This is why the number you see on the scale, in and of itself, is really quite meaningless. What matters is the *direction* that number is going. And for almost everyone with AFib, that direction really needs to be down.

Losing weight can feel like an impossible goal, and for a lot of people it nearly is. Back in the 1950s, researchers learned that up to 98 percent of dieters will regain all of their weight in just two years.[31] And while a lot has changed over the following decades in our understanding of human health, the success rate for people on diets hasn't changed much at all. As the director of the Health and Eating Lab at the University of Minnesota, Traci Mann has led multiple studies on the long-term outcomes of all sorts of calorie-restricting diets. The results are crushingly negative. Sure, people *can* lose weight using almost any diet that regulates caloric intake, but that weight rarely stays off. In fact, while dieters do tend to lose weight on these diets, Mann and her colleagues have learned, almost all of it comes back in the next few years. So while these diets might be able to offer our hearts a temporary reprieve—and that's a start—it's not the secret to putting our metabolism into balance.[32]

As most people can't seem to make weight loss stick, those who have the most to lose, like more than one hundred pounds, sometimes turn to weight-loss surgery, often known as bariatric surgery. There are many different procedures, but among the most common is gastric bypass surgery, in which the stomach is divided into sections and the small intestine is rearranged. If that sounds like a complicated procedure, that's because it is, and there are many potential risks and side effects. However, it can also be tremendously beneficial for those trying to fight AFib—or to keep it from happening in the first place. In a study of Swedish patients who were overweight but had not yet developed AFib, for instance, those who had bariatric surgery were 29 percent less likely to develop AFib.[33] A separate study showed that for those who already have AFib, bariatric surgery can boost the success rate of ablation from 45 to 80 percent.[34] We've even seen cases—quite a few, in fact—in which AFib has gone into complete remission with bariatric surgery alone.

But, to be clear, bariatric surgery is a tremendously drastic step that alters your physiology. Before you go down that road, you should know that most people with AFib can get the results they need in other ways. It takes a combination of food, exercise, and other lifestyle habits to optimize this part of our lives.

## Eat Good Food

Let's start with food. A healthy diet, specifically designed for people with atrial fibrillation, is unquestionably important for losing weight and keeping it off. (Indeed, chapter nine of this book is dedicated to this revolutionary way of eating.) But "health" doesn't mean "low calorie." In fact, when it comes to bringing our metabolism into sync, we really need to stop focusing on calories—because diets that are based on counting calories don't work for most people.

That said, you're not most people—you're you—and everyone is different. That's why, if there's a specific way of eating that is working for you consistently (meaning you are tracking your weight day by day and seeing a steady drop, month by month), then, in most cases, there's really no reason to change what you're doing. Not yet, at least. After all, the initial goal is just to shed a few pounds to give your heart a little breathing room.

Across our big and diverse planet, people have successfully lost weight, and kept it off, with all sorts of diets. Some eat cheese and others eschew the stuff. Some eat meat while others get sick at the thought. Programs like Weight Watchers, Nutrisystem, and Noom don't work for everyone, but they sure do work for some people. The Atkins Diet isn't a good fit for some people, but seems to be a healthy option for others. In recent years, the so-called paleo diet and keto diet have gained a lot of popularity, and research suggests these ways of eating could help many people lose weight and stabilize essential biomarkers,[35] but none of those diets are right for everyone, either.

What should *you* do? Well, if you have siblings who have had success losing weight and keeping it off by using a certain diet, that way of eating may be a good start; they share a lot of your genes and were likely brought up with many of the same social and cultural food influences as you were.

If a spouse has had long-term success with a certain diet, that might be an even better starting place; partners share meals, after all, and have more similar gut microbiomes than siblings do.[36]

Whatever you do, if you're minimizing or avoiding added sugar and flour, eating lots of vegetables, and avoiding processed and fast foods, then you're probably doing a good job for your health and your weight. If that's working for you—and the rest of your biomarkers are responding as they should—don't stop!

If you're struggling with this, you're not alone. The research on this matter is pretty clear: chances are that, at some point long before you reach your goal weight, you're going to plateau. Then, the studies indicate, you'll likely start putting weight back on. At that point, instead of going back to the drawing board and choosing from yet another diet that works for some people but not most, it will be time to head over to chapter nine, where you'll learn about a way of eating specifically designed for people with atrial fibrillation that doesn't rely on counting calories, and that has been proven exceptionally effective at helping people drop weight and get their biomarkers into better shape.

## Follow Other People's Success

It's important to remember that diet alone can't get an out-of-balance metabolism back into sync. For evidence of this, we have merely to look at the habits and lifestyles of people who have been able to take the weight off and *keep* it off. That's what a research team led by Rena Wing and James Hill did, starting in the 1990s, when they created the National Weight Control Registry. After advertising widely, they collected a group of more than 10,000 people who had beaten the weight-loss odds—averaging a drop of sixty-six pounds over more than five years.[37] Some even reported losing up to 300 pounds without the need of drugs or surgeries.

Obviously, to maintain weight loss like that, these people were doing something right. And, as it turns out, it wasn't always some fancy weight loss program or clinic that cost them thousands of dollars. In fact, about half of these people achieved their results at home. And by modeling yourself after these individuals, you too can achieve these same results.

So, how do people like those in the registry lose weight and keep it off?

- 98 percent changed what they were eating.
- 90 percent exercised an hour daily.
- 78 percent started their day with breakfast.
- 75 percent created a habit of regularly weighing themselves.
- 62 percent limited electronic devices (especially TVs) at home.

Have you lost thirty or more pounds and maintained that weight loss for a year or more? If so, the National Weight Control Registry would like you to join their study so they can learn from you. And if you haven't lost that weight yet but intend to follow the instructions in this book, then you are likely to lose quite a bit of weight in the future. And since being able to join the registry is a fine way to give back to others, it could serve as a great motivational goal.

But, of course, it doesn't do much good to make a goal if you don't know where you're currently standing. So, let's talk about that, too.

## Weigh Yourself Every Day

All ten of the blood-based biomarkers we discussed in chapter four are important, and understanding them—and monitoring them over time—is a crucial part of putting AFib into remission. But if a person was limited, for whatever reason, to focusing on just one number, in most cases it should be the number on their bathroom scale.

Yes—in a manner of thinking, weight is the most important biomarker of them all.

Although the benefits of daily weight monitoring are backed by research,[38] it doesn't take a scientific study to understand why this habit tends to work. People who weigh themselves on a daily basis are getting a steady stream of data—and a reminder to take manageable corrective action when the numbers aren't moving in the right direction. Indeed, we've rarely seen an AFib patient in our twenty-plus-year careers who hasn't successfully lost or maintained their weight loss by simply weighing themselves regularly.

Why does this work so well? After seeing a bit of weight gain, "maybe they exercise a little bit more the next day, or they watch what they are eating more carefully," explained University of Georgia exercise and nutrition researcher Jamie Cooper, who led a study showing that people who weigh themselves every day during the holidays either maintain or drop weight during a time when most people pack on a few extra pounds. "The subjects self-select how they are going to modify their behavior, which can be effective because we know that interventions are not one-size-fits-all."[39] Just the simple act of weighing yourself daily almost subconsciously sets off a chain reaction of behaviors that makes maintaining a healthy weight a lot easier.

For some, the thought of stepping on the scale each day is nauseating. There are other options. For example, we have many AFib patients who have successfully maintained their weight loss through the use of a food journal, often in the form of a notebook or an app on their smartphone. Still others have achieved desired results from commercial weight loss programs or fitness coaches. Whatever you do, the key is daily accountability—a regular time in which you must reckon with the choices you've made and those you intend to make moving forward. For most, stepping on a scale is the easiest way to do that.

So, how much do you need to lose? Well, everyone's healthy body weight is different. But let's not sugarcoat this: the vast majority of people we see with atrial fibrillation are significantly above the recommended body mass index. And while BMI isn't a perfect indicator of what a healthy body weight looks like for everyone, it's generally a good target. What's more, most of these individuals have been overweight for many years, and quite often many decades. As such, the amount of weight most people need to lose is usually quite a bit more than they think they can lose.

Rather than be discouraged about how much you need to lose, know this: anything helps. For example, in one study we showed that even patients who lose just 3 percent of their body weight, which could be as little as five pounds, increased their long-term chances of putting AFib into remission.[40] If you are going to take the necessary steps to get your weight in check, however, you have to be 100 percent committed. "Yo-yo dieting," in which your weight constantly goes up and down, is really bad for AFib, with our research[41] and that of other physicians[42] showing that back-and-forth weight changes could be an additional AFib risk factor.

You cannot let that keep you from trying, though, because the data is very clear on this point: if you want to end your affair with AFib, losing weight isn't optional.

Knowing that even a few pounds could help improve her life, when Eileen was diagnosed with AFib, she set a goal of losing one pound every month. That's a very conservative and reasonable goal, and one that we suggest for many of our AFib patients.

Even that, however, can be hard, especially since weight gain is a side effect of some medications and because AFib can make it hard to exercise, which is why it is okay to celebrate an initial month in which you simply don't gain any weight.

If your scale currently tells you that you are 220 pounds, for instance, then that is the number you need to maintain for this month. Do everything possible to keep things from tipping over that point. Next month your goal is 219. After that, it's 218. Is that slow? Sure it is. Will some people need to lose more, and more quickly? Absolutely. But slow and constant progress in one direction is far preferable to erratic shifts this way and that. Moving in the right direction is key to a life without AFib.

Eileen didn't meet her one-pound-less-per-month goal within the time frame she was planning, but her weight loss was nonetheless commendable. On average, she shed a little more than half a pound each month. And while a half a pound might not seem like a lot, over time it adds up. In the first three and a half years after she began her journey toward putting AFib into remission, she dropped twenty-four pounds—mostly by making the sorts of day-to-day adjustments that come with increased daily awareness of "the biggest biomarker of them all."

That resulted in some very big improvements to her condition, "but I didn't want to settle for 'less bad,'" she said.

It was time to take the next step. Or, in another way of thinking, the next few thousand steps.

## GET MORE EXERCISE

Eileen's pedometer wasn't fancy. The basic black band could tell her the time, work as a stopwatch, and count her steps. That was about it. But that's all she needed to jump-start a life full of a lot more activity and exercise.

"Once I started counting my steps, I got competitive with myself," she said. "Every day, I wanted to beat the previous day's score. After I started getting to ten thousand regularly, which was the goal I set with my doctor, I wanted to see how many days I could hit that number in a row."

While research shows exercise to be the number one factor in maintaining a healthy weight, exercise *alone* is rarely effective as a weight-loss tool.[43] That's because even grueling exercise doesn't burn as much fat as we might like to think. For most people, a mile of running might burn about 100 calories. Now, that would be a lot of calories over the course of a 26.2-mile marathon, but most people don't run marathons. The worse news is that even if you did run a marathon tomorrow, you'd likely only shed about a pound of fat in the act.

So, would you like to shed twenty pounds in the next twenty weeks? Just run twenty marathons!

Does that sound like a bad idea to you? It is. Because even if you could do that, what do you think your body would want after all that exercise? Food! The more you exercise, the hungrier you get, so exercise really doesn't help much when it comes to weight loss itself.[44] Rather, exercise is for weight maintenance and to build muscle mass.

In other words, if you're 185 pounds right now, you're not likely to get down to 180 just by exercising. But when healthy food habits result in lost pounds, exercise will help you keep those pounds from coming back.

That was Eileen's experience. After three years of steady but slow weight loss by just dieting, Eileen found that her new exercise regimen helped her drop another twenty pounds—and keep it off.

Since most people who lose weight eventually gain it back, Eileen, like the people in the National Weight Loss Registry, is an outlier. But she's not magical. In study after study researchers have shown that the most effective way to maintain a healthy weight is to not only eat right but also to exercise an hour a day.[45] That might seem like a lot of exercise, but the most common form of exercise among the people on the registry was exactly what Eileen was doing: brisk walking.

If you're able to step up the pace—going from walking to jogging—then you can save some time, too. If you're like many people on the registry, you might only need thirty-five to forty-five minutes of jogging every day to maintain your weight loss.[46] It's important to remember that everyone's needs are different. Some people need more exercise to maintain their weight, while others need only a bit. Until you know, err on the side of more. The best way to move away from the mostly sedentary existence that defines the lives of many AFib sufferers is to simply get up and put one foot in front of the other.

That might sound easy to some people, and we want to make it clear: that's not always the case. Your heart's atria are responsible for 20 to 30 percent of total cardiac performance. It's impossible to have the two upper chambers of your heart not beating, as happens with AFib, and not to have some drop-off in your exercise capacity.

And even if you can overcome that, it can be difficult in our hectic lives to carve out time to exercise. Fortunately, there are a lot of ways to achieve that goal. A half hour in the morning before breakfast and another half hour after dinner will get you there. If you work in an office, a treadmill desk will get you there in no time at all. If you get a daily lunch break, eating a light lunch and then using the remainder of the time to walk briskly can help, too. If you work a standard eight-hour workday and are able to take a five-minute break every hour for a walk, you'll be forty minutes toward that sixty-minute goal by the end of the day.

Of course, not everyone can work short periods of exercise into their workday.

Chris, a heavy equipment operator, was stuck in a seated position in the cabin of a crane for most of his workday. And the copper mine where he worked was hardly a place where, during his breaks, he could simply go for a walk—that could have been dangerous. So when Chris was diagnosed with atrial fibrillation, he had to make extra time before and after work to exercise.

"It only took a little bit of creativity, really," Chris said. "There were opportunities all around me to get more exercise without even going to a gym or taking up a new sport. I just had to start looking."

For starters, on the days when he wasn't responsible for driving in the rideshare, Chris began riding his bicycle to the pickup location. "Pretty soon, some of the other guys were doing that, too, and we all went out and bought bike racks for our cars so that we didn't have to leave our bikes locked up in the parking lot."

As a huge sports fan, Chris spent hours each week watching football and basketball on television. "So the other thing I invested in was a good treadmill for my living room," he said. "I've got to admit, it's ugly. It doesn't really go with the décor of the room, but I get five or six hours of brisk walking in each week just because I've made a rule that when I'm watching sports, I'm moving."

At a manageable pace, sixty minutes of walking equates to about three miles. That, in turn, equates to about 6,000 steps for a person with a fairly average stride. Add that to the few thousand steps that even mostly sedentary people take in an average day, and you're darn near close to the 7,500 steps that researchers from Harvard University have concluded is the place where the health benefits from walking alone begin to level off,[47] and the 10,000 steps that many physicians, including us, suggest is a good daily goal.

Even a short walk can be a frightening proposition for those who are newly suffering from AFib, especially if they are taking medications that make them feel worn down. For these people, a home treadmill like the one

Chris got can be a literal life-saver, offering the opportunity to exercise in short shifts without ever getting far from home.

An hour of moderate exercise each day is a tremendously good start, especially since not everyone is initially able to get vigorous exercise, but ultimately the goal should be to augment your regimen with the sort of exercise that makes you breathe heavy and sweat a bit—if only for a few minutes each day. Research has shown that just a little strenuous exercise each day, like a five- or ten-minute jog around the block, can confer many of the same health benefits as much longer periods of vigorous exercise in terms of longevity and reduced risk of heart disease.[48]

For Chris, that vigorous exercise comes toward the end of every game he watches while on the treadmill. "If it's a good game, it's sort of exciting already, and that gives me a little surge of energy that helps me move faster," he explained.

It's never too late to start toward this goal. Take Joshua, for instance. In the ten years following his AFib diagnosis, he'd had more than a half dozen cardioversions to restore his heart rhythm to normal and had been on so many different medications that he'd lost track of them all. At his worst point, he couldn't walk more than a block or two without having to stop and catch his breath.

"My longtime cardiologist told me that he was running out of options for me," Joshua said. "It's a pretty sobering experience when your cardiologist of ten years starts scratching his head."

That experience was what Joshua finally needed to commit to the process of lifestyle optimization. And while exercise wasn't the only factor in this process, it was certainly a big one. He joined a gym and created a daily exercise routine, determined to go just a little further each day than he did the day before. Within a year, he was a changed man.

"Now I can jog without being exhausted," he explained. "My daily treadmill routine is three miles per hour for one hour each day—and I don't get winded at all."

Most importantly, Joshua said, he has a new appreciation for life. "My heart function has improved 20 percent," he explained. "I still have some issues, but my attitude tells me that things will continue to improve over time. I told my wife I feel like I'm twenty years old. I honestly do not know in my lifetime when I felt better than I do now."

# HOW TO LOSE 100 POUNDS

Have you ever wondered what happens to the "biggest losers" on reality TV shows? When the cameras stop rolling, do their incredible transformations stick? Not usually. Researchers have found, in fact, that these contestants' crash diets send their metabolism into a tailspin, making long-term weight maintenance nearly impossible. In most cases, the weight comes right back[49] and, even six years later, their metabolism is slower than it was before they started filming.

This is what scientists call "metabolic adaptation" and is something you definitely want to avoid. That's why, no matter how much weight you have to lose, and especially if it's a lot, you need to take four big-but-doable, drastic actions that won't crash your metabolism but will result in long-term sustainable loss, even if that loss amounts to just one pound a month. These actions will reengineer your environment to make it far more conducive to weight loss.

First, you need to clean the cupboards and the refrigerator. Throw out the sugar and anything with added sugar. Then throw out the flour and anything made with flour. Finally, throw out anything that is processed.—that's basically anything in a can, box, or bag that doesn't still look like the ingredients from which it came. If it's made by a company, rather than grown by a farmer, it needs to go—even if it "seems" healthy. Like the famed organizing consultant Marie Kondo going through a cluttered home, you need to go through your kitchen with ruthlessness. As Kondo does to sentimental items, you may choose to thank those foods for their service or, if it pleases you, curse them instead. Either way, these foods need to be gone from your home. Once that is done, it's off to the store to shop for veggies, fruits, possibly some intact whole grains, and legumes, nuts, and seeds. Your cupboards and refrigerator should now look like a miniature farmers' market, stocked not with cans, boxes, and frozen meals, but with single ingredients that can be eaten separately or mixed together for meals.

We'll explain the purpose for all of these foods and more later, but for now the important thing is to take action because, in doing this, you are banking willpower—creating a system in which you don't have to go to war with yourself in your own home. Now, junk food binge-eating will be a lot harder. To do that, you'd have to leave your home—giving you precious time to let cooler heads prevail.

Second, now that your kitchen is stocked with healthy foods, it's time to eat. You can eat as many non-starchy vegetables as you want, as much as you possibly can. It's almost impossible to eat too many vegetables. Whenever a vegetable runs out, replace it as soon as you can; in your home, eating something healthy should always be easier than eating something unhealthy.

Third, you need to start tracking your food and weight and face some consequences for bad decisions. There are more things you'll need to learn to track in the future—that's what chapter eight of this book is about—but these two things are vitally important. If you aren't keeping track, you won't make progress. No tracking means no awareness, which is why it's also important to be accountable to someone (like a trainer) or something (like an app). That will help with the "face the consequences" part of this edict. There's no reason for self-flagellation, but putting something on the line can offer a huge boost in willpower. An AFib patient named Heather, for instance, gave her trainer a crisp Benjamin Franklin and instructions to donate it to the election campaign of a politician she abhorred if she failed to make her goals twice in a row. One year down the road, the trainer put the $100 in a card and told Heather to buy herself something nice.

Fourth, exercise. An hour a day. Remember, this is the step that helps you keep weight off. You cannot expect to see changes to your weight from exercise if you're not also making changes to your diet. And yes, an hour each day is a big commitment—one that can be especially difficult for people who are taking drugs that sap them of their strength or for whom exercise is an AFib trigger. But it's also a commitment that will help save your life.

## STOP SMOKING AND VAPING

Cigarette smoking is associated with so many adverse health conditions, it's sometimes hard to keep up. There's coronary heart disease and stroke. There's lung cancer, stomach cancer, and colorectal cancer. There's diabetes, arthritis, and chronic obstructive pulmonary disease.

It should come as no surprise that smoking and AFib go hand in hand. Our lungs and our hearts are intricately connected. When we pollute one, we pollute the other.

It might come as a surprise, then, that until the early 2010s, it wasn't certain whether smoking increases the risk of atrial fibrillation. So researchers from the Mayo Clinic decided to find out, diving into the medical records of 15,000 people to assess the potential connection. Sure enough, they found that smoking was associated with a higher risk of atrial fibrillation—and not just a little bit. For current smokers, the risk is 200 percent higher.

Not that anyone should need yet another reason to quit smoking, but if you have AFib, and you're still smoking, your chances of an AFib remission are very unlikely.

This brings us to vaping. While many have viewed e-cigarettes, or vapes, as "less bad" for you than smoking, that may not be the case. Research shows that e-cigarettes may be every bit as bad as traditional cigarettes, albeit in some different ways.[50] We still largely have no idea what many of the chemicals used in vaping products can do to us in the short and long term. What we do know, as mentioned, is that the heart and lungs are directly connected, and lung diseases can directly impact the pressures in the heart, causing heart chamber enlargement—a key cause of abnormal heart rhythms.

Yet for many AFib sufferers, even those who are aware of the many potential dangers of vaping and very well aware of the association between smoking and heart health, quitting feels almost inconceivable. And, without a doubt, it is really hard to quit.

A lot of people look at smokers who struggle to quit with scorn. That's not fair. The Centers for Disease Control and Prevention estimate that nearly 90 percent of smokers begin before they are eighteen, a time in which almost everyone makes some very bad decisions. The recognition that people should not suffer a lifetime of consequences for childhood mistakes is so deeply ingrained in the culture of the United States that there is a separate justice system for children, specifically focused on rehabilitation and reintegration, and used for all but those who have committed the most heinous of crimes. And yet people who begin consuming a product that is, by some estimates, as difficult to quit as cocaine or heroin, are often shamed and shunned for a vice that captured them before they were old enough to vote.[51]

But let's be very clear: no matter who is to blame, and no matter what else you are doing to improve your health, if you don't quit, you stand little chance of seeing any measurably positive effect on your AFib.

Most smokers want to quit. Most have tried. Those who are successful often need several attempts to do so. That's because most smokers try to quit without using one of the treatments that research has demonstrated to be most effective, including working with a doctor who can prescribe medications that help break the cycle of addiction, and engaging in addiction-specific counseling.

Quitting smoking has a multiplicative effect. Not only does it lower the risk of AFib, but it also lowers the risk of other diseases that can aggravate AFib or make it harder to fight. It also, quite simply, makes it easier to breathe—making exercise easier, too.

All of that is to say that smoking is one stressor you absolutely need to eliminate from your life. But, of course, it's not the only source of stress that you'd be better without.

# STRESS LESS

If there was a lifetime achievement award for artwork that exemplifies the expression "easier said than done," it would almost certainly go to the ineffably talented Bobby McFerrin, whose 1988 hit song put into the global consciousness a philosophy that was often espoused by the Indian mystic Meher Baba: "Don't Worry, Be Happy."

In reality, it's not enough to just tell yourself not to worry. Our lives are complicated. They can be hard. They can be full of suffering. Buddhism teaches that suffering is innate to life. All of this can bring us negative stress, which often manifests as worry.

And that's simply not good for us. One study showed that the impact of chronic stress is as damaging as smoking five cigarettes a day.[52] That tracks with another study that showed lots of stress is enough to cut your life shorter by ten years.[53] It should come as no surprise, then, that stress can be a key cause of atrial fibrillation. A team led by Yale University cardiologist Rachel Lampert found that stress and anxiety can lead to up to a fourfold increase in episodes of atrial fibrillation.[54]

But if we can't just sing it away, what should we do about it?

Well, for starters, we can follow the examples of people like Angelica, who you might recall was diagnosed with AFib while she was working multiple jobs, dealing with significant life changes, and trying to help her youngest child navigate the challenges of middle school. After recognizing that stress was a key aggravator in her life, she took an assessment of stressors and began working on ways to address each one, starting with one stressor nearly everyone shares: work.

## Reevaluate Work

When Swedish researchers reviewed the research connecting work stress and AFib, they came upon findings that should make anyone who suffers from negative stress at work pay close attention. People who experienced negative job-related stress were 37 percent more likely to develop atrial fibrillation. That's frightening enough. What is worse is that women were at particular risk: the researcher found that female workers who suffered from a lot of negative stress at work had a resounding 79 percent increased risk of AFib.[55]

That's important information to have, but it certainly doesn't help people who feel "stuck" in high-stress jobs. And that's the situation that Angelica was in while managing a grocery store and working a rideshare gig. She knew she wasn't in a position to leave her full-time job, which felt very secure and came with decent healthcare benefits—which she absolutely needed given her AFib diagnosis—even if her overall pay was lower than she wished.

She did, however, know that she had long been taking on responsibilities that managers at other stores had delegated to other employees, reasoning that "if you want something done right, you have to do it yourself." After her diagnosis, she recognized that these extra tasks were adding negative stress to her life, and she finally did what those other managers had done.

She also kept her eye on the job listings. Just exploring other options for work can make a big difference in the way we perceive stress at work. If you know that there are some fallback plans, even if those plans aren't perfect, it can help make tough days a little easier to handle. "My father was a pilot in the Air Force," Angelica said, "and I remember asking him once if he ever had to use his parachute. He laughed and told me that nobody ever wants to 'punch out,' but it's always nice to know that the ejection seat is there if you ever really need it. That's how it felt to explore my options."

That exploration led to a change in her side hustle. Angelica couldn't see a viable financial path to stop working part-time alongside her managerial position, but given how much stress the rideshare work was bringing her, she took a harder look at what she was making. She concluded that, after factoring in expenses, she was only taking home a bit more than minimum wage.[56] "It suddenly hit me that I could pretty much choose any other minimum wage job I wanted, as long as it was fairly flexible," she said. "I hadn't babysat since I was in high school, but I love children, and I realized that there were a lot of people in our neighborhood who would like to have someone reliable to watch their small children so they could have an occasional date."

Angelica had been driving three or four hours a night, and often was far from home when she took on her final fare of the evening. This meant she needed to drive another thirty minutes or so to get home, for a total of up to four and a half hours each evening behind the wheel. In that same amount of time, the parents in her neighborhood could fit in a dinner and a movie, and all Angelica had to do when they returned was walk back to her own home.

It wasn't hard to drum up business, either. "I was a teenaged babysitter once, so I say this with all due respect, but the parents in my neighborhood were all really happy to have someone a little older and more maternal to watch their kids, and they were quite generous in the way they paid me," she said. "And I had no expenses, so I was actually making better money than I had been making sitting in traffic and driving strangers to the airport."

## Change Your Media Habits

Good, bad, or otherwise, the news used to come to us in far more manageable doses—a bit in the morning when the newspaper hit the doorstep and a bit in the evening when Walter Cronkite, or another seemingly trustworthy person, sat behind the desk with the evening news.

Nowadays, news is a twenty-four-hour affair. And what often *passes* for news—angry people screaming over one another, blowhard commentators spewing politically predictable talking points, and celebrity news aimed at exposing the embarrassing secrets of the not-so-rich and only-so-famous— is so ubiquitous via the internet and social media that it can take a pretty heroic effort to stay informed (as all citizens of a democracy should be) without going mad.

We've known for decades that a constant flow of negative news can cause people to feel sadness and anxiety, exacerbating worries that news consumers already have about their own lives.[57] Research now shows that unremitting psychosocial stressors can have physiological repercussions, too, with copious studies showing a link between stress and heart problems,[58] and "profound effects on electrophysiology of the cardiomyocytes and the cardiac rhythm."[59]

What's the most common emotion you associate with consuming news content? If you said "anger," you should know that researchers have found that the likelihood of an atrial fibrillation episode goes up nearly six times following an experience with anger. By contrast, according to the same study, on the days you are feeling "happy," your risk of an AFib episode is decreased by 85 percent.[60]

It's not just "hard news" that can start a chemical chain reaction that pushes our hearts out of rhythm. We've grown increasingly tribal when it comes to our sports allegiances, too.[61] (If you've ever yelled at a referee through your television, this applies to you.) And while social media can be a way to spread all kinds of emotions—from joy and humor to sadness and empathy—nothing goes viral like anger. "Anger is a high-arousal emotion, which drives people to take action," Jonah Berger, a professor of marketing at the University of Pennsylvania's Wharton School, told *Smithsonian Magazine* in 2014. "It makes you feel fired up, which makes you more likely to pass things on."[62] In a world in which clicks equal cash for savvy social media marketers, what emotion do you think is most likely to be pushed in your direction when you open that app?

What should you do if your media habits are adding stress to your life? Well, you don't need to completely tune out, although that might not be a bad idea for a while. There isn't a lot of hard research yet on what is often called "social media fasting," but it's not hard to find plenty of personal anecdotes about how it made people feel more productive, more clear-headed, and less stressed.[63] By contrast, it's not nearly so easy to find people who took a break from social media and didn't feel like it was a worthwhile break, even if they ultimately returned to their old ways.

While you're considering a social media fast, you might as well consider a more general media fast as well. Indeed, we've seen many people decrease their AFib episodes just by getting rid of social media and the news. Or you might simply consider consuming your media the way people did a few decades ago. That doesn't necessarily mean subscribing to a morning newspaper and only watching one network news show, but spending a little time each morning and evening checking the latest state of the world, sports updates, and celebrity gossip—and keeping away from that content throughout the rest of the day—can do wonders for your psychological and physical health.

## Reconsider Stress

Next time you're stuck in traffic, standing in a long line at the grocery store, or waiting for a colleague who didn't arrive at a meeting on time, take note of your emotional state. Why? Because studies clearly show that your risk of an AFib episode is much greater on days when you're feeling impatient. By some estimates, the increased risk is threefold.[64]

Impatience is one of many emotions connected to life's negative stressors. And while it's important to do what you can to reduce these stressors, the truth is that few people have complete control over their schedules, surroundings, and circumstances. Sometimes doctors' schedules run late. Sometimes planes get delayed. Sometimes coworkers don't get their work done and it affects us. So what do you do about the things you can't change?

Well, a few years ago, in an effort to answer questions like that, researchers at the University of Wisconsin began digging into research from the National Health Interview Survey, which has been used to monitor the health of people in the United States since 1957. Two questions in particular stood out to them: "Are you under a lot of stress?" and "Do you believe stress is harming you?"

Not surprisingly, those who reported high levels of stress in their lives were more likely to suffer from health problems and die early. But what was quite astounding is that this didn't hold true for people who didn't believe their stress was harmful. It was almost as though their mindset about stress inoculated them against bad health outcomes.[65] This finding was further emphasized a few years later when an interdisciplinary team of researchers found significant geographic and racial differences in the risk of stroke among AFib patients, and concluded that the way different groups of people perceive stress was a big factor in the disparities.[66]

How can you change your mindset about stress? By embracing the fact that we actually *need* some stress in our lives. In fact, it's good for us! Scientists call this "hormesis," the idea that a reasonable "dose" of various stressors can evoke a favorable biological response. With limitations, it really is true that "what doesn't kill you makes you stronger."

The other way is to "give stress away" in the sort of way that the religious studies professor Reinhold Niebuhr invoked when he wrote the Serenity Prayer, the most common modern version of which goes: "God, grant me the serenity to accept the things I cannot change, the courage to change the things I can, and the wisdom to know the difference."

When we remind ourselves that some stress is good—and remember that, good or bad, there are parts of life that we can't always control—stress loses its power to ruin our lives. This isn't an easy conceptual shift to make. It takes time and practice. But given how easily stress can trigger AFib, and knowing that perception is a powerful force when it comes to stress, it's absolutely worth the effort. (And a great place to start is your doctor's office.)

## Become a Yogi

At the confluence of mindfulness and exercise, you'll find the ancient Indian practice of stretches, postures, and meditation called yoga. You'll also find one of the best therapies for atrial fibrillation in the world.

That's the considered opinion of Dr. Dhanunjaya Lakkireddy, from the University of Kansas Medical Center, who has demonstrated that yoga can reduce a person's AFib burden by a whopping 24 percent.[67] The same study found tremendously positive impacts on blood pressure, anxiety, and depression among patients with AFib.

That's better than any drug, and it's a lot more enjoyable, too. Just about everyone who is taking a form of AFib medication will share with you some sort of complaint about how the medicine makes them feel. Yet it's hard to find anyone who will tell you that yoga makes them feel bad.

The idea of yoga intimidates a lot of people at first, but that's usually before they give it "the old college try." Find a yoga studio, join a gym with yoga classes, purchase a series of instructional videos, or just go online (the internet is chock-full of free yoga videos for people at every level of practice). Try it before you dismiss it as "not for you."

How will you know if it's working for you? To some extent, certainly, some patients are simply able to "feel the difference." For others, more concrete evidence is needed. By simply checking your heart rate variability on your smartwatch or smartphone on the days you engage in yoga versus the days you do not, you can get a good idea of whether all that stretching and posing is working for you. (We'll discuss this in greater detail in chapter eight.)

But yes, it's true; yoga isn't for everyone. If yoga doesn't work for you, other forms of mindful engagement, like meditation, tai chi, prayer, nature walks, or daily exercise, can be just as effective. The key is turning distress into "eustress," a moderate state of psychological stress that is beneficial for us.

## A LONG-TERM COMMITMENT

Nobody optimizes their lifestyle overnight. It takes real dedication to block out the necessary time to become a healthy sleeper. It requires true devotion to balance your diet and exercise in a way that ensures pounds come off and stay off. It takes a lot of work to quit smoking or vaping. And as for our relationship with stress? Even the most Zen-like of Zen masters will tell you it takes a lifelong effort to keep negative stress away and accept the role of the stress that remains as a positive force in our lives.

But Paula has done it. So have Eileen and Joshua. So have Peri and Angelica. They all took different paths to significantly reducing their AFib events or putting it completely into remission. Some have struggled in one area while excelling in others. But all have increased their healthy sleep, adopted a healthy diet, dedicated themselves to an hour or more of exercise every day, and adjusted their lives to avoid negative stress.

Each of these individuals was alike in another way, though: while they were all able to put their AFib into remission with biomarker and lifestyle optimization, as the years (sometimes decades) have passed, they all required additional intervention to keep them in remission. Each of their paths to beating back AFib included an ablation.

## LIFESTYLE OPTIMIZATION

| "Life Op" | Specific Steps |
|---|---|
| **Get better sleep** | • Maintain a strict sleep schedule<br>• Get a total of seven to nine hours of sleep each day, including naps<br>• Get tested for and treat sleep apnea |
| **Maintain a healthy body weight** | • Weigh yourself daily<br>• Follow a way of eating that works for your metabolism (see chapter nine)<br>• Take a minimum of 10,000 steps daily<br>• Get some daily exercise that breaks a sweat (in addition to 10,000 steps)<br>• Shoot for an hour of exercise daily, even once you've hit your target weight |
| **Stop smoking/vaping now** | • Engage in addiction-specific therapy<br>• Talk to your doctor about medications that can help break the cycle of addiction |
| **Stress less** | • Change your work environment<br>• Change the way you consume media and technology<br>• Minimize or avoid toxic relationships<br>• Engage in daily stress-reducing activity (yoga, meditation, nature walks, etc.) |

## Chapter Six

## ᴧᴧ ABLATION ᴧᴧ

Why the procedure is safer, easier, and more
successful than you may think

D iagnosed in the early 2000s when he was in his late forties, Jose was
never comfortable with the idea that medication would solve his
condition. And, of course, he was right. He started a daily exercise
program and adopted a version of the paleo diet that helped him drop some
weight. He took up yoga to help manage stress. Whenever he would have
an AFib episode, no matter where he was at the time, he would stop what
he was doing and take a walk.

Jose was doing just about everything right, and it worked for a long time.

Over the years, though, his AFib worsened, and not even the drugs he
was taking were helping keep his heart in rhythm. The next antiarrhythmic
his doctor suggested was amiodarone, and he definitely didn't want to go
down that road, given all of its long-term toxicities.

It was time for an ablation.

Accepting ablation is not accepting that you weren't "good enough" to cure your AFib in other ways. After all, many of our patients are endurance athletes, often in their thirties or forties, who are a picture of health. As most of these athletes can't compete on medications, and have already optimized many aspects of their lives, many end up getting their AFib ablated. And, with that, because so many aspects of their health have already been optimized, almost all are able to return to full physical activity, including competitions, without any medications and without any further AFib episodes.

We cannot emphasize this enough: ablation isn't what you do when all other options fail, any more than a cast is something you put on a broken arm when all other options fail. Ablation is a procedure that can often be avoided with early and aggressive lifestyle changes—and it's nothing to rush into lightly—but for many people, it's an absolutely necessary treatment that should be discussed with an expert EP sooner rather than later.

That's what Jose did. And that's what finally gave him back control of his life.

In a catheter ablation, an electrophysiologist controls the movement of several catheters—specialized tools designed to work in the heart that are gently inserted into a patient's body through a large inner thigh vein or sometimes a neck vein. A lot of people are surprised to learn that doctors can reach the heart in this way, but cardiac catheterization is nearly a century old, having been first completed by the German physician Werner Forssmann, who slid a twenty-four-inch catheter from his own arm to his right ventricular cavity in 1929.[1] In the decades that have passed, doctors have learned to guide catheters toward malfunctioning heart cells in the atria. Those cells are destroyed with either radiofrequency or cryo energy (sometimes informally referred to as "fire" and "ice"), creating a barrier of scar tissue to prevent abnormal electrical signals from triggering AFib (such as electrically isolating heart tissue near the pulmonary veins) or directly eliminating misfiring cells in the heart. Either way, the end goal is to stop AFib from happening again. As no cutting or stitches are needed, patients often are able to go home the same day.

Now, it might seem counterintuitive that purposefully creating more cardiac scar tissue is one of the ways to fight a condition that is partly *caused* by scar tissue, but when you consider what the newly scarred tissue does—or rather, what it doesn't do—it makes a lot of sense. The process creates a sort of electrical bypass that takes malfunctioning heart cells out of the equation. The electrical currents that run through a patient's heart have no choice but to move through the remaining healthy tissue. Or, in another way of thinking, the currents can no longer get "lost" in a jumbled maze of bad cells. What's more, studies show that when these "bad cells" are eliminated, it can strengthen the rest of the heart so much that both the atria and ventricles are stronger after the procedure, since they are now working in harmony with one another.[2]

The result can seem miraculous. Patients who felt doomed to a life of atrial fibrillation with all of the accompanying medications, cardioversions, and hospitalizations are suddenly free from this affliction. Thus, if getting off of medications is their goal (as we'll discuss further in the next chapter), it can be a tremendously important step in that direction.

But this isn't a miracle at all. It's a medical procedure—and a very serious one, at that. And if you're going to decide if it's right for you, you should have as much information as possible about what it is.

## WHAT HAPPENS DURING AN ABLATION

Ablation patients are usually instructed to begin fasting from food and water the night before the procedure. Antiarrhythmics and rate-controlling medications are usually discontinued, too—sometimes for several days before the ablation—but that should only be done under a doctor's direction. However, most electrophysiologists will have you continue your blood thinner to minimize your risk of stroke, as part of the anticoagulation strategy we discussed in chapter three.

After checking into the hospital, ablation patients change into a gown and meet with a lineup of hospital staff and the medical personnel who will be on hand for the procedure, including the electrophysiologist and the anesthesiologist.

Some ablations are done under local anesthesia and sedation, meaning a patient is awake but drowsy (also known as conscious sedation). Others are done under general anesthesia, meaning you are completely asleep and require a breathing tube and respirator during the procedure. In the United States, general anesthesia is more common, whereas in Europe and Asia, where it can be difficult to get an anesthesiologist, conscious sedation is usually used. There are obviously pros and cons of both approaches. With general anesthesia, you are totally asleep and motionless, so the 3D maps created to identify the areas of the heart that need treatment tend to be more accurate. Also, it is a very relaxed working environment for your EP, as they can focus on your heart and not have to worry about their patients either waking up in the middle of the procedure from too little sedation or stopping breathing from too much sedation. The downside to general anesthesia, however, is that the first twenty-four hours of recovery can be more difficult.

Before the procedure begins, each catheter—multiple in the inner thigh and possibly one in the neck—must be placed into a vein via a small sheath, which is a larger and longer IV that holds the vein open so the catheter can move easily in and out of the vein.

Once all of these catheters have made their way to the heart, the EP goes to work. The triggers for atrial fibrillation are most often on the left side of the heart, and the catheters are inserted through the veins to the right side of the heart. Once in the right atrium, the catheters are passed through a thin membrane (the septum) into the left atrium. The opening this creates typically closes three to four weeks after the procedure is complete. EPs generally map out the areas of the heart that need treatment and apply point-by-point radiofrequency energy to isolate the pulmonary veins, as well as treat any other problem area. If, however, the EP is using a cryoballoon, then the mapping part will probably be skipped and they will just electrically isolate the pulmonary veins with the cryoballoon. Because of the bulky size of the cryoballoon, however, it is difficult to treat any additional arrhythmias, and if these are present, additional catheters are often used to map and ablate these areas.

Having trouble visualizing all of that? Here again is the "before" voltage map of the forty-two-year-old man with familial paroxysmal AFib we showed you in chapter two.

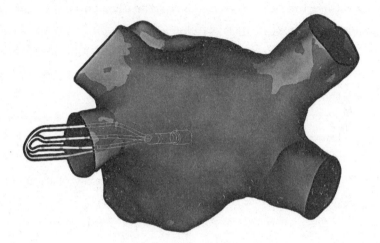

This is a posterior (backside) view of the left atrium, where the four pulmonary veins are entering the heart. The map shows high electrical voltages evenly dispersed throughout the left atrium and a few centimeters up each pulmonary vein.

Now, compare that map to this one:

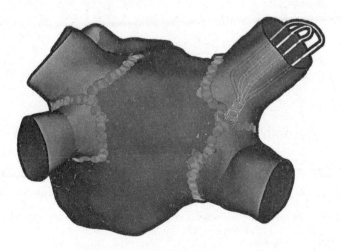

On this "after" voltage map, the circles show where ablations were performed, leaving the resulting discoloration, indicating lack of any voltage, in the electrically isolated four problematic pulmonary vein areas. Now, any premature atrial contractions from this patient's pulmonary veins will no longer be able to put his heart into AFib.

If all of this sounds like an exacting process, it's because it is. Even with the best technology available, it takes exceptional patience and meticulous action to successfully perform an ablation. Healthy and unhealthy areas of tissue, after all, are often jumbled together in very small areas, being moved this way and that by the flow of blood and the normal contractions of the heart. Imagine trying to hit basketball shots, again and again, in the middle of a tropical storm; that's what it's like. As such, it takes time. A catheter ablation usually takes at least two hours, and sometimes four hours or more, depending on the state of a person's heart, the complexity of the needed treatment, and the experience level of your EP.

Once the procedure has been completed and the catheters have been removed, patients will be monitored as they come out of anesthesia. And in many cases these days, healthier and younger patients can head home on the same day, and others the day after the procedure; all hospitals have different approaches to how they care for their ablation patients immediately after the procedure.

This is generally what to expect if you are getting any of the most common types of ablation. But there are some differences in approach, so let's talk about those next.

## RADIOFREQUENCY VERSUS CRYOBALLOON: WHICH IS BEST?

Anyone with AFib who has spent some time on the internet or has participated in the various online forums sooner or later encounters the radiofrequency versus cryoballoon debate. And while this is a fast-moving area, with both technologies getting better every year, the research thus far suggests that the overall success and complication rates are almost identical.

In the biggest head-to-head study, the "Fire and Ice Trial," research-ers concluded that "cryoballoon ablation was noninferior to radiofrequency ablation with respect to efficacy for the treatment of patients with drug-refractory paroxysmal atrial fibrillation, and there was no significant dif-ference between the two methods with regard to overall safety."[3] It bears noting that the trial reviewed by this study, and the various substudies, was funded by the maker of the cryoballoon, which obviously has an interest in demonstrating the superiority of "ice." And while they have found a few minor areas in which to possibly claim a victory, at the end of the day the results are almost the same. Basically, as long as you perform a durable pul-monary vein isolation (PVI) procedure and complete the procedure in a safe manner, it really doesn't matter if you get there by fire or ice. Thus, from a patient perspective, as both technologies are equivalent in outcomes, you want your EP to use the technology they feel most comfortable with and have the most experience with as a tool.

One other consideration when debating radiofrequency versus cryo-balloon is radiation. In the process of doing an ablation procedure, most EPs use some degree of real-time X-ray, called fluoroscopy, to help them with this procedure. And, as you likely know, the more radiation you receive, the higher your lifetime risk of cancer. With technological advances in 3D arrhythmia mapping, many EPs can now do radiofrequency ablations with either no radiation or less radiation than what you get in a standard X-ray, while cryoballoon ablation may require more radiation.

While the fire-versus-ice debate always draws a lively crowd at the AFib medical meetings, the truth is that, in about five years, there is a good chance we won't be using either of these technologies. There is exciting research showing that pulsed field ablation, or electroporation, may offer a far more durable and safer procedure that can be done in minutes, rather than the hours needed today.[4] Right on the tail of pulsed field ablation is external beam radiotherapy, which would treat AFib with the same highly focused radiation therapy that oncologists use to treat cancer.[5] The best part of external beam radiotherapy is that we won't even need to put a cath-eter into the heart. Before you rush to have either of these procedures for your AFib, though, you need to know that both of these new technologies are still very experimental and not approved for routine use anywhere in the world. The current procedures will certainly get better over time, but most people with AFib don't have any time to waste.

## CATHETER VERSUS SURGICAL ABLATION: WHICH IS BEST?

Along with the other common debates that take place at any major AFib medical meeting, you'll also hear EPs and cardiac surgeons discussing— sometimes quite passionately—whether catheter ablation is better than surgery for treating AFib.

Surgical ablation, often known as the "mini MAZE," is far more invasive than a catheter-based approach. While surgeons once held an advantage in that their pulmonary vein isolation procedures for AFib were more durable and better tailored for treating areas beyond pulmonary vein isolation in persistent atrial fibrillation, recent advances in catheter ablation have eliminated this advantage.[6] That's not to mention the fact that the risks of surgery will always be much higher than that of the less invasive catheter.

The one area where surgery does offer a clear advantage is in the opportunity to quite easily eliminate the left atrial appendage at the time of the surgery. (The left atrial appendage can also be occluded with a catheter-based technique at the same time as a catheter ablation.[7]) You will recall that the left atrial appendage is a pouch in the left atrium where blood clots can develop from the stagnant blood flow there when the heart is in AFib. While eliminating the left atrial appendage may improve ablation success rates, it also comes with some serious risks, as we described in a 2017 *Journal of Thoracic Disease* article.[8] For example, eliminating the left atrial appendage may increase the risk of stiff left atrial syndrome[9] (which can lead to fluid retention, pulmonary hypertension, and heart failure), significantly impair the pumping function of the left atrium,[10] and forever alter the balance of brain-heart hormones, such as atrial natriuretic peptide.[11] And, unfortunately, if the appendage is not removed completely and a small communication remains, the risk of stroke actually increases.

So should you opt for a catheter- or surgery-based ablation procedure? That depends. If the EPs in your area aren't very experienced, but you have a surgeon who is, then the surgical approach is the way to go. Also, if you need open heart surgery, such as bypass surgery for blocked arteries or valve surgery, then it is very easy for your cardiac surgeon to do a traditional MAZE surgery for AFib while your chest is already open.

Finally, there is a "hybrid" ablation approach in which both the EP and the surgeon work on the heart together. The hybrid ablation approach has never really made much sense to us. After all, why would you want to expose yourself to the risks and recovery of both a catheter ablation and a surgery when there is an excellent chance that either one alone will get rid of your AFib? But there are still pockets around the United States where the hybrid approach is actively promoted.

One thing to bear in mind: there's nothing prohibitive about the surgical approach. If it doesn't work, you can always have a catheter ablation afterward.

## PULMONARY VEIN ISOLATION ALONE OR PVI PLUS SOMETHING ELSE?

If you are suffering from paroxysmal atrial fibrillation, you probably want your EP to perform only a PVI procedure. Of course, if your EP finds other arrhythmias, such as atrial flutter or a supraventricular tachycardia, you'll want those treated at the same time. But for AFib ablation strategies, less is more. Pulmonary vein isolation alone for paroxysmal atrial fibrillation offers a 70 to 80 percent chance of being free from AFib, without the need of an antiarrhythmic, for at least one to two years—offering the vital time needed to optimize your lifestyle in all of the other ways described in this book.

While PVI alone is the best approach for paroxysmal atrial fibrillation, what should be done for persistent atrial fibrillation? The challenge with answering that question is that not all persistent AFib is the same. Studies

## RADIOFREQUENCY VERSUS CRYO VERSUS SURGICAL ABLATION OF ATRIAL FIBRILLATION

| | Radiofrequency | Cryo | Surgery |
|---|---|---|---|
| Outpatient Procedure | Yes | Yes | No |
| Complication Risk | Low at experienced hospitals | Low at experienced hospitals | Higher than radio-frequency or cryo |
| Left Atrial Appendage Elimination | Possible, but rarely done at same time | Possible, but rarely done at same time | Yes |
| Able to Treat Other Arrhythmias | Yes | Yes, if another expensive catheter is used (many hospitals discourage due to costs) | No |
| Success Rate | Equivalent to surgery at experienced hospitals | Equivalent to surgery at experienced hospitals | High |

show that even if you have persistent AFib, but with minimal fibrosis, your success rate with PVI is likely to be similar to that of paroxysmal atrial fibrillation ablations.[12] But, unfortunately, even the best EP in the world, using the best technology available, can only offer about a 60 percent success rate (as indicated by no antiarrhythmics and no AFib recurrences for one to two years) from PVI alone.[13] As such, many EPs will want to do "PVI plus something else," and currently the most popular technique is to electrically isolate the posterior wall of the left atrium in addition to PVI. One study looking at all the research done to date reports that isolating the posterior wall, which isolates additional heart scar tissue, may boost the success rate. In other studies, though, it appears it could make things worse. It also comes at the cost of increasing your risk of a massive and potentially fatal thermal injury to the esophagus, known as an atrio-esophageal fistula.[14]

It's important to remember, though, that the research and development picture changes for the better each year. Indeed, our ongoing research into targeting atrial fibrillation drivers in persistent AFib, or specific areas of the atria that seem to cause atrial fibrillation when the pulmonary veins aren't the cause of AFib, looks very promising with improved success rates. Meanwhile, countless biotech companies are looking for ways to improve ablation success rates and, as part of that investment, many companies are developing new 3D AFib mapping techniques to see the actual source of persistent AFib wavefronts, which may increase future success rates. In the meantime, nothing has been conclusively proven to increase ablation success rates above PVI alone.

What that means is that, if you have persistent AFib, you need to buy yourself time. And there is a proven way to do that, because, as you know, the better your daily health decisions regarding weight management, food choices, exercise, stress management, and sleep optimization, the slower your heart will age and the less fibrosis you'll pick up. Indeed, lifestyle optimization improves the chance of ablation success by up to 42 percent. And not only does this increase your one- to two-year ablation success rate, it could also keep you from developing new AFib circuits three, five, or ten years in the future.

Now that you know your options about ablation, the biggest decision ahead is when it makes sense to have one.

## DRUGS VERSUS ABLATION

As you know, atrial fibrillation tends to get worse with time: AFib begets AFib.

But something remarkable happens when the heart can maintain normal sinus rhythm for prolonged periods of time: rhythm begets rhythm! The heart can actually heal itself.

In a fascinating study, Australian researchers using MRI and high-tech 3D mapping technologies of the heart were able to show that by eliminating AFib with an ablation, non-ablated diseased areas of the heart were able to heal themselves over the following two years.[15] Remarkably, inflamed and fibrotic areas of both the atria and the ventricles healed. It was as if the heart repaired what could be repaired and replaced what needed to go—structurally the cells were healthy again, and electrically most of the "electrical shorts" went away.

A lot of other problems can be reduced by ablation. In our study of nearly 38,000 patients, for instance, we showed that ablation didn't just reduce AFib, but also reduced the risk of premature death, stroke, and dementia.[16] Further research has demonstrated that patients getting an ablation also enjoy much better kidney function, which makes sense because AFib may compromise blood flow to vital organs.[17] The greatest benefits seem to come for the sickest patients—those who are fighting both AFib and heart failure. After ablation, research shows, their risk of death, stroke, bleeding, or cardiac arrest plummeted by half.[18]

Of course, results like these are always met with skepticism. And they should be. That's why dozens of researchers from around the world aided in the nearly decade-long Catheter Ablation vs. Antiarrhythmic Drug Therapy for Atrial Fibrillation trial, also known as the CABANA study,[19] the biggest ablation study ever done. Researchers enrolled more than 2,200 mostly older AFib patients worldwide and randomized them to either medications or an ablation. They then followed these patients for about four years to see what happened next.

Now, there was a problem with this simple study design. More than a quarter of patients who were assigned to the "drugs group" ended up requiring an ablation before the four years were up. Meanwhile, 9 percent of the patients who were assigned to the "ablation group" decided not to have the procedure done. This muddied the statistical waters.

Some statisticians will argue that the "pure" way to conduct a study is to count the results based on how patients were *assigned* rather than what therapy they ultimately *received*. Under this way of analyzing the data,

patients who were assigned to medications, but who really had an ablation, would be counted as "medication patients." Likewise, those patients
assigned to ablation, but who never had the procedure, would be counted
as if they really did have a procedure. And if you analyze the results in this
way, the primary end points of the study—strokes, bleeding, cardiac arrest,
or death—were similar between the groups.

And yet, even when looked at in this way, the advantages of an ablation
over drugs are clear, with the study showing the following:

- If your goal is normal sinus rhythm, then ablation is significantly better than drugs at keeping your heart in rhythm. And
  sinus rhythm has now been convincingly shown to decrease
  your risk of cardiovascular death, stroke, worsening heart failure, and heart attack.[20]
- If your goal is a better quality of life, then ablation may be your
  answer.
- If your goal is to stay out of the hospital, then once again ablation offers you a potentially lower risk.
- If you have heart failure, ablation may be a better option, as
  also suggested by additional research.[21]
- There's a possible benefit to youth: people who were fifty-five
  to sixty-four when they received an ablation did better than
  those who were sixty-five to seventy-five, who in turn did better
  than those who were older than seventy-five.

Perhaps most importantly, particularly given the unease with invasive
procedures (revealed by the fact that many people assigned to the ablation
group did not go through with the procedure), the CABANA study found
that ablations are very safe when done at the experienced hospitals partici-
pating in this study. In fact, medications—which are often viewed as being
the easier and safer option—did not result in any less risk.

If you're considering receiving an ablation, though, you may not care
about proper statistical procedures. Rather, you likely want to know what
happens when someone is actually treated with ablation or actually treated

with medications. And here, the answer is clearer: patients who were actually treated with ablation had a much lower risk of stroke, bleeding, cardiac arrest, and death.

But ablation is not, as many have suggested, a "cure" for atrial fibrillation.[22] Not by itself, at least. AFib recurs after ablation in up to 40 percent of patients,[23] in no small part because, as you'll recall, AFib is a whole-body condition that will progress if other actions are not taken. When patients treat ablation as a cure, they are far less likely to engage in the lifestyle optimization strategies that help keep AFib in remission.

In a way, ablation is like getting a cavity "fixed" by your dentist. Sure, it might be possible that some people have a genetic tendency toward cavities, but research demonstrates that tooth decay is far more likely the result of poor food choices or personal dental care.[24] And while your dentist can get rid of the cavity, if you don't change your lifestyle, then sooner or later you'll have another cavity to contend with. The same is true in the heart. EPs can get rid of these "faulty" heart cells with ablation, but if you don't change the lifestyle factors that brought about AFib in the first place, sooner or later the AFib will be back.

But the risk of AFib coming back isn't the only thing that keeps some people from seeking an ablation. After all, even temporary relief from arrhythmia can be life-changing. Rather, the prospect of something going wrong, even in a procedure that is minimally invasive and usually has a quick recovery time, is enough to keep many people from pursuing this procedure.

You'll recall from the beginning of this chapter that Jose waited for some time before having an ablation, and complications are the reason why. Even though he was quite young relative to most AFib patients, and thus was far more likely to have a successful outcome, he was unnerved by the prospect of any complication, including inadvertent esophageal injury, nerve damage, cardiac perforation, stroke, pulmonary vein stenosis, and even death. This was in the early 2000s, which might not feel like it was so long ago, but the procedure—first developed in the 1980s—was still evolving at that time. It wasn't until the late 1990s, in fact, that doctors began using it for complex conditions like atrial fibrillation, which previously they had treated through surgeries that targeted the heart in a shotgun approach, rather than discerning how electrical currents were passing through that organ. Today's technology and overwhelmingly positive outcomes are light-years ahead of the situation Jose faced back then.

There are still risks, of course. No medical procedure or medication is without risk, and anyone who tells you otherwise is either a charlatan or a fool. Today, when electrophysiologists meet with patients before a catheter ablation, they are compelled by ethics, the rules of the hospitals where they practice, and the standards of their field—not to mention common decency—to engage in a series of conversations about the potential risks. (And to complete, with their patients, a bit of paperwork confirming those conversations have taken place.)

Jose eventually had those conversations, but first—like many people— he chose to wait. Fortunately, he was advised by a forward-thinking cardiologist that while an ablation should remain on the table for the future, there were lifestyle changes he could implement immediately to manage his condition. Even still, Jose needed some medications to help keep his heart in rhythm; despite his initial reservations, he accepted those drugs and their side effects as necessary evils.

The progression of Jose's AFib slowed, but it didn't stop. As the years went by, his AFib slowly got worse, with more and longer arrhythmic events. Meanwhile, the procedure was quickly getting better, with more doctors trained to do it, more research and development dedicated to doing it safely and effectively, and more positive outcomes. By the time Jose made an appointment to see us in the early 2010s, the potential for a successful outcome in a single procedure was much better, even though he was a decade older.

"Ablation had never fallen off my radar completely," Jose said, "but I hadn't thought about it a lot and wasn't actively researching it, because for the most part the other things I was doing with my diet and exercise especially, but the drugs too, were keeping my AFib from getting completely out of control. I don't know why I assumed the risks of ablation would be the same as they had been a decade earlier, but when I looked back into it, I was impressed by the advances that had been made. At that point, it was almost a no-brainer. It was clear to me that the situation has really changed, and it was time for me to have an ablation."

A few weeks after meeting with us, Jose was checking into the hospital. And nearly a decade more down the road, his life with AFib had become something of a distant memory. "Sometimes I wonder if I should have waited as long as I did. Like maybe I could have spared myself a bit of continued suffering if I'd been a little less cautious and a little more attentive to the way the procedure was improving," he said. "Other than that, though, I have no regrets. The ablation absolutely changed my life, and it feels like it has given me the energy and confidence I need to double-down on my diet, regular exercise, and all of the other things I need to do to make sure AFib stays in my past."

Ultimately, as we'll see in chapter seven, ablation also helped him reduce his medications—to almost none at all.

Given his age, the state of the biomedical technology, and his determination to engage in a process of lifestyle optimization, Jose might have made the right decision in waiting to have an ablation. These days, though, the research is clear: for many patients eligible for ablation, waiting may be the wrong strategy.

## THE TIPPING POINT

Around the same time Jose was reconsidering his ablation options, we embarked on a study of more than 4,500 of our patients who had undergone an ablation procedure as a treatment for atrial fibrillation.[25] Going into this study we knew that many patients who develop AFib experience worsening of their arrhythmia over time. In other words, at some point you develop so much atrial fibrosis that nothing will work to keep you out of AFib, not even ablation. (This was the case of the seventy-four-year-old woman suffering from obesity, hypertension, diabetes, and long-standing persistent AFib that we showed you in the fibrosis map included in chapter two.) What we didn't know—what no one knew, in fact—was the optimal point at which catheter ablation could be most successful in changing outcomes for the better. Should cardiologists tell their patients that they have some time to make lifestyle changes before recommending ablation? Should patients wait and see if drugs are effective before taking on a procedure that, even today, has some risks?

When we looked at outcomes that included the one-year rate of recurrence, stroke, hospitalization due to heart failure, and death, we learned that ablation success rates slightly decreased with each year people live with atrial fibrillation. Part of the failure in success rates was because with time, people spent more of each day, on average, in atrial fibrillation. However, the influence of time was relatively modest and the data coalesced behind a clear conclusion: in much the same way that the causes of AFib are different for everyone, so is the tipping point. It can come at any time.[26] Moreover, since the technique is usually effective for treating the forms of AFib that generally turn up earlier (paroxysmal or intermittent atrial fibrillation), ablation is less effective at treating more advanced, persistent forms.

The study made it clear: for many patients, the sooner an ablation can happen, the better. In our experience, the only people who should wait are those who are still holding normal sinus rhythm the vast majority of the time. And getting your AFib treated earlier rather than later has recently been shown to decrease your long-term risk of cardiovascular death, stroke, worsening heart failure, or heart attack.[27] So if you have symptomatic AFib, and especially if medications aren't working for you, you need to do everything possible to get a consultation with an electrophysiologist about whether ablation is right for you. That's true even if you are older. Although the CABANA trial seems to suggest that people over the age of seventy-five may do better if started on medications first,[28] this isn't a hard-and-fast rule. There's a big difference between active and sedentary octogenarians, after all. Indeed, our five-year outcome study of eighty-year-olds who have had an ablation led us to conclude that the procedure is safe and effective even for octogenarians. And even though it seems clear that better success rates could be obtained if the procedure was done earlier in life,[29] we have plenty of examples of individuals who got an ablation in their eighties who have said goodbye to AFib, many for the rest of their lives.

The corollary to the fact that much older individuals tend to have less successful outcomes with ablation (which is true for nearly every medical procedure you can imagine) is that those who are diagnosed at a relatively early age can enjoy vast benefits, since they tend to respond much better to the procedure. In fact, an argument can certainly be made that younger patients should be offered ablation as a first-line treatment for their atrial fibrillation, rather than a step to be taken only after other remedies have failed.

We must note, however, that no one should rush into an ablation procedure unless they absolutely have to. And not everyone has to. Some people, especially older and sedentary people, don't experience many symptoms with atrial fibrillation. For these people, there is generally no immediate reason to have an ablation, especially given the fact that, according to the CABANA study, some people over age seventy-five might have a worse outcome with an ablation. Likewise, if medications are working great for you, and you don't mind taking them, then there is also no immediate reason to have an ablation.

But if AFib symptoms or antiarrhythmic medications are compromising your quality of life, you can't beat AFib with lifestyle interventions alone, and you are in a condition to undergo a procedure that requires work in the heart under anesthesia, then getting an ablation is probably your best option. And yes, in these cases, sooner is often better.

## PREDICTING THE TIPPING POINT

How well your heart responds to an ablation has a lot to do with how much scar tissue has already formed. You want your ablation done before you've passed the "tipping point," when there is just too much fibrosis for an ablation to have any benefit. Research shows, after all, that the amount of fibrosis has consistently predicted the likelihood of a successful ablation.[30]

But how do you know how much fibrosis has already occurred? While you could certainly get a cardiac MRI or an expensive blood test to evaluate for atrial fibrosis, a far simpler approach is to quickly calculate your "APPLE score,"[31] which includes:

**A**ge over sixty-five (1 point)
**P**ersistent AFib (1 point)
**P**oor kidney function (1 point)
**L**eft atrial enlargement: left atrial diameter more than 4.3 cm as measured on an echocardiogram (1 point)
**E**jection fraction below 50 percent (1 point)

To add up your points, you will need your most recent echo (cardiac ultrasound) test results. If you haven't yet had an echo, or your results aren't readily available, there is a "quick and dirty" way of determining your left atrial size and ejection fraction. If you're under age sixty-five, have paroxysmal rather than persistent AFib, are not overweight, and don't have high blood pressure, then your left atrial size is probably normal to just mildly enlarged. If any of these factors are present, you may have moderate or even severe left atrial enlargement. For ejection fraction, if you've never been told you have heart failure before, then your ejection fraction is likely above 50 percent.

If your APPLE fibrosis score is 0 or 1, then your fibrosis levels are typically very low and your ablation success probability is very high. In contrast, if you scored a 4 or 5, then your left atrium is probably full of scar tissue and your ablation success probability is quite low.[32] Obviously, if your APPLE fibrosis score is a 2 or 3, then the chances of an ablation working is somewhere in between these two extremes.

It's important to note, however, that ablation outcomes aren't limited to total success and complete failure. Sometimes a few cells are missed or are incompletely treated. In these cases, the procedure can be repeated. The overall success rate is improving, and is approximately 70 to 80 percent for paroxysmal atrial fibrillation and 50 to 60 percent for persistent atrial fibrillation. But even when the procedure is not completely successful, the amount or burden of atrial fibrillation is often decreased, the rhythm is more often paroxysmal rather than persistent, and the downward spiral of "AFib begets AFib" may be stopped.

## WHEN IS AN ABLATION MEDICALLY INDICATED?

The medical world is increasingly moving toward "evidence-based medicine," which is a fancy way of saying that physicians, hospitals, government officials, and insurers want to know that medical decisions are based on the best available data from high-quality studies. AFib ablations are no exception. In the heart rhythm field, the document that establishes the conditions under which ablation is "medically indicated" is called the "Expert Consensus Statement on Catheter and Surgical Ablation of Atrial Fibrillation." This document, which comes out about every five years, reviews the latest research and sets the standard for EPs around the world on how best to perform these procedures, and our studies and expertise were used to establish the standard in the latest document.[33]

Since 2007, when the first such document appeared, the indications for an AFib ablation have remained essentially the same. The document might be 169 pages long, but it all comes down to two criteria. While there are other factors, including age, paroxysmal versus persistent, and having other medical conditions, that might make you a better or worse candidate for the procedure, the basic standard is very simple. You should at least be considered for an ablation if

1. AFib is causing you symptoms, and
2. antiarrhythmics either fail to control your AFib symptoms or cause intolerable side effects.

What symptoms? The most common is fatigue, but there are many others. Feeling mentally or cognitively slow is another relatively common symptom of atrial fibrillation. Another is feeling less enthusiastic about or interested in things your previously enjoyed. These symptoms are just as important as those traditionally thought to reflect a heart problem such as palpitations, dizziness, shortness of breath, or chest discomfort.

As for the second criterion, there is some wiggle room, because insurance companies generally don't specify the duration of drug use before moving on to an ablation. But while some patients have come to see even a short trial of antiarrhythmic medications as something negative, aggressive lifestyle changes sometimes result in a situation in which the person needs neither the antiarrhythmic nor the ablation. And if money is a factor—and for most people it is—at least trying an antiarrhythmic first can minimize the risk of getting stuck with a big bill when an insurer declines to pay.

## TWELVE QUESTIONS TO ASK YOUR EP

In the most experienced hands, serious complications from an ablation are rare and the chance of death is very low. That's actually quite remarkable, considering most AFib patients are older and are contending with a lot of other medical conditions.

But mind that caveat: "in experienced hands." That's very important. While expertise and experience are mounting, as recently as 2013 one study reported an unacceptable mortality risk from EPs and hospital teams that don't have enough experience ablating AFib.[34] As such, the decision on who you should let touch your heart for this procedure shouldn't be taken lightly.

How do you find an electrophysiologist with the right combination of expertise and experience? By asking a lot of questions.

What questions? Start with these:

*What ablation approach do you use?*
Not all catheter ablations are created equal, particularly when it comes to the technology and techniques used, but there is also no one procedure that is best for every patient in every situation. Your electrophysiologist should be able to speak, in a way you can understand, about why they have chosen the kind of ablation they perform, how it compares to other types of this procedure, and why they believe it is right for you specifically.

While it can be tempting to want your EP to use the "latest and greatest" technology, that can be a recipe for danger. Often, the new technology may in fact be *too* new, without enough evidence to establish long-term outcomes. You want your doctor to use the technology they are most comfortable with and have used successfully with many previous procedures.

*How many of these precise procedures have you done?*
It is not unusual, at this point, to be able to find a doctor who has done thousands and thousands of catheter ablations. But this statistic alone actually doesn't tell you much about how successful those procedures have been. Perhaps it can be said that electrophysiologists who have done thousands and thousands of these procedures would probably not be permitted to continue doing catheter ablations if they were routinely losing patients, but with the exception of patients who die on the table—an exceptionally rare event—longer-term outcomes are much harder to track.

Even long-term outcomes don't tell you much because different doctors work with different groups of patients. It shouldn't be surprising if an electrophysiologist whose practice targets younger AFib patients has a higher rate of success after a single ablation. It also shouldn't come as any surprise that a doctor whose patients are predominantly geriatric or have many other heart diseases might have a significantly lower rate of success.

Also, because there are different kinds of catheter ablation, and because new innovations are being made all the time (as we will discuss in the next section), a doctor who has done thousands of ablations using one specific set of tools may have far less experience, and a very different rate of success, with a newer technique.

So why should you even ask this question at all? Because of the answer it should elicit.

If that answer is simply "I have done thousands of these with a high rate of success" or "I have done fewer of these procedures relative to my peers, but am updated on the latest technology and techniques that many of them are not using yet," then you are not being provided with the deep nuance that an answer to this question requires. At the very least, that should color the process you use to make decisions about which electrophysiologist you will work with.

*What do you do to minimize complications?*
Good electrophysiologists should prepare themselves for each and every case. This means having detailed conversations with their patients, reviewing files ahead of time, and staying up to date on the latest updates and technologies in the field, even if those updates are not immediately adopted. Like all tech users, some electrophysiologists are "early adopters" while others are "wait-and-seers."

Regardless, your EP should be able to tell you exactly what they do to avoid the biggest complications like esophageal injury, pulmonary vein stenosis, nerve injury, cardiac perforation, or stroke. Also, an EP who has encountered some of these complications will likely recognize them early if they develop, have experience in their treatment, and hopefully will have learned or changed their approach to avoid them.

*How do you track your ablation outcomes?*
While any doctor can quote you success and complication rates from any procedure in general, you don't want to know those outcomes. What you want to know is the actual outcomes of the EP you are considering for your procedure.

Does this EP keep a database of all ablation results, good and bad? Who in their office or hospital is tracking these data? Do they participate in an atrial fibrillation ablation registry? Do they get regular feedback from this AFib ablation registry? If not, then chances are that this EP probably doesn't really know how successful or how safe their procedure really is. And if you don't know your outcomes, then how can you improve your procedure?

*What do you do to ensure you are rested and not distracted?*
Just like an Olympic athlete would never be up all night the night before their event, answering phone calls during their competition, or trying to compete when they aren't feeling their best, you should

also expect the same of your EP. For the optimal ablation outcome, at a minimum, every EP should get enough sleep the night before your procedure. Studies have shown that the effect of sleep deprivation on our mental judgment and fine motor skills may be worse than alcohol intoxication.[35]

To maximize the chances of this happening, you probably don't want to do the procedure the day after your EP was on call, unless they have many buffers to protect their sleep, like residents, fellows, hospitalists, and nurse practitioners who have tended to those middle-of-the-night phone calls.

Just as getting good sleep should be the goal for anyone trying to optimize their lifestyle to beat back AFib, it should also be the goal for anyone who works anywhere near an EP ablation suite. If your doctor doesn't understand why you are asking about sleep, they are unaware of a simple and well-researched truth: good sleep makes us better at what we do, no matter what we do.

Time of the day is also important. Some studies suggest that having your procedure somewhere between eight and ten in the morning might offer you the lowest risk of a complication and the lowest chance that your procedure will be delayed.[36]

Likewise, distractions make us worse at what we do, no matter what we do. Just as you don't want your doctor on call the night before your procedure, you also don't want your doctor on call while you are having your procedure done, unless, once again, there is a series of buffers in place. Someone else should be responsible for any situations that might arise during your procedure so that your EP can focus on you and you alone. This is serious stuff, after all, and the distractions of our modern world have been shown to affect cardiac surgery.[37]

*How do you avoid esophageal perforations?*
Now that your prospective electrophysiologist knows you're serious about minimizing complications—and has responded with eagerness and positivity to that concern—you can dive into

more technical territory. Here's the key: you don't actually have to have technical knowledge to ask technical questions—good doctors should be able to meet you with an answer that you can understand.

One good way of setting this particular question up, for instance, is to say, "I don't understand all of the reasons, but I do understand that excessive ablation near the esophagus can be a life-threatening complication. Can you tell me why that is and what you do to avoid it?" Don't be afraid, by the way, to write questions like this down—a doctor who cannot be patient with your questions may be one who will not be patient during the procedure.

Because the backside of the left atrium, the posterior wall, is just millimeters from the esophagus, collateral damage to the esophagus can occur—and that can lead to dire injury and even death. For this reason, a good electrophysiologist will have a tried-and-true plan to protect your esophagus from damage via radiofrequency or cryo energy.

Also, don't be afraid to ask your EP if they have ever had this complication before, what they learned from it, and what specific steps they have taken to prevent it from happening again.

*How do you decide which areas of the heart to treat with an ablation?* As you know from chapter two, regardless of how your AFib is classified, the pulmonary vein is the most important area of the heart your doctor can target. This part of the procedure is called pulmonary vein isolation, or PVI. As such, the first thing you want to hear when you ask your EP this question is that they will electrically isolate your pulmonary veins from your left atrium.

There was a time in which isolation was often only temporary, a condition called pulmonary vein reconnection, but research now suggests that with experienced EPs using the best technology, reconnection no longer occurs in the majority of patients after PVI.[38] That's good, but reconnection remains one of the big causes of needing a second ablation procedure, so you should follow up on this question by asking your EP how they ensure that the PVI procedure they perform is durable enough that nothing grows back.

The fibrotic cells that cause AFib aren't just near the pulmonary veins. What you therefore also want to hear is that your EP will look for—and treat—any unique AFib triggers you may have, like atrial flutter, supraventricular tachycardia, or repetitive premature atrial contractions.

This question is particularly important for EPs using cryo energy, because the high cost of cryoballoons, the tools used to deliver the "ice" treatment, might make doctors hesitant to use a cryoballoon to treat your AFib and then another expensive ablation catheter to treat other areas of your heart. They might want to get it all done while they are in there with the balloon. The problem is that this can result in damaging more cells than necessary. Remember, ablation solves a problem created by scar tissue with new scar tissue. And this new "good" scar tissue is created to isolate or separate the "bad" scar tissue from the healthy parts of the atrium. But too much scarring can prevent your left atrium from stretching properly, which can lead to stiff left atrial syndrome, as described earlier.

*What is your anticoagulation strategy?*
This is a slightly less technical question, but one of paramount importance. As a basic defense mechanism, our bodies form clots on any foreign object or tool that comes in contact with our blood. That's why strokes are a key risk during atrial fibrillation in general and ablation specifically.

The key to lowering risk is to stop the body from doing what it naturally wants to do. Anticoagulation is such a built-in part of the ablation process that some EPs don't give it much thought. But it's of such vital importance that you want to make sure your EP is indeed thinking about it, which is why it's good to ask them to explain to you how they are going to minimize the clotting risk, as well as the bleeding risk, before, during, and after the procedure.

*Will you be gentle when you manipulate the catheters, and who will be doing the actual procedure?*

This might seem like a question that "tough" patients wouldn't ask. You'll be asleep during this procedure, after all, so what does it matter?

The answer is that it matters to the utmost, because the top cause of death from catheter ablation is cardiac perforation (a situation in which the catheter pushes through the heart wall and creates a hole) and heart compression that results from an accumulation of blood in the membrane enclosing the heart, known as the pericardium, when those tears occur. Inexperienced operators carry higher risk of this.

Therefore, if a fellow (an EP doctor in training) will also be touching the catheter, you want to know how many of these procedures they have done and how the supervising doctor works with the fellow.

The risk of a cardiac perforation may be further increased by the use of sheaths, which make catheter movement easier but put an added, stiffer element into areas of the body that are in some places quite sturdy and in other places quite delicate. Similarly, when an operator uses a stiffer catheter that may have more technology packed in it, the risk of a perforation may increase. The left atrium, for instance, is a very thin-walled part of the heart, susceptible to tears. Likewise, prolonged and repeated ablation in the same location can cause a rupture of the atrial wall.

You can't always prevent these eventualities, but you can be ready to deal with them. Your doctor should assure you that they will have everything they need to treat this complication ready to go, that they have managed the complication in the past, and that a cardiac surgeon can be very quickly summoned in the rare chance surgery is required to repair a life-threatening tear that won't stop bleeding.

*Would you tell me about a time when something went wrong?*

Every time you step into a car there is a risk of a life-threatening accident. Good drivers know how to reduce the risk. Great drivers are vigilant about what could go wrong at any time and have a plan to respond. But you can't ever make that risk zero. Drive long enough, and you'll eventually run into a situation that puts your life at risk.

Medicine is similar. There is a common saying among doctors that if you haven't had a complication, then you haven't done enough cases. And since you want the most experienced EP you can find, you actually want someone who has faced some complications along the way.

Now, there isn't a doctor in the world who has gotten everything right, every time, with every patient. All of us experience good and bad days. What's more, every patient's body is different, which means that a technique that works a hundred times on a hundred patients might not work for the 101st. If your doctor cannot own that fact, and speak about it clearly without making excuses, then they lack the humility that separates good doctors from great ones.

Admitting error and acknowledging negative results is not a sign of a bad doctor. Not being honest about those outcomes—and, even worse, not caring—is a strong sign that someone might have their interests in mind over yours. All doctors make mistakes, suffer setbacks, meet with disappointment, and sometimes even lose patients. The ones you want to trust with your heart are those who are willing to speak to you about this part of the job.

*How do you help me ensure that there will be no surprises when it comes to costs?*
This is an important question. It does no good to save your life if, in the wake of a procedure, your inability to keep up with your medical bills drives you to want to end your life. (This is, unfortunately, not a hypothetical situation. The phenomenon of people taking their lives when confronted with medical bills they cannot pay has been well documented.)

Your electrophysiologist may not have the answers to this question, but if they are dismissive of this concern, and the rest of the people in their office are, too, then you are absolutely in the wrong office.

While you will certainly get a bill from your EP, and an anesthesiologist if one is used, these doctor bills are just a small fraction of the total bill you will see in the mail. The bill from the disposable technology used to do your ablation could easily top tens of thousands of dollars. That's not to mention all of the other hospital costs associated with the procedure. Until there is better medical cost transparency in the United States, your best bet is to ask your EP's office for all of the billing codes they use in a typical ablation procedure and any others that are common for their practice. With these codes in hand, call your insurance company and ask them what your copay will be for each one.

If you're lucky, you may have already hit your out-of-pocket deductible for the year so your procedure will cost you next to nothing. Even if you believe that to be the case, insurers and hospitals are quite good at passing the buck back and forth if it seems like the ultimate person who will pay the tab is you. For most of our patients, whatever is left of their deductible is what they personally will pay for the procedure. Regardless, do your homework.

*How do you help me minimize the chances of AFib ever coming back?* This question may elicit two different answers. First, as we've discussed, a good EP will be able to explain to you the strategies they use to minimize electrical reconnection after the ablation procedure. But while this is important, what you really want to hear is that they recognize that ablation isn't an endgame; they should not only realize that lifestyle factors play a critical role in preventing a second ablation, but also have a plan and resources available to help you succeed in this important part of your treatment.

Indeed, studies show that having an integrated atrial fibrillation clinic—one that offers not just ablation but also the long-term support you'll need after the procedure—decreases the risk of premature death by 54 percent.[39]

Below, you'll find a tidy list of these questions that you can copy down or photograph with your smartphone, so that you'll have them all on hand when you visit your doctor. Remember: if an EP isn't willing to address your questions and concerns, that doctor isn't the right doctor for you.

---

## TWELVE QUESTIONS TO ASK YOUR DOCTOR BEFORE AN AFIB ABLATION/SURGERY

1. What approach do you use?
2. How many of these procedures have you done?
3. What do you do to minimize complications?
4. How do you track your procedure outcomes?
5. What do you do to ensure you are rested and not distracted during the procedure?
6. How do you avoid esophageal perforations?
7. How do you decide which areas of the heart to treat?
8. What is your anticoagulation strategy?
9. Who will actually be doing the procedure?
10. Would you tell me about a time when something went wrong?
11. How do you help me ensure that there will be no surprises when it comes to costs?
12. How do you help me minimize the chances of AFib ever coming back?

---

Ultimately, the choices you make will be led by a combination of the information you collect from asking lots of questions and your perception of trust. And while some very talented academics have homed in on the factors that compel one human being to trust another, the act of giving someone trust often rests in our gut.

By all means, consult with your family and close friends, but when it is time for the final decision to be made, their advice, and all of the information you have collected, should feed into a decision you make for yourself, for you know yourself better than anyone else in the world. Fear is very natural. Feelings of mistrust are not. If you're not feeling confident about your decision, take a break and reassess.

Once you've made a decision, however, the best thing you can do is get onto your electrophysiologist's schedule as soon as possible. As we have discussed, your AFib tipping point may come upon you at any time. So, once you've made a well-informed decision, the sooner you can make your ablation happen, the better.

## POST-PROCEDURE RECOVERY SYMPTOMS AND THE DREADED "BLANKING PERIOD"

Just about everyone feels some nausea and grogginess from general anesthesia after they wake from a procedure. This usually subsides within a few hours. After that, throat soreness from the breathing tube can last for a few days. If, however, your EP opted for conscious sedation, where you were never fully put to sleep for the ablation, then you probably won't experience nausea and you definitely won't have a sore throat.

After your procedure, you may notice a few small bandages, about the size of Band-Aids, on your inner thigh and sometimes on your neck, where the catheters were inserted in the veins. In contrast to arteries, which are used for procedures like heart stents, veins heal fast and are at low risk of any significant bleeding, so only two to four hours of bedrest after the procedure are typically needed. To protect your veins, however, most EPs will ask that you wait five to seven days before resuming your daily exercise routine.

A lot of people assume that means they'll be up and active in a matter of days, and exercising again soon thereafter. After all, this is a very noninvasive procedure that doesn't even require a stitch. And while some patients "pop right up" after a catheter ablation, that's not always the case. In fact, an ablation can be very hard on the body, especially if general anesthesia is used, and some patients need several weeks of recovery time.

Additionally, medications are often given during the procedure to stimulate the heart to look for AFib triggers, and these can also produce fatigue after the procedure.

Beyond that, in our twenty-plus-year history of performing these catheter ablation procedures, there are three things that commonly send patients back to the emergency room after being discharged from what appeared to be a successful procedure.

The first is pericarditis chest pain. Because small areas of the heart are burned or frozen in an ablation, some degree of chest discomfort should be expected. Yet many patients initially go home feeling fine, then wake up with chest pain sometime during the first or second night after the procedure. This is normal; up to 75 percent of patients will experience chest discomfort in the first few days after the procedure. Most feel a somewhat sharp chest pain when taking a deep breath or while lying down. The pain typically diminishes with more shallow breathing or by sitting up, and, fortunately, it's generally gone within seventy-two hours after the procedure. Regardless of how common it is, or even how bad you think it is, you will still need to report your symptoms to your EP, as chest pain can be a life-threatening warning sign. In most cases, however, it can be addressed with a few days of an anti-inflammatory gout drug called colchicine, as well as NSAIDs like ibuprofen or naproxen.

The second common post-procedure problem is fluid retention, which can lead to shortness of breath. If you've never had a problem with swollen legs before, you probably won't experience many fluid retention issues with your ablation. But, since most AFib ablation patients tend to be a little older and heavier, it is common for them to retain fluid and feel shortness of breath even before the procedure. That can be exacerbated by the fact that most radiofrequency ablation tools deliver continuous fluid irrigation from their tip to improve efficiency and minimize injury to the inner surface of the heart. As a consequence, it isn't uncommon for a patient to pick up two or three liters of saline during a procedure. So, whatever tendency they have to retain fluid prior to the procedure is magnified for the first week or two afterward, with some fluid also building up in the lungs, resulting in shortness of breath. This can be dangerous, though, which is why it is important to weigh yourself before your ablation and then each day at the same time after the procedure. If your weight goes up more than two or three pounds, call your EP and report this finding. Assuming your EP determines the cause is just benign fluid retention, better to take a diuretic for a few days at home at their direction than to ignore fluid retention until your family rushes you to the emergency room with your weight up ten or twenty pounds and you gasping for air.

The final common post-procedure problem is ongoing arrhythmias, including atrial fibrillation or atrial flutter. It can take your heart up to three months to heal from an ablation. Indeed, arrhythmias are expected during this period, due to healing and inflammation, so most EPs will keep you on your antiarrhythmic. These episodes aren't counted as a procedure failure, which is why EPs call the first three months after the ablation the "blanking period."

These are not signs of failure. Weird things can happen during the blanking period, so don't get depressed if the immediate results aren't what you hoped for. Our research shows that most people who have arrhythmias during this time, and especially in the first month after the procedure, won't have them in the long run.[40]

So what should you do if your heart goes out of rhythm after the procedure? We usually tell our patients that if they are feeling okay and are taking a blood thinner, they can give their heart twenty-four to forty-eight hours to see if it will correct on its own. If not, we schedule them for a cardioversion—and that isn't a sign of failure, either. Especially if it happens early in the blanking period, these arrhythmias will often eventually go away without further treatment.

Sometimes, though, the arrhythmias don't go away. And once the blanking period has passed, it may be time for another ablation.

## IS ANOTHER ABLATION NEEDED?

In the past, AFib ablations got a bad reputation for requiring multiple procedures to get the job done. This was because the technology EPs had at the time was more primitive by today's standards, we still had a lot to learn about how to perform the best procedure possible, and we didn't realize the importance of lifestyle optimization. All of these things added up to the electrical reconnection of the pulmonary veins. Fortunately, this is now very uncommon, as EPs have better technologies and a better understanding of what is needed to achieve durable pulmonary vein isolation. So more recently, the first-time success rate has skyrocketed.

But even if you have selected the best EP in the world and have optimized your lifestyle in every way possible, sometimes another ablation is still needed to make the arrhythmias go away for good.

In many cases, a second ablation may be needed to treat atrial flutter. The two arrhythmias, atrial fibrillation and atrial flutter, often coexist in the same person. But whereas AFib represents total electrical chaos of the upper chambers of the heart, atrial flutter often has an organized circuit. Doctors classify flutters as typical or atypical. Most atypical atrial flutters are from the left atrium, whereas typical atrial flutters are from the right atrium. The typical atrial flutter is an organized arrhythmia that commonly makes the heart beat more than 100 times per minute. An atypical flutter, on the other hand, results from abnormal circuits that can develop in or around previous ablation sites or atrial scarring. These atypical flutters may even be more bothersome than the original AFib, and are often less responsive to medications. Fortunately, if you do develop either type of atrial flutter after your AFib ablation, most can be treated easily and effectively with another ablation procedure. And while it's no fun to go back to the hospital, most patients accept this proposition for the chance of ending their arrhythmia.

Other times, a second ablation is needed because a new AFib circuit has developed. And this is why lifestyle optimization, and especially weight management, is so critical after your ablation. You don't want to keep coming back for another ablation every few years because you haven't addressed the underlying problem causing your AFib in the first place.

# AV NODE ABLATION/PACEMAKER: WHEN EVERYTHING ELSE HAS FAILED?

Sadly, not every heart can be fixed with an ablation. Sometimes there is too much atrial fibrosis, the AFib has been persistent for too many years, or there are too many other conditions going on with the heart or body that an ablation just won't hold. What then? Is there any hope?

If there isn't too much fibrosis, and an ablation didn't achieve the desired results, you might consider using antiarrhythmics until the next technological breakthrough in ablation that may improve success rates comes along.

But if that also fails, your heart won't ever slow down, and you can't take the unpredictable rapid heartbeat anymore, you might be a candidate for an AV node ablation with pacemaker insertion. This is an option we advise for older patients with AFib who suffer 24/7 from a fast and irregular pulse when antiarrhythmics, cardioversions, and ablations have all failed or aren't an option.

The AV node is the main electrical relay station of the heart. All electrical signals from the atria have to pass through the AV node before getting to the ventricles. Thus, if you ablate the AV node, which is incredibly easy to do, the ventricles will no longer beat fast and wild. However, without an AV node, your heart rate will probably be stuck at about thirty beats per minute, or slower, for the rest of your life. Thus, pacemaker insertion always accompanies an AV node ablation.

The end result is that your heart never races or beats irregularly again, as the pacemaker is 100 percent in control of your heart rate. While this was the desired end point of the procedure, it comes with some risk as you will also be what we call "pacemaker dependent." In other words, your heart rate relies 100 percent on your pacemaker functioning properly—if it goes out, you're in trouble.

Fortunately, pacemakers have come a long way technologically. Many pacemakers now can be entirely inserted within the heart itself, so there is no scar on the chest and it is impossible to know someone even has a pacemaker unless a chest X-ray is done. Surgeries are quick, often less than an hour, and most patients go home the next day. Some pacemakers are now miniaturized and can be inserted directly into the heart through a vein without surgery. Also, pacemakers can now be checked on from afar, meaning patients don't have to do anything to make sure they are functioning properly. What's more, many pacemakers come with a battery that may last ten or more years before it needs to be replaced. If only our smartphones had a battery that lasted that long!

This might seem like a really good option, and for many people it is, but an AV node ablation/pacemaker procedure isn't a cure for AFib. In fact, the upper heart chambers may even be out of rhythm all the time. All pacemakers do is speed up a slow heart. The only difference is that, for most of our patients, the AFib is no longer perceptible, because their heart rate is regular and controlled. So, while you will no longer need rate-controlling drugs or antiarrhythmics, you will still probably need to take a blood thinner.

So, unless you are a patient with slowly conducting AFib that results in a slow heart rate, your heart slows down too much from the medications used to steady the rhythm or decrease the rate, or you opt for an AV node ablation, then odds are that you won't ever need a pacemaker as part of your AFib therapy.

## THE BIG RESET

It is common for people who have been newly diagnosed with atrial fibrillation, or who have recently learned that they are at risk, to discover inside of them a deep resolve to take the steps they need to drive their disease into remission through lifestyle optimization. This is also the preferable approach, and it is a road that many of the patients in this book have successfully navigated.

Alas, that does not mean it is a very common story. For some patients, as gallantly as they might try, the combination of better sleep, a balanced metabolism, avoiding pollutants, and preventing negative stress isn't quite enough to move all of their AFib-connected biomarkers in the direction of remission. For a greater number of people with AFib, it's not that these strategies couldn't work, but that—for one reason or another—it is simply too hard to implement each and every one of these approaches as faithfully as needed. However resolved they might feel to meet their health challenges with a fight worthy of Hercules, they wind up stumbling. Biomarkers that have fallen in a promising way begin to rise again. Biomarkers that have risen in a way indicative of better heart health begin to fall. The biggest biomarker of all, their weight, slowly climbs upward. And once again, their hearts begin to pound away.

It is then that they often turn to ablation. And it is immediately after that procedure that they often feel as if they have been injected with another mighty dose of resolve.

It is important that this moment not be wasted. Ablation, after all, can only "fix" your current misfiring AFib circuits—it does nothing to prevent them from future misfires. You have to address the underlying cause of your AFib to minimize your chances of ever needing another ablation procedure. To be fair, yes, we have seen 400-plus-pound AFib patients undergo a successful ablation and then never have another episode of AFib again, even though their weight never comes down. This is, by far, the exception. An ablation is a chance to give your heart a new start. It is a reset. It is an opportunity.

This is the opportunity you have been waiting for. This is the moment you need.

That was how Paula beat her AFib. She had done a commendable job prioritizing her sleep, reliably getting seven or more hours every night in regularly scheduled intervals. She was stressing less. She had done everything she could, short of moving to another city, to surround herself with a clean environment.

"Even still, when I was trying to address those last few steps, and particularly when it came to what I was eating, I just felt so powerless and self-defeating," she said. "I knew how I was supposed to eat and exercise, but I was still feeling quite tired, I think as a result of the medications I was on, and it felt like the more tired I got, the less willpower I had to get outside for a jog and to address my mostly good—but sometimes really bad—eating decisions. However, even when I was eating clean, my weight still wouldn't go down, which I think was due to the AFib medications I was on."

After her ablation, something clicked.

"For the first few days I was tired and hurting. For a few weeks, it felt like, although I wasn't having any more AFib episodes, my energy hadn't come back to even the level it was before the ablation. But then it happened."

A surge of energy. An easier time walking, and even running, from here to there. Deeper breaths, which filled her lungs with air and filled her heart with confidence. And, with all of that, a renewed sense that she could truly win her lifelong fight with obesity.

This was the "Big Reset"—a moment many patients experience post-ablation. Paula gathered her family and asked for their help in doing something profound. Together, she asked, could they commit to a 95 percent unprocessed plant-based diet with no added sugars? The only exception would be Sunday dinner when they would have meat and a dessert. Together, she pleaded, could they decide on an exercise regimen, like a commitment to the gym and a brisk walk or bike ride after dinner each evening, that they could do together, as a family?

She looked at her teenage children and her husband. "I was crying a little," she recalled, "and I said, 'Please, if we can, I think my life depends on this.' I love my family, but I would have never had the resolve to be that vulnerable with them. But there I was."

Her youngest daughter, eight, was the first to respond. "Mommy," she said, "of course."

Her middle son, thirteen, was next. "You know, I didn't really like junk food anyway," he lied.

Her oldest daughter, sixteen, didn't hesitate. "Anything," she said.

And her husband, married to her for eighteen years and in love with her since the day they met in high school, made it unanimous. "What will we do first? Go on a walk or head to the market?"

There might not be anything particularly magical about walking, cycling, or going to the gym with your family, or about committing to a mostly plant-based diet free of added sugars and processed foods. These are, however, objectives related to a balanced metabolism that are specific, measurable, attainable, realistic, and timely—so-called SMART goals, as first described by the writer George T. Doran in 1981. Paula could just as easily have asked her family to commit to an every-afternoon game of street soccer and any of a number of other diets that prioritize eating truly healthy foods instead of counting calories.

There is, however, something that feels quite magical about moments like this, for ablation isn't just an opportunity for a Big Reset for AFib patients—it is an opportunity for everyone around that person to recognize that nobody can walk this path alone.

And maybe there's something symbolic about going to sleep and waking up with a heart that works better than it did before. This is a symbol that cannot be wasted, a moment that cannot be allowed to pass.

For the next year, Paula's family maintained their promise to one another. The kids sometimes grabbed a burger when they were out with friends. Her husband, who often worked nights, wasn't always there for the family walks. But whenever they were in the family home, the rules they'd committed to remained sacred.

A year later, Paula's weight was down by thirty-two pounds, and every one of her biomarkers had moved into the territory close to, or indicative of, AFib remission. Every other way in which she had already optimized her lifestyle was sticking.

It was time to take the next step. Paula called her doctor—the same person who had convinced her that it would take more than a handful of drugs each day to save her life.

"Can I come in for a consultation?" she asked. "I'd like to talk about getting off of my medications."

# Chapter Seven

## STOP UNNECESSARY DRUGS

Why most AFib medications can be reduced, and many can be eliminated, and why some patients can look forward to a completely drug-free life

The car crash was frightening enough.

It had been raining that morning, and Annabel was on her way to see the cardiologist, who had recently increased her dose of the anti-arrhythmic sotalol and wanted to see her again. She was rounding a turn when everything went black. Really black. When she regained consciousness, her car was in a ditch next to the road.

Annabel had hit her head on the driver's-side window, and it was clear that her wrist was broken, too. But she still remembers her first thought as she stepped out of the car: *It could have been so much worse.*

Just like that, things *did* get worse. First, her chest felt tight. Then, she began having trouble breathing. Her heart began beating so hard that it felt like a drum in her ears. She fainted again. The next thing Annabel could recall with any sort of clarity were the faces of two paramedics who had arrived on the scene of the crash. They had just shocked her heart out of cardiac arrest. Soon, she was in the hospital.

Other than a minor concussion and her fractured radius, the crash itself did not appear to have caused Annabel any greater harm. This was especially remarkable considering that she was also on a blood thinner in addition to the sotalol she was taking for her AFib. But emergency room doctors quickly recognized the cause of her blackout, the car crash, and the cardiac arrest: the higher sotalol dose had caused the QT interval on her EKG to become dangerously long.

You may recall that a QT interval is a measurement of the time it takes for the ventricles to be electrically stimulated and then recover. When it gets too long, it can cause the ventricles to become unstable and go into a lethal arrhythmia called ventricular tachycardia or ventricular fibrillation. While the higher dose of sotalol had kept her heart free from atrial arrhythmias, she almost died from a lethal ventricular arrhythmia (the most dangerous antiarrhythmic-induced proarrhythmia, as we discussed in chapter three).

Fortunately, Annabel survived this terrifying event. Within twenty-four hours of stopping her sotalol, her QT interval returned to normal and she was out of danger. But, of course, without the sotalol it was just a matter of time before the AFib would be back. Her cardiologist was aware of this as well and wanted to try a different antiarrhythmic.

But by the time Annabel was sitting face-to-face with the cardiologist in her hospital room, she'd had enough. She wanted to get off the drugs for good. That, she had learned in the days after the crash, was what her Aunt Claire had done. After several years of conventional treatment, and suffering from a lot of truly terrible side effects from her medication, Claire had shed all of her atrial fibrillation medications following a fastidious attentiveness to her biomarkers, a successful catheter ablation, and a near-religious dedication to lifestyle changes aimed at the causes of her condition.

"I already know the diet that worked for my aunt," Annabel told the doctor. "I'll exercise every day and, as soon as you say it's okay, I'll get the ablation. I'm willing to do whatever it takes."

Her cardiologist was impressed—but also concerned. Annabel's heart was back in normal sinus rhythm for now, but the AFib could return at any time. If it did, he told her, it could also be deadly.

"I'd like you to try amiodarone instead of sotalol," her doctor explained.

"But aren't these antiarrhythmic medications all terrible?" Annabel asked.

"Yeah, some of them really are," the doctor told her. "But they're also really good at what they're intended for. And that's what you need right now."

Annabel was distraught. "How long will I have to take these for?" she asked. "I really don't want to take them at all."

"Hard to say," her doctor said. "Perhaps for the rest of your life."

Just a decade or two ago, conversations like these often did result in people like Annabel taking amiodarone for the rest of their lives—or at least until they began experiencing significant side effects such as a loss of vision, breathing struggles, thyroid problems, liver inflammation and failure, and bluish skin discoloration. That's to say nothing of the other drugs that are most often prescribed in various combinations depending on an individual patient's perceived needs. Back then, AFib patients didn't have as much information about AFib, let alone a plan of attack for putting it into remission, so they took what they could get.

What a difference a few years make. Today, thanks to easier access to information and the increasingly common stories of people who have successfully put their AFib into remission, like Annabel's Aunt Claire, a small but growing number of patients are becoming active advocates for themselves, especially when it comes to getting off AFib medications. Doctors, meanwhile, are slowly becoming more open to the idea that "here are your drugs, have a nice life" might not be the best approach to treating this condition.

But old habits die hard.

Even patients with the best of intentions can quickly be lulled into a sense of complacency once they get on AFib medications. Sometimes these medications aid in this complacency by lowering energy levels and increasing feelings of depression and despair. Without the constant drumbeat of an arrhythmia to remind them of how important it is to scrupulously stick to a good diet and exercise habits, patients become prone to lapses in decision-making. One lapse can easily turn into two. From there it can be hard to get back on track. All too often, the result is that patients don't just stop dreaming about having a life like the one they had before their AFib diagnosis; they forget that such a life ever existed.

Once a prescription has been written, even doctors who are forward-thinking when it comes to AFib treatment can lose track of which patients have expressed a desire to avoid medications. They turn their attention to the important tasks of drug monitoring and vigilance for side effects—especially if their patients don't continue to actively advocate for themselves.

But Annabel was clear: she didn't want to spend the rest of her life on drugs.

If you feel the same way, this chapter is for you.

## HOW TO APPROACH YOUR DOCTOR

If your goal is normal sinus rhythm, without drugs, the expert and advocate you need is an electrophysiologist. Even if you think there's a chance that you might not need an ablation (and there is), most general practitioners, and even many general cardiologists, are still of the school of thought that the best way to deal with AFib is with drugs. For most people, this means multiple medications.

Even among doctors who tend to prescribe lots of medications for AFib, though, there aren't many who would not be *willing* to at least have a conversation about the possibility of getting a patient off medications. If you have a physician who won't engage in that discussion, then you probably need a new doctor.

But don't jump the gun on this. Indeed, in many circumstances—especially when private insurance is involved—your general practitioner or general cardiologist is the best pathway to an EP. Many of these physicians have an interest in promoting general health and preventing heart disease, and they can start you on your path toward health. They can also write the referral that will help ensure your treatment is covered by your insurer, help you find an EP with a good reputation among their peers, and even help you get an appointment with that specialist faster. As such, even if their immediate impulse isn't what you have in mind for treatment, your non-EP doctor can be an important part of your team, and you should approach them with that in mind. Tell them you appreciate their advice, but that you would also at least like the opportunity to meet with an EP to evaluate all of your treatment options.

Not all of these doctors will come around to your way of thinking, but most will respect your desire to seek additional understanding and treatment options and help you find the specialist you need. If your experience is anything different than that, be polite but firm: you'd like to see an EP, and you'd like them to help you find a good one that has an interest in helping you with important lifestyle changes in addition to performing different types of treatment. If, after all of that, your doctor won't help, then you're not going to change their mind.

This is where the internet comes in. The Heart Rhythm Society, the world's largest network of EPs, is a good resource for finding a respected doctor who specializes in this field. Social media can be helpful, too. Ask your friends and family for help identifying a good electrophysiologist; you'll be amazed how many people you know have met with an EP, were treated with an ablation, and can point you in the direction of the doctor who helped them.

Ideally, the EP you choose will be part of an integrated AFib clinic that addresses all of the contributing factors to AFib, along with dieticians, cardiac rehab, pharmacists, heart failure specialists, weight loss specialists, hypertension clinics, sleep clinics, stress reduction specialists, and others on staff who are dedicated to a holistic approach to fighting AFib. The Heart Rhythm Society recently published a guide highlighting what these centers do to promote AFib care that is integrated, team based, and patient centered.[1] Research suggests that clinics like these may cut your risk of premature death in half,[2] in no small part because, as you know, it isn't just the AFib that has put your life at risk, but rather all of the other medical conditions that led to your AFib in the first place.[3] One day, we believe, integrated AFib clinics will be everywhere and become the standard of care. For now, they're generally located in larger cities. If you can afford it, these places are worth a long drive, train trip, or plane ticket.

If your goal is to beat back your AFib without ablation, the people at these clinics are going to be a tremendously important resource. But you shouldn't be surprised if, after expressing a desire to end your relationship with AFib drugs, the ablation discussion comes up a few times. And while you've already learned about the power of ablation in chapter six, it's important to point out that for people who have made it their goal to go drug free, ablation can be a powerful force multiplier.

## THE POWER OF ABLATION

Lanny's atrial fibrillation made him feel horrible. His AFib drugs made him feel even worse.

The avid outdoorsman and owner of a car-repair shop desperately wanted a drug-free solution to his condition. Moreover, he believed, he needed one. There was no way that he could do the things he loved, let alone the work that sustained his family, if the one-two combo of AFib and AFib medications was sapping him of his strength.

At the age of forty-two, Lanny set to work monitoring his biomarkers and optimizing his lifestyle. The pounds fell pretty quickly. Ten. Then twenty. By the time he'd "leveled off," Lanny had lost seventy pounds.

But he still had AFib.

That, of course, isn't great news. But it's an experience that a lot of people share. About half of our patients can't reach a drug-free goal with lifestyle and biomarker optimization strategies alone. For these folks, if antiarrhythmics aren't working or result in intolerable side effects, ablation is the next step. For Lanny, the chance of living without AFib drugs was all he needed to convince himself the procedure was his best option. And so he had it done.

And he *still* had AFib. A year later, he was still suffering from some arrhythmias. That might be the point at which some people would give up and accept a life of at least some drugs. But Lanny wasn't willing to compromise.

The irregular electrical currents, we told him, might still be coming from an electrical reconnection of one or more of the pulmonary veins entering his left atrium. Together, we decided that the best course of action would be to go back and try one more time.

This time it worked. A few months after the procedure—with his heart in a steady state of normal sinus rhythm and with all his biomarkers stable in "safe" zones—he took his last dose of meds. Years have passed, and he's healthier than ever.

"I completely eliminated three daily medications, the side effects of which added to the terrible way I felt," Lanny said. "Nowadays, my energy is abundant—even to the point I can't find enough things to do some days. There literally isn't a day that goes by that someone I know doesn't stop and ask me my secret, and for those who really want to know, I love to share the concepts that are now a part of my daily life. It is a pleasure for me to share my newfound health and happiness with everyone I know."

Lanny's story is certainly an homage to the power of persistence, but it's also a testament to the potential for ablation to be the procedure that tips the scales toward an AFib drug–free life. Lanny, after all, had done pretty much everything right in terms of lifestyle and biomarker optimization, but that alone wasn't enough to quiet his heart. Even then, it took two ablations to achieve durable pulmonary vein isolation. But Lanny will tell you it was all worth it.

"I am able to put in a full day's work and still want to find something to do to keep going when I get home," he said. "I am able to play basketball with my kids, hike the mountains, and haul hay, all without worrying about what might happen if I overdo it. I truly feel like I have my life back."

It is important to note that even among EPs, there is a diversity of viewpoints on the most realistic approach to keeping AFib in remission after an ablation. Some are very supportive of patients who want to use lifestyle optimization to work toward the goal of getting off drugs. Others aren't quite so open-minded. As more research comes along to support the idea that patients can indeed go drug free after AFib with the right steps and support, more doctors will come around. However, a dose of realism is also needed here. Far too often we see a new patient who hasn't had a day of normal sinus rhythm in the last five or ten years but yet still wants a drug-free AFib solution. Sadly, for these people, the AFib tipping point has come and gone, and meds will likely be required. That doesn't mean, however, that they can't see a tremendous improvement in their condition by following the steps offered in this book.

Even if you're a very good candidate for a drug-free-after-AFib life, you might have to do some work to find a supportive EP. And, in a way, this can be a good test of your resolve. If you're not willing to do that work, then there's a good chance that you won't be able to do the even harder work it takes to actually keep AFib in remission anyway.

Whether your doctor is highly supportive, cautiously optimistic, or skeptical but willing to reserve judgment, you're eventually going to need to demonstrate to them that it is not only your desire to live without medications, but that you truly no longer need them. Because, to be very frank, the people who are willing to change their eating habits, lose fifty pounds, and commit to a lifetime of daily exercise are sort of like unicorns. Or, at least, they are right now. That can begin to change with every new patient who proves to their doctor that they have what it takes to get off and stay off the drugs.

You cannot put the cart in front of this horse. A desire to live without drugs and the ability to live without drugs are two different things. What this means is that you are best equipped to talk to a doctor about getting off AFib medications if you have the data to prove that you have done the hard work necessary to live a life off the meds.

That's what Annabel had with her when she came to see us, after getting a referral from her aunt. "Here are my numbers," she said as she handed us a spreadsheet. "My weight is down ten pounds. And you can see from this graph that my blood pressures have gone from about 140/90 down to 130/80. And my blood glucose, hemoglobin A1C, and CRP numbers are also coming down, too. And even though I have been off sotalol for a month now, my smartwatch hasn't detected any AFib—see here? It's right there on the printout. And I know that my biomarkers aren't anywhere close to where they need to be, but I wanted to show you that I'm keeping track. I'm committed, and with your help I'll get there."

When she finally took a breath, we told her what she wanted to hear: her goal of a drug-free life was our goal. And we'd do everything we could to make it happen.

Of course, we also discussed ablation. Given her aunt's experience, Annabel was eager to get it done. Having learned about the AFib "tipping point," she figured the sooner the better. In fact, we were the ones who pumped the brakes on that line of treatment.

"We definitely don't want to wait too long," we said, "but if these numbers all move in the right direction and your heart stays in rhythm, as confirmed by your watch, there's no reason to rush into a procedure."

## THE RIGHT DOSE

Once you have found a doctor who is willing to work with you toward the goal of getting off drugs, the next step is to work together to develop a plan for each medication.

In some cases, especially if you are already on a small dose, the plan can be relatively simple: the drugs can stop when your biomarkers indicate that your lifestyle changes (with or without ablation) have reached the point where you are at a significantly reduced risk of recurrence.

In most cases, however, the plan will likely be a bit more involved. Doctors are usually, and very reasonably, quite wary about taking patients off medications "cold turkey." Their concern only increases with the risk of a lawsuit if something goes wrong. So, instead of agreeing to a plan to eliminate drugs at a certain point, your doctor might prefer to wean you from the medications over time. This can be an effective strategy, allowing patients to hit waypoints while approaching their goal that result in a lowered dosage and, in doing so, possibly alleviating some of the side effects of these med-ications that make them a barrier to further progress.

This is also a strategy that can help patients who can't eliminate every drug get to the goal of a minimally effective dose. For while "drug free" is a great goal, even patients who do everything right might nonetheless find they still need a little pharmaceutical help. If you wind up in this situation, the goal is to put no more drugs into your body than you absolutely must in order to have the effect you need.

Whatever strategy you embrace, it's helpful to know what you're work-ing toward. Doctors, ever conscious of the fact that there are always more X factors than anyone can account for, are fond of saying things like, "Let's see where you're at in six months and go from there." But as studies into the factors leading to weight loss among people with obesity and diabetes have long shown, setting precise and realistic goals leads to greater long-term success.[4] Having hard targets to work toward is powerful.

There is no magic combination of numbers that will prompt every doctor, in every instance, to sign off on the reduction or elimination of any particular drug, let alone every medication in the colorful cocktails prescribed to many AFib patients. These specific goals are best built in consultation between patients and their doctors. In building those goals, however, it will be helpful if you understand a few more things about each kind of medication.

## GETTING OFF ANTIARRHYTHMICS

You now know that even though antiarrhythmics help you to stay in rhythm, they won't make you live any longer. What's more, after first diagnosis, anti-arrhythmics only have a fifty-fifty chance of keeping your heart perfectly in rhythm for a year.

So why on Earth would you ever want to take an antiarrhythmic? To buy you time. A little time—a short window of opportunity for getting your weight down, controlling your blood pressure, eating right, exercising daily, optimizing your sleep, and reducing your negative stress—can make a world of difference in your long-term outcomes if you use that time wisely. The faster these things happen, the better, and patients who can show big improvements in the amount of time their heart is staying in rhythm, as measured by wearable technology (which we'll discuss further in the next chapter), are those who can rightfully find themselves talking to their doctors about reducing or eliminating their antiarrhythmic use, sometimes even within a few months.

As with most things, the more data, the better. A patient who can *show* (rather than just claim) that their heart has stayed in rhythm for several months has a better chance of getting their doctor's support to reduce or eliminate their antiarrhythmic prescription.

Even with that level of evidence, though, doctors might be wary of letting their patients go completely without an antiarrhythmic, and some might discuss a strategy that has informally been called the "pill in the pocket" approach, in which they don't take an antiarrhythmic day to day, but instead keep the drug immediately available in case their heart goes out of rhythm.

For many patients who optimize their lives in such a way as to drastically reduce their AFib incidents, an episode may just be a once- or twice-a-year occurrence. Others, after a successful ablation, may be AFib free except in times of a confluence of bad luck, like if they are struggling with a bronchitis infection at the same time as things are really stressful at work. In both of these situations, a better option than using an antiarrhythmic 365 days a year may be to use it only when it is absolutely needed.

If you are on an antiarrhythmic and you are no longer having any AFib episodes, or the attacks you got were quite rare even before you started the medication, it's worthwhile to talk with your EP about dropping the daily antiarrhythmic and instead switching to a pill in the pocket. You won't take an antiarrhythmic every day, but you'll always have one ready to use—in your pocket, your wallet, your purse, or somewhere else always available—in case you really need it.

Not every antiarrhythmic has been well tested for the pill-in-the-pocket approach. The best studied are flecainide and propafenone,[5] and there is still a long way to go before we have a complete picture of how this dosing strategy works in various populations. As such, caution is paramount, as is selectivity about who is right for this tactic. Patients who choose this strategy are typically younger and more motivated to minimize drugs. They also know how to use their technology to correctly diagnose and treat AFib attacks. (Again, this is something we'll dive into in the next chapter.) After all, it does you no good to have a pill ready to go for an AFib episode if you don't realize you are having an episode—and, as you know, it is not uncommon for people to be in AFib and not know it.

When some patients move to this strategy, they ultimately find they don't need the antiarrhythmic whatsoever. Others find that they end up using their pill often, in which case they need to either go back to the daily dosing schedule or explore a different option for treating their AFib. But when the practice proves to be effective—and even if you need a pill once in a while—it is a blessing in multiple ways. Foremost, there may be an additional safety benefit in taking antiarrhythmics only when you absolutely need them, because side effects tend to increase over time with daily use and at higher doses. The fewer drugs you put into your body over time, the less likely you are to accumulate these negative reactions. Also, it's cheaper to use a drug occasionally than it is to use it regularly, although that should definitely be seen as an added bonus, rather than a decision-making factor. Cost should not be a factor in what medications people use and how they use them, although, alas, it would be tremendously disingenuous to pretend it isn't.

When helping patients transition to a pill in the pocket, EPs will often also prescribe a beta-blocker or calcium channel blocker to go along with the antiarrhythmic, even if you weren't on these drugs before. In other words, for a while you may be advised to keep multiple pills in your pocket rather than just one. Yes, this is more drugs, but it is important to take these pills as directed to make sure your heart doesn't go too fast during an AFib attack. It's also important to know that, if you aren't on a blood thinner and your AFib doesn't stop within twenty-four to forty-eight hours, your risk of stroke will go up—and fast.

# GETTING OFF RATE-CONTROLLING DRUGS

If, with the help of your EP, you have been able to successfully get off your antiarrhythmics, the next step is to say goodbye to the rate-controlling drugs.

You already know that if your heart beats too fast for too long, AFib can cause heart failure. Rate-controlling drugs like beta-blockers (usually metoprolol) or calcium channel blockers (mainly diltiazem), and, rarely, digoxin, are intended to keep that from happening. Additionally, beta-blockers and calcium channel blockers can help keep your blood pressure in check. So, if you are going to get off of these drugs, the obvious goal is to keep your heart in rhythm and your blood pressure down. This is why, once again, it is important to keep accurate records confirming normal sinus rhythm, without any abnormal heart rate spikes, and well-controlled blood pressure.

Since we've already discussed how to keep your heart in rhythm, let's take a minute to review eight ways to keep your blood pressure in the normal range naturally, without the need for medications. (If you're reading this book in chapter order, some of this will sound familiar to what we discussed in the chapter about lifestyle optimization. If you're reading this book out of order, and have already read chapter nine, you've seen some of this there, too. Either way, though, it's worth a refresher.)

First, you're going to need to eat a low-sodium diet. This can offer a four-point reduction in your systolic blood pressure, an effect equivalent to about half a typical blood pressure–lowering medication.[6]

Second, you'll need to eliminate any added sugars. That's generally worth a seven-point reduction.[7]

Third, it's time to commit to a daily workout for a six- to seven-point reduction.[8]

The fourth thing is really hard to do by itself, but it's a ton easier if you've done the first three things: if you're overweight, you've got to drop some weight. How much? Broadly speaking, twenty pounds gets you a ten-point reduction.[9]

Fifth, you'll want to embrace a high-fiber diet. That could be worth another six-point reduction.[10]

Sixth, follow the US National Heart, Lung, and Blood Institute's Dietary Approaches to Stop Hypertension plan, also known as the DASH diet. This is a mostly plant-based dietary pattern (and one that squares nicely with the diet we'll outline in chapter nine) that is high in potassium and magnesium with limited saturated fats, and it's worth a six-point reduction.[11]

Seventh, you need to get some more nitric oxide from greens and root vegetables. Eat enough of that molecule, the intake of which causes blood vessels to relax and dilate, and you could enjoy a five-point reduction in your systolic blood pressure.[12]

Last, you've got to do something about your stress, which you already know is a key driver of high blood pressure. That can help drive a five-point reduction in your systolic blood pressure.[13]

Yes, that's a lot, but it's also a plan that falls almost perfectly in line with the rest of the strategies in this book. In fact, if you've even gotten to the point where you can start thinking about how to eliminate one or more medications from your life, you're likely already well on your way.

## GETTING OFF BLOOD THINNERS

Even if you're successful at reducing or completely eliminating rate controllers and antiarrhythmics, getting off blood thinners might not be an option. That's because, according to medical society guidelines, it's all about the CHADS-VASc, the stroke-risk scoring system we detailed in chapter three.

As a quick refresher, the CHADS-VASc factors are as follows:

Congestive heart failure: One point.
Hypertension: One point.
Age: Being over sixty-five adds one point. Over seventy-five adds two.
Diabetes: One point.
Stroke or transient ischemic attack: Two points.
Vascular disease: Any arterial blockage adds one point.
Sex category: Women over the age of sixty-five get one point.

When you recognize that the guidelines call for strict lifelong blood thinners for a CHADS-VASc score of 2 or higher, something quickly becomes clear: for some people, it's impossible to reach a "good" score of less than 2. If you're over seventy-five, you're already at 2 points. If you're over the age of sixty-five and female, you've reached the mark by default. You can't control your age and biological sex.

That doesn't mean there is nothing that can be done, though. While some of the CHADS-VASc criteria can't be changed, like age, other things, like heart failure, hypertension, diabetes, and vascular disease, may be reversed through lifestyle and biomarker optimization. And for the people who can reverse these conditions, we no longer count these points when determining their CHADS-VASc score. (Please note that some doctors don't believe you can ever reverse these conditions by completely changing your lifestyle, so they may not be willing to "lower" your CHADS-VASc score. We strongly believe these doctors are uninformed and, if you end up with a physician who holds firm to this point of view, it's time to seek a second opinion.)

And then there's ablation. Our research in tens of thousands of patients,[14] along with many other studies from around the world,[15] presents a strong evidentiary picture that people who have an ablation have a much lower AFib stroke risk, but this isn't factored into the CHADS-VASc scoring system.[16]

Now, for the first two months after an ablation, medical societies recommend a blood thinner for everyone, regardless of their CHADS-VASc score.[17] This recommendation largely reflects the higher stroke rates in the early ablation era, when warfarin levels were not adequate. Studies with newer anticoagulants and ablation tools don't indicate a similarly high stroke rate in the months immediately following a procedure, so this could change over time. Our research has shown that patients at low risk for stroke can safely avoid mandatory anticoagulation following an ablation procedure provided they are taking aspirin, maintain normal sinus rhythm in the month prior to their ablation, and continue to maintain normal sinus rhythm after their ablation.[18] Because the definitive study on this approach has yet to be done, though, and because it is common to experience recurrent atrial fibrillation and flutter during the blanking period, most EPs continue to advocate for the use of anticoagulation for the first two months.

And since what many of our patients are seeking isn't a couple months of freedom from thinners, but a lifetime of such freedom, it's the bigger picture we'll focus on here.

Starting in the third month following an ablation, ongoing needs for blood thinners are typically determined by a patient's CHADS-VASc score, with a score of 2 or higher meaning lifelong blood thinners regardless of whether or not the ablation fixed the AFib. Should ablation be considered a negative point? Perhaps. After all, the drug widely considered to be the safest blood thinner when it comes to bleeding, apixaban (Eliquis), still carries at least a 2 percent annual risk of life-threatening bleeding,[19] while warfarin (Coumadin) carries an even higher risk (3.09 percent).[20] So yes, a less traditional interpretation of the CHADS-VASc could come with an increased risk of stroke, but staying on blood thinners comes with a risk, too.

It is also critically important to realize that not all "points" are truly created equal. For example, in our experience, a prior stroke should count for more than 2 points and female gender should count for less than a point. Even if we stick to the scoring system as it is, however, our research from more than 56,000 patients suggests that warfarin offers few benefits to patients until they reach a CHADS-VASc score of 3 or higher.[21] None of that might ultimately change your doctor's mind about whether you need a thinner, but it's a good place for starting a conversation about what the CHADS-VASc means in your case.

And whatever your score is, it's not the only way to understand your risk of stroke. As you recall from chapter four, your hemoglobin A1C is an incredibly important biomarker when it comes to stroke risk: the lower the better. Your thyroid and lipid panels are also key, as are your BNP and troponin levels. Indeed, a different model for predicting stroke using just age, history of prior stroke or transient ischemic attack, and the two biomarkers BNP and troponin, was shown to be much more accurate in predicting strokes and bleeds than CHADS-VASc.[22] Move all of those numbers in the right direction—and document it all—and you'll be in far better shape to make a decision with your doctor about what is best for your long-term health through the process of shared decision making, in which patients, considering the guidelines and their doctor's advice, are the ultimate arbiters of what is best for them.

## Left Atrial Appendage Closure/Excision

There's one more way to potentially get off blood thinners: having your left atrial appendage closed or removed.

Intuitively, it seems this should be an enormously effective solution. After all, approximately 90 percent of all AFib strokes arise from blood clots forming in the left atrial appendage, a small sac in the muscle wall of the left atrium. Many doctors believe closing off this part of the heart, by having the appendage either tied, clipped, or cut off, or through the insertion of a closure device that plugs the sac's opening, can keep clots from coming loose and heading toward the brain, where they can get stuck and cause a stroke.

But what seems intuitive and what happens in real life can, in some patients, be two different things. Studies show that a left atrial appendage closure device, along with a daily aspirin, offers a survival rate about as good as warfarin, which is great if you consider the risk that comes with that medication. Warfarin, however, is the blood thinner with the highest risk of bleeding. And, if you were to dig into the research, you'd see that a big reason why an appendage closure device and aspirin did just as well as warfarin is because there was a lot less bleeding. However, with these left atrial appendage closure devices, there is a small chance that you could develop a blood clot on the device itself. This is intuitive, too, because any time you stick a foreign object into the circulatory system, the body wants to form a clot, so you may be trading one potential cause of stroke for another.

We still don't know how an appendage closure device and aspirin will stack up against one of the newer blood thinners, which may be more effective in preventing strokes with a much lower bleeding risk than warfarin. We also don't know how these devices compare to aspirin alone, or even to taking nothing at all. What we do know is that, regardless of whether you choose a closure device or have your appendage tied, clipped, or cut off, there is also a small chance that your cardiologist or surgeon will leave you with a left atrial appendage leak (which means blood can still get in and out of your appendage) or stump (which means you now have a new "dead-end pouch" in your left atrium where blood clots can form). Either way, that's not a good thing—a leak or stump can increase your stroke risk as much as twenty-two-fold.[23] Fortunately, as the technology has improved over the years, the chances of these complications have fallen.[24]

These rare complications haven't stopped patients from wanting to know about this procedure—especially those who have been admitted to the hospital multiple times with life-threatening bleeds. Take Phil, for instance. With a CHADS-VASc score of 4, he knew he needed some sort of stroke protection. But blood thinners were really hard on him, and he didn't want to keep going to the emergency room every few weeks with another nose or gastrointestinal bleed.

Desperate for an alternative, he approached us to ask about the left atrial appendage closure device he'd seen on a television commercial. We offered him the information we just offered you.

"Well, I haven't had a stroke, and I definitely don't want to sit around and wait for one to happen," Phil said, "but it sounds like there is a risk either way, so I've got a lot more to chew on."

That was a good outcome, because this was a big decision—and Phil deserved to know the facts. If he did opt for a left atrial appendage closure or excision, we told him, it would be imperative that he get a transesophageal echocardiogram done after the procedure to make sure there were no clots, leaks, or stumps. Often, ongoing blood thinners or additional procedures may be helpful in treating these issues.

Bringing up the risk of a clot, leak, or stump might make you think we're pessimistic about this approach. That's absolutely not the case. In fact, the vast majority of our patients who have had one of these procedures done will attest that eliminating the left atrial appendage, and then getting off blood thinners, was the best thing in the world they could have done for their AFib. But we also need to be clear: this procedure, like any other procedure or medication, does come with risks. In the long term, though, we very much believe these procedures, and the technologies that enable them, will keep getting better. We're also confident that, at some point, a technology will be developed that doesn't put you at risk for blood clots, leaks, or stumps.

Even then, however, we wouldn't have a perfect procedure to prevent the potential of stroke, because left atrial clots represent just a fraction of the different ways in which you could get a stroke—yet another factor that emphasizes the importance of treating the entire heart and body.

## Alternative Dosing Strategies for Blood Thinners

One might assume that a lower dose of a blood thinner could offer a "middle of the road" compromise between the risk of bleeding and the risk of stroke, especially for those who have had an ablation and committed to steadfast lifestyle optimization.

Unfortunately, the studies aren't promising when it comes to this approach. Research has demonstrated that low-dose warfarin isn't protective against AFib strokes and doesn't even lower the bleeding risk.[25] And while studies evaluating low doses of the newer blood thinners have shown better results, it's still not optimal.[26] What's more, with newer blood thinners, nonadherence to prescribed doses or missing doses has been shown to increase the risk of stroke by 50 to 70 percent.[27] This, however, was in a cohort study of AFib patients from the US Veterans Health Administration, all of whom have vastly different lifestyles and treatment backgrounds. What isn't known is what the results might look like among a cohort of patients who have had a successful ablation and have optimized their lifestyles to keep AFib in remission.

Anecdotally speaking, we haven't seen any strokes in our patients who are taking a lower dose of one of the newer blood thinners if they have also had a successful ablation, have optimized their lifestyles and biomarkers, and are checking their rhythm every day. But, as you know, anecdotal evidence is never a substitute for real data to guide your decision-making process, and that's important to keep in mind as we talk about another option—a pill-in-the-pocket blood-thinner approach similar to what some patients use with antiarrhythmics.

This approach is truly only for highly motivated AFib patients who are at low to intermediate risk of stroke, and even then, your doctor may not approve, because it is not part of the official guidelines for treating AFib. But in the era of AFib-detecting smartwatches, lifestyle and biomarker optimization, newer blood thinners, and ablations, we do believe there is a role for the pill-in-the-pocket approach to protect patients from a "once in a blue moon" AFib attack.

Just like pill-in-the-pocket antiarrhythmics, this "on demand" approach means you would only take a blood thinner when you need it—like when you're having an AFib attack—and not when your heart rhythm is perfectly normal. Dr. Rod Passman, a cardiologist from Northwestern University in Chicago, has been a champion of this approach, and he hasn't been shy about sharing his opinion on its merits, going so far as to say the way we typically administer blood thinners is "stupid."

"We know that only about half the patients who should be receiving an anticoagulant are actually prescribed one and when we do prescribe it, probably only half are still taking it after a year or two," he told TCTMD, a comprehensive online resource focused on interventional cardiology. "People simply do not want to be on these drugs long-term and if they can minimize their exposure to it without compromising stroke risk, well that's a win-win."[28]

Passman not only has a good point, he might in fact have understated patient disgust for these drugs. Studies show that as many as two in three patients have quit their blood thinners on their own within a year.[29] But, unfortunately, the vast majority of these patients are stopping them the wrong way—going against the wishes of their doctors, instead of working with those doctors to come to consensus about what is prudent.

Patients who familiarize themselves with the latest research, as best they can given the sometimes esoteric language used in scientific studies, are better armed to have those conversations. As of the writing of this book, there have been four studies published on pill-in-the-pocket blood thinners in patients with lower CHADS-VASc scores,[30] and the results were very promising. All of these studies showed that it may be a reasonable alternative to the daily blood thinner, protecting patients from side effects and saving them money without increasing risk.[31]

But, to put things into perspective, altogether these four studies involved fewer than 3,000 patients. By way of contrast, the study that resulted in FDA approval for Eliquis included more than 18,000 patients. A lot is at risk here—especially considering that an AFib stroke could put you in a nursing home for the rest of your life.

There are a few other things that need to be said about this approach. First, all of the studies that have been completed so far have used one of the newer blood thinners. Warfarin cannot be used "on demand," as it takes a few days before it has an effect; by then, a stroke could have already happened.

Second, there is no consensus on how long an AFib episode should be before it triggers the use of a pill, or how long you should continue taking the pill after the episode ends. Intuitively, though, most EPs who are open to this pill-in-the-pocket approach would probably recommend a month of blood thinners after an AFib attack.

Third, studies show that there is no direct relationship in timing between when the AFib attack starts and when the AFib stroke occurs.[32] Strokes don't always happen around the time of an AFib attack. This is because, as you know, AFib sufferers are almost always dealing with other medical conditions, including diabetes, hypertension, heart failure, and coronary artery disease, that also raise the risk of stroke. It would be delusional to think that a blood thinner, taken only in the aftermath of an AFib episode, could work for anyone except those people who are completely healthy other than their AFib.

Fourth, if you don't have a pacemaker or use an implantable continuous heart monitor, you'll have to rely, to some degree, on perceivable symptoms. That's because many wearable heart monitors don't measure the heart continuously (as it would drain the battery quite quickly) and can miss periods of atrial fibrillation. But after a bit of experience with AFib, most people get pretty good at knowing when it's happening—with self-reported symptoms correlating to actual episodes about 70 percent of the time.[33]

Don't be discouraged. This approach might not be right for you just yet, but there are studies ongoing that are evaluating whether implanted or wearable heart monitors can make the pill-in-the-pocket blood-thinner approach work even better for even more people.

For those who are highly motivated, though, we do believe this can be a viable option right now, provided a patient is 100 percent committed to optimizing their lifestyle and to using the latest AFib monitoring technology to guide their use of blood thinners. (We'll discuss tech in greater detail in the next chapter.)

## CUTTING HEART FAILURE MEDICATIONS

Sometimes heart failure causes AFib. Sometimes, though, it's the other way around.

When a very fast arrhythmia, like atrial fibrillation or atrial flutter, causes heart failure, we call that tachycardia cardiomyopathy, which means "a fast heartbeat causing heart muscle weakening." And, in one way of thinking, tachycardia cardiomyopathy is a good thing, because if you can put AFib into remission, then your heart failure will probably go away as well. But even if both the AFib and the heart failure are gone, your doctor might still want you to be on a beta-blocker, ACE inhibitor, or ARB medication, as well as a diuretic or two. Can you also get rid of these drugs?

While your cardiologist probably won't have a problem getting you off diuretics if you're not retaining fluids, convincing them to get you off the other meds may be a greater challenge, because there is a chance the beta-blocker, ACE inhibitor, or ARB medication also played a role in healing your heart failure. The trick, then, is figuring out whether it was a normalization of sinus rhythm, the meds, or both that helped you get rid of the heart failure. And while it can sometimes be difficult to tell, in most cases there are some clues.

Mo's case is a great example of how those clues were identified and used to determine whether he still needed to be taking heart failure medications. It all started one day when, seemingly out of the blue, the fifty-two-year-old postal clerk started feeling fatigued. Soon thereafter he noticed that even light exertion was leaving him short of breath. Like a lot of people, he ignored it. It was, he figured, just age. But when Mo's wife saw him huffing and puffing while they climbed a single flight of stairs, she insisted he go to the emergency room to get things checked out. He resisted, but she eventually won the argument—and it's a good thing she did. In the ER, staff members detected an irregular pulse of 150 beats per minute, and Mo was immediately fast-tracked to see the doctor.

After just one EKG, the first diagnosis was obvious—Mo was in rapid AFib. After an echocardiogram showed he had an ejection fraction of 20 percent (normal is 50 to 70 percent), the second diagnosis was also obvious—he was in heart failure.

The double diagnosis seemed to have come out of nowhere, since he'd never had a heart problem before. In fact, as part of his usual workup, Mo had a stress test the previous year, which showed no signs of any blockages in his heart and no heart failure. What's more, his coronary calcium score, a measurement of calcified plaque in the coronary arteries, was 0—there wasn't even a hint of atherosclerosis detected.

But Mo didn't have much time to dwell on any of that. After a transesophageal guided echocardiogram (an ultrasound done with a probe placed down the esophagus) confirmed there were no blood clots that had developed in the left atrial appendage, Mo's heart was shocked back into normal sinus rhythm with a cardioversion.

So, did Mo's heart failure cause his AFib, or was he suffering from tachycardia cardiomyopathy, in which the AFib was the instigator of the heart failure? The next few weeks would offer the answer. In a tachycardia cardiomyopathy, the atrial fibrillation or flutter is quite fast (a resting rate of 120 beats per minute or more) and the ejection fraction quickly normalizes once normal sinus rhythm is restored. That's what happened in Mo's case. Within a month of maintaining normal sinus rhythm, Mo's ejection fraction was back in the normal range at 58 percent. Once the AFib was gone, the heat failure was, too.

Sometimes, it's not so cut and dry. When it is unclear whether an arrhythmia caused a case of heart failure, doctors may order a cardiac MRI.

If the ventricular fibrosis is less than 10 percent, it's probably a tachycardia cardiomyopathy.[34] And that's important for the question of whether to continue on heart failure medications, because if the cause of the heart failure was from a fast arrhythmia, doctors won't generally have any problems stopping the meds unless the patient also has high blood pressure.

Of course, Mo's story wasn't over. A cardioversion doesn't fix AFib, after all, and if other changes weren't made, he could look forward to the return of his arrhythmia—and with it, most likely, the heart failure. So Mo's new challenge was ensuring the AFib went away forever, making it likely the heart failure would, too.

## CUTTING YOUR OTHER MEDICATIONS

It should come as no surprise that Mo had to work very hard to keep his AFib and heart failure from coming back. But we're pleased to report that he is among the growing number of people who only talk about these conditions in the past tense.

"Being told that I had both AFib and heart failure at the same time turned out to be a real blessing," Mo recalled. "I shot past fifty acting just like I had when I was forty and thirty and twenty. I didn't focus on my health. I literally got shocked into making a change, and everything about the way I live my life is healthier now."

That means better food, consistent daily exercise, and well-managed stress, of course. But Mo hasn't stopped there. Having narrowly avoided two conditions that could have resulted in a lifetime of medications and a premature death—and recognizing how much those medications would have changed his life—he began considering the other meds he was on. And he resolved to get rid of those, too.

And why not? Why stop after you have eliminated the AFib and heart failure meds? Can you keep going? Can you also eliminate everything else while you are at it? Fortunately, for many of our patients, the answer is "yes."

This makes perfect sense. If you drop weight to put your hypertension and AFib into remission, after all, then there's a really good chance your acid reflux, back pain, and knee pain will probably go away as well, so you can also get rid of your stomach acid–reducing medication and pain pills. Likewise, lifestyle optimization leaves people feeling so good that many of our patients can also get off their antidepressant (under the direction of the prescribing doctor, of course).

Indeed, if you are motivated enough, in many cases there's reason to be hopeful for a life free of medications of any kind.

## NEVER TOO OLD

There are cases in which patients are very successful at bringing their biomarkers to levels that indicate the lowest possible risk for AFib, in which they optimize their lifestyles to what seems like the cusp of perfection, in which they get an ablation from a skilled electrophysiologist, and in which they work with their doctors to wean themselves off drugs—only to find that, even after all that work, they simply can't go completely drug free.

These people are not failures. Not in the least. Just as many cancer patients can benefit from a lifetime of low-level "maintenance therapy" once their disease is in remission, some AFib patients are better off when they have found the minimally effective dose of one or more medications to keep their arrhythmia at bay. The end goal, after all, is the best possible life. Often that can be achieved without drugs, but sometimes medications are still part of the equation that allow for that goal to be reached.

There are few people, though, who can't benefit from trying to reduce their reliance on medications, and there is almost always something left to try—one last effort to eat a little healthier, one more attempt to exercise a bit more, or one final biomarker to move.

And it's only "too late" if you don't want to try anymore.

Jake is proof of that. The accountant from Utah was in his seventies when he was diagnosed. He tried flecainide without success, and although the chances of antiarrhythmic success go down if the first one doesn't work, he got lucky: sotalol kept his heart in rhythm.

And then, like a lot of people, he got complacent. A life in rhythm was good enough, even if some of the side effects of the drug made him feel lousy sometimes.

He was in his early eighties when he decided he'd had enough of that. He wholeheartedly embraced the Mediterranean diet, adopting mostly plant-based eating habits, getting rid of processed foods, cutting his sugar down to nearly nothing, and eliminating all fried and fast foods. He also started running, biking, and swimming every day. He volunteered as an accountant for a nonprofit organization and frequently traveled to developing countries to help that group build schools—keeping plenty of "good stress" in his life while eliminating the negative stressors that had been present throughout much of his career.

As a result, Jake's diabetes and hypertension went into remission. His CHADS-VASc score fell to 2—with both points coming from his chronological age being over seventy-five. Biologically, it would appear, he was twenty years younger.

Day by day, Jake's AFib went away, and as it did, he decided to go after the sotalol. Working with us, he cut his dose in half. After six months without incident, he cut it again. A year later, still AFib free, he took his final pill.

"And then I just figured, 'why stop there?'" Jake recalled. "If I could get off the antiarrhythmics, could I get off the blood thinners, too? And really, what did I have to lose?"

With a CHADS-VASc score of 2, his annual stroke risk according to the AFib guidelines was 2 percent.[35] But on Eliquis, his bleeding risk was also 2 percent.[36] "That seemed like more or less an even trade," he said. "So I decided to go for it. I tracked my pulse twice every day to confirm normal sinus rhythm. I never missed doing that. I also promised my EP I'd call immediately if anything was amiss."

And nothing was amiss. Not in those first weeks. Not in the following months. Not in the years to come.

No, it's never too late.

And it's never too early, either.

## HOW TO STOP THAT RARE AFIB EPISODE

If you find yourself experiencing a very occasional incident of AFib, you need not panic. And the off chance that such an attack might happen in a very inconvenient time—like when you're on a long international flight, taking a cruise, or in a very remote area of the world—absolutely shouldn't stop you from living your life.

Lots of people travel with a first aid kit. That doesn't mean they intend to use it—it simply means they are ready in case something happens. No matter how long your AFib has been in remission, we suggest having a plan of response ready to go, especially when you know you're going to be away from a hospital or doctor for a while. As the Boy Scout motto goes: "Be prepared."

First, keep an antiarrhythmic medication on hand for an emergency. Even though many of our patients haven't had an AFib episode in years, they still keep an antiarrhythmic in their wallet, purse, or car just in case their heart ever starts fibrillating again. If nothing else, it gives them peace of mind and a sense of control should anything ever change.

Next, always be ready to rehydrate. As dehydration is a big AFib trigger, many of our patients report that they are able to quickly get back to sinus rhythm simply by rehydrating. Always travel with clean water at arm's reach.

Third, keep your electrolytes up. Low levels of magnesium and potassium are another common AFib trigger. A quick boost through electrolyte-heavy foods, or drinks like tomato juice or low-sodium vegetable juices, is always a good bet. But if you're going to be away from a place where you can access these foods and drinks, supplements are a good idea, especially in the case of magnesium.

Fourth, exercise. While it may seem very counterintuitive, many of our patients, like Jose from chapter six, report that all they need to do is to overtake their AFib heart rate with an elevated exercise heart rate to get back in normal sinus rhythm. When their heart slows after the exercise, their normal sinus rhythm is restored.

Fifth, lie down. If an exercise-induced increased heart rate doesn't work for you, the opposite might do the trick. Many of our patients report that taking a nap or going to bed early when they are in AFib is the trick to getting back in rhythm.

Sixth, stimulate your vagus nerve. As you learned in chapters one and two, sometimes autonomic nervous system imbalances can trigger AFib. One way to quickly correct this is through vagal maneuvers, like slow deep breathing, bearing down like you are trying to have a bowel movement, tightening your abdominal muscles, inverting your body by raising your legs or standing on your head, coughing, or taking a cold shower.

Finally, if all else fails, it's time to contact your EP and consider visiting a medical facility for a cardioversion to restore normal rhythm. With that in mind, even if you think you absolutely won't need it, it's worthwhile to do a little planning before you travel so that you know where the best medical care is relative to where you are going to be along the way.

This isn't admitting defeat. Sometimes life just throws us a curveball. Let bad experiences become good data that can help you prevent another such experience. After all, this is a lifetime fight.

## TAKE A STEP

You'll remember that Annabel, who we met at the beginning of this chapter, was determined from the moment of her diagnosis to live a life free of AFib medications. Following the advice of her doctor, though, she consented to a prescription for the usual cocktail.

But she never got complacent. Just as she pledged, Annabel began to follow the diet her aunt had adopted when she went to battle with AFib. Annabel also joined a gym and got heavily into the fast-growing sport of pickleball, playing with friends at least three times a week. She tracked her biomarkers as though her life depended on it, "because, the way I saw it, my life absolutely did depend on it," she said.

The first drug to go was her antiarrhythmic medication. It wasn't long after that she was able to say in good faith that her CHADS-VASc score was down to 1—a single point that she couldn't shed because she is a woman—so she was able to get off the blood thinner.

She kept a flecainide in her purse, just in case, but never needed it. "It feels good to have it there," she said. "But really, though, I don't even think much about it anymore. I'm AFib drug–free. That was my goal from the start, and it feels good to know I reached it."

That doesn't mean she was done, though. Not by a longshot. Because putting AFib into remission and keeping it there are two different things. And the people who are able to keep their atrial fibrillation at bay are those who never stop tracking the messages they're receiving from their bodies.

## HOW TO GET OFF YOUR MEDS SAFELY

1. Antiarrhythmics
   a. As-needed dosing with close AFib monitoring may be possible
   b. Lifestyle optimization may eliminate need by putting AFib into remission
   c. Ablation may eliminate need

2. Rate-Controlling Medications
   a. As-needed dosing with close AFib monitoring may be possible
   b. Lifestyle optimization may eliminate need by putting AFib into remission
   c. Ablation may eliminate need

3. Blood Thinners
   a. As-needed dosing with close AFib monitoring may be possible but not yet proven
   b. Left atrial appendage elimination may eliminate need

    c.  Lifestyle optimization may lower CHADS-VASc score enough to eliminate need

    d.  Ablation may eliminate need in low- to moderate-risk patients with close AFib monitoring but not yet proven

4.  Heart Failure Meds

    a.  Lifestyle optimization may normalize ejection fraction and eliminate need

    b.  Sinus rhythm maintenance may normalize ejection fraction and eliminate need

## Chapter Eight

## ∿ TRACKING WELLNESS ∿

How a lifetime commitment to data collection and analysis
is the final step toward a potential cure for AFib

She calls him "Doctor Fancypants." And if you ever hear Debbe McCall talk about him, you'll realize quite quickly that's actually a pretty kind nickname.

He was a general cardiologist, fresh out of med school, and he was probably very well meaning. But when Debbe arrived in his clinic after experiencing heart palpitations and trouble breathing, he wrote her off before she could even start explaining all of her symptoms.

"It's either anxiety or menopause," he said.

Debbe didn't think that was right. She knew her body—and she knew that something *else* was off.

But there was a problem: she was paroxysmal. Her palpitations had come and gone, and the doctor wasn't convinced that what she'd faced was anything to worry about.

"Just like your car doesn't make the funny noise when you bring it to the mechanic, my heart wasn't doing the funny thing when I was in front of the doctor," she said, "so he didn't believe me."

Another general practitioner did, though, and she wrote Debbe a standing order to have an EKG at any time she was having palpitations. "Finally it happened," Debbe said. "I went in and the doctor's physician's assistant diagnosed it as AFib."

It was time to go see Dr. Fancypants again.

His solution, as you might expect by now, was drugs.

Debbe didn't like that. By this time, she'd done quite a bit of research on atrial fibrillation and its treatment options. She also understood the CHADS-VASc and had already assessed her own score—and she was concerned when the cardiologist didn't do that before ordering up an anticoagulant.

"So I very nicely asked him, 'Please explain your thought process,'" she said. "He was insulted. He said, 'I'm the doctor; you're the patient,' and I said, 'I understand, but it's my heart.'"

Debbe wasn't against blood thinners. She just wanted to know that the drugs she was being prescribed were right for her. That's never too much to ask.

She does give Dr. Fancypants credit for one thing: he referred her to an electrophysiologist. That set her on the course to get the treatment she needed, including an ablation.

Today, Debbe is one of the world's foremost advocates for AFib patients. As the facilitator of the AFib Patient Support Forum on Facebook,* which has more than 16,000 international members, she helps connect people to information they can understand about their condition.

She's also one of the greatest examples of someone who has perfected the final piece of the BLAST model for putting AFib into remission: she is a meticulous tracker.

"I have spreadsheets from here to eternity," she laughs.

---

*https://www.facebook.com/groups/AtrialFibrillationSupportForum.

That might seem funny. But if you want the best chance of keeping your AFib in remission, you'll follow her lead.

In this chapter, we'll talk about the different tools you'll use—and habits you'll want to develop—for tracking your health. This includes keeping tabs on your exercise, sleep, food, and stress. It also includes paying close attention to your medications, especially if you're using a pill-in-the-pocket strategy. We're also going to discuss how to track and analyze all of your biomarkers, from common metrics like weight and blood pressure to lesser-known numbers like A1C and CRP.

All of this should go into a "heart rhythm portfolio." In this portfolio, you'll keep your test results, track your biomarkers, and watch—hopefully with a good deal of awe and glee—the way your decisions and actions often result in health outcomes that you can see in the numbers and feel in your life. Over time, based on your personal needs and goals, you may see opportunities to track other parts of your life that could affect your AFib. If you're like many people, it will become part of your daily routine—a part that you don't even have to think about all that much. Eventually, you'll be able to delegate a lot of this to an app running in the background.

If you're like some people, though, you might end up obsessing a bit. And that's okay. It's possible to overdo anything, of course. But we're talking about your health, here. If you've got to obsess over something, that's a pretty good thing to obsess over.

## WATCH IT

Remember when watches used to keep time—and that was pretty much all they did? Even then, a timepiece could be a powerful tool for keeping track of heart health. All you had to do to check your heart rate was to find your pulse, count your beats for fifteen seconds, and multiply by four.

Your resting heart rate and your heart rate during exercise are still really great pieces of data to track. But these days you don't need to find your pulse, or do any math whatsoever. Smartwatches can do that for us. And that's not all. It turns out that smartwatches are also pretty good at detecting AFib.

When Mick bought the first FDA-approved EKG smartwatch, the Apple Watch 4, he didn't do it for the AFib and EKG features. He just happened to be a really big fan of Apple products.

But thank goodness he was, because in the year before he made that purchase, he had noticed that occasionally it was getting harder to exercise and that he felt tired more often. "I just figured that was just what happens when you get older," he said. "You have some good days and some bad days, right?"

He did think the smartwatch would help him get back in shape through apps that track exercise and steps. But soon after his purchase, his watch notified him of a potential arrhythmia. Although he ignored the first few alerts, Mick eventually reached out to his family doctor, who referred him to a local cardiologist. After an EKG and a stress test, the doctor confirmed that Mick had AFib, prescribed the usual meds, and sent him on his way.

But Mick kept getting the AFib alerts. "And this time I took it more serious," he said. "The watch had been right the first time—it alerted me to a possible arrhythmia and, sure enough, that's what the doctor confirmed. So now that it was basically saying that the meds weren't keeping my heart in rhythm any more than it had been before, I was pretty concerned."

When Mick returned to his local cardiologist with that information in hand, the doctor agreed it was time to get him in to see us.

Just think about this: because Mick's symptoms were so subtle and intermittent, he would likely have not known he had atrial fibrillation for many months, if not years, if he had not had the watch. Fortunately, with his early smartwatch diagnosis, his AFib was easily treated—long before any significant atrial fibrosis developed. So, it isn't hyperbole to say that Mick's watch might have saved him from a devastating AFib stroke.

Now, some people don't think they need an AFib-detecting watch. They think they can feel every episode. Studies clearly show, however, that many people with AFib experience episodes that they can't feel.[1]

What's more, waiting until an episode is strong enough that it can be felt may mean you've waited too long. Complicating matters even further, studies also show that symptoms perceived to be AFib are something else at least 50 percent of the time.[2] And, to make things even more challenging, if you've had an AFib ablation, many of the cardiac nerves that once helped you perceive your AFib symptoms may have also been treated as part of the procedure, so all bets are off as to whether your symptoms will still reliably flag future episodes of AFib.[3]

All of this is why it's important to have a watch that can detect AFib episodes—and to be able to understand what it is telling you.

Remember, AFib is usually a fast and irregular rhythm—so much so that you won't be able to detect any pattern to the beats. That's not a hard rule, though. We have seen plenty of cases over the years where people have had a very slow heart rate with their AFib, so don't rule AFib out simply because your heart isn't beating quickly.

On the other hand, atrial flutter is usually fast and regular, with a steady, patterned beat. However, just as with AFib, atrial flutter can also come with a heart rate that isn't fast, although this is less common.

And then there are premature beats, premature atrial contractions, and premature ventricular contractions, which usually cause a normal to somewhat lower heart rate, but with a detectable pattern to the irregularity. In other words, you may have three or four beats with normal timing and then one beat that is off.

But why do you need to know this? Isn't that what the smartwatch is for, after all?

While these devices are getting better, and some manufacturers claim an accuracy of close to 100 percent, we have seen a number of cases where even top-of-the-line AFib-detecting watches offer the wrong diagnosis.

What bothers our smartwatch-wearing patients the most is when their watch can't "figure out" their rhythm. When this happens, the watch calls the EKG "unclassified" or "inconclusive." Usually, unclassified or inconclusive means that you were moving too much during the EKG and this movement made your EKG uninterpretable. However, it could also mean that your heart rate is too high or too low, that there are too many premature beats, or that your heart is in some other rhythm.

With all that in mind, let's look at some charts, starting with what normal sinus rhythm looks like:

**Sinus Rhythm — ♥ 94 BPM Average**
This EKG does not show signs of atrial
fibrillation.

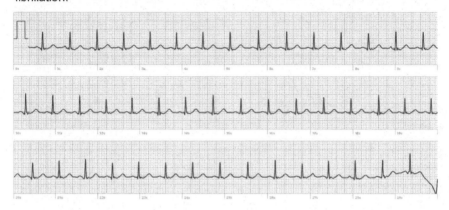

On this smartwatch-recorded EKG, the watch correctly diagnosed its owner as being in normal sinus rhythm at ninety beats per minute. This is a high-quality recording; the watch's owner was sitting perfectly still when it was taken. Each beat is perfectly timed and the heart rate is within the normal range.

Now, let's look at an EKG chart for this same person at a different time:

**Atrial Fibrillation — ♥ 113 BPM Average**
This EKG does show signs of AFib.
If this is an unexpected result, you should
talk to your doctor.

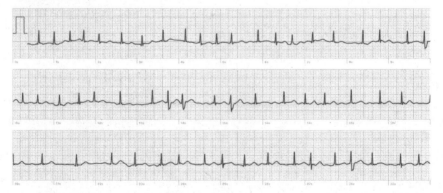

In this tracing, you'll notice that this individual's resting heart rate is elevated at 113 bpm, and that the distance between every beat is completely different. We call this being "irregularly irregular," and, once again, the watch has made the correct diagnosis: she is in AFib.

There are some limitations to these devices, of course. Take this tracing, for instance:

**Heart Rate Over 120 — ♥ 143 BPM Average**

This EKG was not checked for AFib because your heart rate was over 120 BPM.

If you repeatedly get this result or you're not feeling well, you should talk to your doctor.

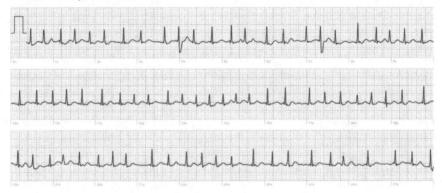

In this case, the user knew she was out of rhythm. Indeed, her resting heart rate was 143 bpm and her pulse was very irregular. However, because her resting heart rate is above 120 bpm, this particular watch wouldn't even venture a "guess" as to whether she was in AFib. But as an astute observer of AFib, you can easily make the call. Once again, we see that the rhythm is fast and the distance between every heartbeat is "irregularly irregular." This is another episode of AFib.

Now, how about a challenge?

**Sinus Rhythm — ♥ 86 BPM Average**
This EKG does not show signs of atrial
fibrillation.

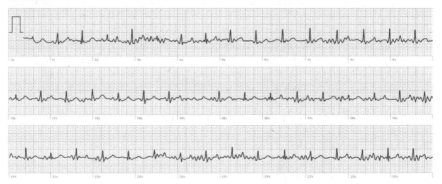

In this case, the rhythm is mostly regular. The heart rate is not elevated. But there are lots of jagged lines between each heartbeat. What's happening?

Well, in this situation, the watch is correct. This is normal sinus rhythm. The distance between each beat is mostly constant. But what are all those jagged lines? Those are from "movement artifact," which happens when the electrodes aren't making stable contact with the skin.

Now, all smartwatches are not created equal. Technology will change over time. But if you have AFib, or if you are at risk of developing AFib, there's really no better investment than a watch that will, at a minimum, be able to detect AFib with reliability and record an EKG. Watches that just record your heart rate, or try to record an "artificial EKG" through the light sensor based on the regularity of your pulse on your smartphone, are not as accurate for detecting AFib. We will refrain from making brand endorsements, but it's not hard to find a good one. Forums like the one Debbe facilitates on social media are a great place to go to learn about the latest products that people with AFib are using and learn about their experiences with those products, both good and bad.

And watches aren't the only tech that can help you track your AFib. Many of our patients use less expensive Bluetooth-enabled electrodes that work with many different types of smartphones. Still others use a pulse oximeter, stethoscope, and blood pressure machine with built-in rhythm checks. Outside of an implanted heart monitor, though, we have found that for many of our patients, wearing a watch is the most reliable method to keep a more frequent vigil for AFib events.

Now, these devices are not continuous monitors, so they can miss short events. In most cases, what you get from a smartwatch is a "fingerprint" of what your heart rate is supposed to look like. Then, by tracking the graphs each day, you can quickly identify when things change. Even still, your doctor may not think that the symptoms you describe are from AFib unless you provide a real EKG for them to review. And that's not a bad thing: you don't want your doctor prescribing new medications or ordering up procedures unless they are 100 percent certain that you are indeed experiencing AFib.

But just because smartwatches aren't perfect doesn't mean they can't be a tremendously important tool for catching early incidents of AFib, tracking incidents over time, and alerting pill-in-the-pocket patients to potential incidents that might warrant the use of medications.

If we only use smartwatches as AFib warning or EKG devices, though, we're not tapping into their true power. Most of these devices collect daily heart rhythm reports that can, and should, be downloaded and stored as part of your heart rhythm portfolio. This is also very powerful data, as it offers an opportunity to see how daily, weekly, and monthly actions impact rhythm. Eventually, these smartwatches will also be able to accurately monitor blood pressure, among other biomarkers that will add to our ability to monitor for diseases.

But even now, there is more these devices can do to help put AFib into remission and keep it there. So, over the next few pages we'll discuss the other parts of your life that a smartwatch can help you track with ease: sleep, exercise, and stress.

## TRACKING SLEEP

When you wake up in the morning, what is the first thing you usually do? Do you kiss your partner? Reach for your phone? Click on the TV news?

When you go to bed at night, what's the last thing you usually do? Do you say a prayer? Count sheep? Listen to Mozart?

Whatever your habits, it's time to add a couple of new ones. As one of your first and last actions of the day, you should be tracking your sleep.

Let's start at the end of the day. What time did you go to bed? Of course, this doesn't tell you what time you actually went to sleep. (Some people end the night with a book, for instance, and, there are other things that can happen between the time the lights go out and the time that you're drifting to sleep.) But recording your bedtime, with fidelity, allows you to better understand the process by which you sleep.

Then, when you wake the next morning, you should be recording how much REM sleep you got. The early apps that purported to record REM were often unreliable. Today, however, both devices and programs are getting much better and are absolutely worth using, as REM is a good indicator of quality of sleep, and quality of sleep is strongly correlated with atrial fibrillation. In general, REM sleep should make up about 50 percent of the sleep you get each night.

It's not enough to just look at those numbers. You need to make sure you keep a log that you're able to reference from time to time. Without that, it will be hard to know whether things are improving, and even harder to find the nuances that can help people not just reduce but truly eliminate AFib episodes.

Once you've recorded those big numbers, which are fairly objective measures, it can be very helpful to jot down a few notes about your sleep. Did you wake naturally or to an alarm? The long-term goal should be to wake naturally, so if this is not happening on a regular basis, it is a strong indication that you need to adjust your bedtime or other conditions that impact your sleep. Also, did you awake several times during the night? Did you have to get up to use the bathroom? Were these trips to the bathroom affected by evening fluid consumption? Does exercising later in the day help reduce bathroom trips and improve sleep quality? Did tackling emails or work assignments after dinner make it hard to fall asleep? Do television programs after dinner impact bedtimes or the ease with which you fall asleep? Did you have nightmares, and do these nightmares correlate with when you started a particular medication or personal stressor? These are subjective metrics, of course, but since *you* are the subject, the quality of the data is largely up to you. And that's especially true when it comes to something that people lie to themselves about all the time—exercise.

## TRACKING EXERCISE

There are endless ways to track exercise, but the best first step might be to just take a step, and then another, and then another, and make sure your smartwatch or phone is counting as you go.

Tracking your steps is a research-proven way to get healthier in all sorts of ways. It's also one of the areas that is hardest to fudge, and that's important because research has shown that, time and time again, people tend to lie to themselves about the amount of exercise they get—egregiously overestimating both the amount of time they spend exercising and the vigor of that exercise.

And vigor is important, which is why it's usually not enough to just take a lot of steps every day, even if you walked all day long.[4] At some point, you might also hit a point of diminishing returns.[5] That's why it's also important to track the number of calories you burn throughout the day from the smartwatch or smartphone. As you might suspect, a device's estimate of burned calories is not actual burned calories. Everyone is different. But whatever number your device comes up with will be derived the same way today as yesterday, and the same way tomorrow as today. Don't worry so much about the number itself as what is says about how you've been doing over time. Nonetheless, it's not a bad idea to make sure your personal information— height, weight, age, and gender, among other factors—are up to date on the device to improve the accuracy of the collection algorithm. Likewise, indicating to your watch or phone whether you are walking, cycling, or running, for example, can also dramatically improve the exercise-tracking accuracy.

## TRACKING STRESS

Stress is one of the most common reported triggers for AFib. It's also a tremendously subjective metric. What is mentally or emotionally stressful to one person isn't stressful to everyone. And what is stressful to you today isn't the same as what might be stressful to you tomorrow. What's more, it isn't just mental and emotional stress that we need to worry about. Physical stress can trigger AFib episodes, too.

But you can get a very accurate measure of how much of all types of stress are being felt in your heart by tracking your heart rate variability, or HRV. Indeed, studies show that the higher your HRV number, the lower your risk of AFib.[6]

Even when in perfect sinus rhythm, there will always be some beat-to-beat variability—so slight that only an app can detect it. This variability is important, though, because it is there as a result of the constant tug-of-war between the two opposing ends of the autonomic nervous system. On one side is the sympathetic response, which is the "fight-or-flight" response, there to "rev up" your heart when you need it. On the other side is the parasympathetic response, which is the "rest-and-digest" response, present to slow things down. Both responses are important, depending on what you are doing during the day, and you want both in proper balance to minimize your risk of AFib.

It's quite easy, these days, to take a significantly accurate assessment of HRV with a smartwatch, although it's important to remember that studies indicate it should be a manual measurement at rest to optimize the accuracy of the test.[7] The automatic HRV recordings that may be running in the background while you are moving around throughout the day are simply not reliable.[8]

What HRV number should you shoot for? Of the various ways to measure HRV, probably the best studied is the standard deviation of beat-to-beat changes, which are known as N to N intervals, and thus this is called the SDNN. When your SDNN is above 50 milliseconds, your chances of getting an arrhythmia, having a heart attack, or prematurely dying go way down. Ideally, though, you'd like to shoot for something over 100 milliseconds. One study showed that maintaining an HRV above 100 milliseconds decreased the risk of a premature death by more than fivefold.[9]

One single score won't tell you much. By tracking this number over time, however, you'll be able to see how stress waxes and wanes from day to day. If your HRV is constantly running low, your heart is probably being crushed from too much physical, mental, or emotional stress. For example, if you're stressed out at work, not sleeping well, not exercising like you should, and your food choices aren't the best, then your HRV will probably be low. And when your HRV is low, you are more prone to AFib episodes, heart attacks, illnesses, and injuries. Indeed, consistently low HRV readings have been shown to predict future AFib episodes even twenty years into the future.[10]

When your HRV is running high, however, it tells you that your heart is responding well to the physical and emotional stress in your life. Your life is in balance and your heart is happy.

It's important to know that arrhythmias will falsely elevate your HRV number. A reliable HRV measurement cannot be ascertained during premature atrial contractions, premature ventricular contractions, atrial fibrillation, or atrial flutter. This test needs to be done when your heart is in normal sinus rhythm without too many premature beats.

Also, any medications that slow your heart or affect the response of the heart to adrenaline—drugs like antiarrhythmics, beta-blockers, calcium blockers, or digoxin—will change your HRV measurement. So, if you're on any of these drugs, a goal of 100 milliseconds isn't viable. Rather, your goal is to increase your HRV number from wherever your baseline is right now. Over time, you will come to learn what HRV number puts you at risk for an AFib attack.

As we discussed in chapter five, there are many ways to reduce stress in your life. Some of the ways that offer a great "bang for your buck" when it comes to HRV are mindfulness, meditation, relaxation techniques,[11] sleep optimization,[12] and the reduction or elimination of alcohol.[13] Moderate levels of daily physical exercise are also good for raising HRV,[14] while extreme, excessive levels of exercise may decrease this number.[15] The elimination of toxic relationships,[16] work environments,[17] and communities[18] from your life can offer a huge boost to your HRV, too. And there's one more source of stress that, as you've no doubt noticed, is part of a recurrent theme in this book: your diet. Diet optimization[19] and weight loss[20] are also research-proven ways to lower all-cause stress in your life.

## TRACKING FOOD

So far, we've discussed things that you track with very little effort—just by wearing a smartwatch. Now, let's discuss some things that take a little more effort, but which will pay big dividends if you get in the habit of tracking, starting with food.

In the next chapter, we're going to talk about a way of eating that is research-backed and designed specifically for people at risk of AFib, who have AFib, or who have pushed back their AFib and want to keep it in remission.

But, as we've previously noted, just about any diet that helps you drop weight and keep it off—without causing other damage to your body—can be part of a successful strategy for those battling atrial fibrillation.

No matter how you eat, though, if you're not tracking *what* you eat, you're missing out on a major opportunity to build a heart rhythm portfolio that can truly help you understand and control your condition. That's because different foods impact people in different ways. What a few "cheat meals" do psychologically or physically to one person won't be the same as what those meals do to another person. That doesn't make unhealthy foods a great choice for anyone, but most people have finite willpower, and there is significant currency in knowing the foods that are most likely to impact your weight, AFib episodes, and other biomarkers. And you don't have a hope of learning that stuff without tracking.

Now, let's be clear: food tracking is not calorie counting.

For some people, counting calories brings awareness and accountability. And that's fine. But calories, first conceptualized in the mid-1800s and originally based on the energy needed to raise the temperature of 1 gram of water by 1 degree Celsius, are an exceptionally imperfect measure of nutrition. In fact, if *all* you're doing is counting calories, you're likely eating in a way that is counterproductive to your goals, and which might even be dangerous.

Not all calories are alike, after all. It's easy to see this when we look at 100 calories of any food. For example, 100 calories of a processed breakfast cereal is almost guaranteed to spike your blood glucose and insulin levels in such a way that you won't feel full for long while the cereal metabolically wreaks havoc on your body. In contrast, 100 calories of almonds will set your body to work processing an order of nutrients that takes hours to digest, keeps you metabolically healthy, and results in a feeling of fullness that well exceeds that of processed foods,[21] helping to prevent over-snacking. Even when eating natural, non-processed foods, though, a calorie is not a calorie is not a calorie. Almonds aren't carrots. Carrots aren't fish. Fish isn't broccoli. You get the point.

Complicating matters even further, we've known for a very long time that humans tend to significantly underestimate their food calories and overestimate their burned calories,[22] rendering this method of balancing metabolism virtually useless.

Here's the caveat: if, by counting calories, you have managed to buck the odds by dropping weight and maintaining a very healthy BMI, there's no reason to stop now. Don't mess with success. What's more, you already have a little bit of experience with tracking food. That's a good start. But don't stop there.

What should you track, then? Nutrients. Not so many years ago, this would have been a very tall order, if not an impossible one, for most people. Scientists generally agree that humans require two specific fatty acids, nine amino acids, thirteen vitamins, and fifteen minerals from food to survive.[23] Plus there are numerous other molecules with health benefits—not to mention all the chemicals that are unhealthy. It would take a supercomputer to crunch the numbers created by all of those chemical combinations.

Today, though, what would have been considered a supercomputer just a few decades back can fit neatly into your pocket or purse. And apps that are specifically designed to help you track and balance your food choices are inexpensive, plentiful, and increasingly user-friendly. Just open the app, type in the food you're about to eat, and let the computer take it from there.

That's the input side of things. What should you be looking for in the data? It might surprise you to learn that, if you had to pick just one food nutrient to monitor, it should be fiber. That's because fiber intake from real food sources is a tremendously strong predictor of the quality of your diet and your risk for cardiovascular disease. Studies show that for every gram of fiber you eat daily above the recommended amount, which is approximately 30 grams daily, you can decrease your risk of cardiovascular disease by 1 percent.[24]

But, of course, if you're going to enter your daily food choices into an app, you might as well review more nutrients than just your daily fiber intake, and it likely won't surprise you at all to learn that sugar is the other most important thing to track. Of course, the goal here should be as close to zero as humanly possible, but keeping your added sugars at zero is no small feat, since food manufacturers have put sugar in everything. But there is absolutely no health benefit that comes from added sugars, so knowing what you're putting in your body from day to day is an essential metric for understanding how much unnecessary risk you're allowing to persist in your diet.

Beyond fiber and sugar, how many nutrients should your app track? A measure of your major macronutrient intake—including carbohydrates, fats, and protein—would be a good start. Vitamins and minerals are the next level, and can offer tremendous depth to the data. With the aid of a nutrient-tracking app, most people can meaningfully keep a watch on vitamins A, $B_{12}$, C, and D, along with calcium, folate, iron, and zinc. And, as so many AFib patients don't get enough magnesium and potassium in their diets, these can be great nutrients to track as well. As you optimize these nutrients over time, you may decide to start tracking more. That can build a lot of added "noise" into the data picture you're creating of your life. Nonetheless, many people find the challenge of associating nutrients and nutrient combinations to specific health outcomes to be a stimulating and worthwhile challenge.

The goal, of course, is to track your nutrition in a way that helps inform what you are eating, specifically in relation to how it impacts any AFib episodes.

But while food is often called "the best medicine," it's not the only medicine.

## TRACKING MEDICATIONS

While it's true that some people who effectively optimize their lifestyles before long-term damage sets in won't ever have to start any AFib medications, most people diagnosed with atrial fibrillation will be encouraged by their doctors to take at least some drugs for a time. And in many cases, that's the exact right advice—when your life is at stake, sometimes drugs can be necessary.

But as you work toward the fourth goal of the BLAST strategy, stopping unnecessary drugs, tracking your meds isn't just going to be helpful—it's going to be vital, especially as you're moving toward the minimal effective dose.

Fortunately, medication tracking is usually easier than food tracking. That's because while there are endless types of food, patients are typically only taking a few types of AFib medications at a time, and those drugs are prescribed in very specific dosages. So, as long as you take your meds the same way every day, the effect of changes should be easy to see, right?

There is one big problem with this. Most people don't take drugs the way they are prescribed. They forget on one day and may "double up" the next. They let their prescription lapse or, in all too many cases, lack the money to pay for a refill when it's needed. And even those who do take their medications reliably every day sometimes don't do it at the same time every day. Just a few hours can make a big difference in how your body responds to your medications.

What's the cure for all of this chaos? Once again, a smartwatch may be your very best friend. Drug-tracking apps with "push reminders" can be very effective at helping you take the right amount of medication every day, at the same time every day, thus giving you the best possible chance of seeing the real impact of those meds in your daily, weekly, and monthly data.

And just as you shouldn't only track one type of food, you shouldn't only track your AFib medications. There are, after all, dozens of classes of drugs—and hundreds of individual medications, including many common ones—that have been shown to affect heart rhythm,[25] even if that is not their intended purpose. Whether it's a once-in-a-while aspirin for a headache or a daily prescription of an anti-asthmatic, keeping track of the chemicals that you put into your body is of the utmost importance.

And remember, those chemicals don't just come in the form of prescribed and over-the-counter medications. For many people, they also come in the form of over-the-counter supplements, including any vitamins, minerals, herbal products, amino acids, and enzymes that aren't included in our food or regular diet. These products can also have an effect on heart rhythm, and may even induce an episode of AFib.[26] The bottom line is that anything you take, prescription medication or supplement, has side effects—and if you haven't noticed any side effects, then you simply may not have discovered them yet. Tracking can help you learn what these drugs and supplements are really doing to your body.

## TRACKING WEIGHT

Let's move now to a discussion of biomarkers, starting with the biggest one of them all: your weight.

Knowing that keeping your weight at a healthy level is probably the best thing you can do for your AFib, it should come as no surprise that you should also be tracking your weight every day.

Yes, every day, for this number will be one of the best indicators you'll have of the net effect of all the other things you're doing to fight your AFib.

A lot of people are afraid to do this. But whatever the scale says is what it says. There is no use beating yourself up over it or lamenting how far you have to go. What will do you some good—and likely a lot of good—is tracking or keeping a record of that number over time.

Many of our patients use Bluetooth- or Wi-Fi-enabled smart scales that record this for you. That's fine, but for many of the reasons we discussed in chapter five, it is important for you to be generally aware of what this number is and the direction it's headed.

Why not just track your weight "as needed" or on a weekly or monthly basis? There are two reasons.

First, the act of stepping on a scale and taking a daily account of your weight can offer a powerful boost of self-control, because it gives you a regular opportunity for reflection, self-correction, and personal accountability. Will the mere knowledge that you are going to be stepping on a scale in less than 24 hours magically keep you from grabbing a donut from the break room at work, or steering your car into a drive-through for a burger and fries when you know you should head to the market for some carrots and nuts? Absolutely not. But it can help. And since we make decisions like these all day long, we should do every little thing we can do to help give ourselves the immediate feedback and willpower to make better health decisions. Everything we can do to increase our odds, we should be doing.

Second, daily tracking is the single best thing you can do to optimize your weight. Studies show that just the act of stepping on a scale every day triples your weight loss[27] and is one of the best predictors of maintaining that weight loss.[28]

Of course, not everyone with atrial fibrillation is overweight. You'll recall, for instance, that AFib is surprisingly common among endurance athletes, many of whom maintain very healthy body weights. Also, many of those with familial AFib may also be very lean but yet still suffer from periodic bouts of AFib. Even if you are at your target weight, though, this is a daily habit that can do you a lot of good, as a sudden drop or increase in weight can be an early warning sign of other troubles that could trigger AFib.

## TRACKING BLOOD PRESSURE

In most of our studies of atrial fibrillation, 70 to 80 percent of the patients had high blood pressure as one of their AFib risk factors. This is not surprising, as high blood pressure (or hypertension) significantly increases your risk of atrial fibrillation.[29] Thus it makes plenty of sense that this is a number you should add to your heart rhythm portfolio.

There are two main reasons for this. The first is obvious: you want to make sure your blood pressure doesn't get so high that it taxes your heart, leading to more fibrosis, heart failure, and future AFib electrical circuits. The second is that, as you optimize your lifestyle, it's quite likely that (unless you have already had high blood pressure for decades) your high blood pressure will go away—making this a great indicator of improving health. It's also an important piece of information for people taking blood pressure medications. Indeed, we've seen many patients over the years who actually pass out because they are still taking their blood pressure meds even though they've lowered their blood pressure naturally from a healthy lifestyle.

There are quite a few relatively inexpensive at-home monitoring kits. If you get one, it's best to check your blood pressure when you are relaxed—and to do it the same way every time. After five minutes of relaxation and with the cuff around your arm at, or near, the level of your heart, take the measurement and, if you have irregular readings, repeat the measurement after waiting three minutes.

Many of our patients like to use a blood pressure machine that can also detect an irregular pulse. As long as you are consistent in checking, twice daily, this is an effective way of tracking both your AFib and your blood pressure. However you choose to do it, tracking this number as part of your portfolio can help you make decisions over time that will protect your health.

For instance, if you see your blood pressure starting to creep up over time—but it's still below 130/80—this is a good sign that you may need to drop a few pounds, work harder on your diet, bump up your daily exercise, get a little more high-quality sleep at night, or concentrate on keeping the bad stress out of your life. If, however, you're consistently running above 130/80, it's time to let your doctor know, as you may need medications until you can bring it down naturally.

## TRACKING BLOOD BIOMARKERS

Let's say you were training for a track-and-field decathlon: ten intense Olympic-level feats in one event. If you wanted to know if you were training right, you'd want to measure your times and distances in each of those events, right?

And let's suppose you did that on the first day of each month. On that day, a coach would stand next to the track with a stopwatch, or next to the high-jump bar with a tape measure, and shout out your scores at the completion of each event.

At the end of the day, would you remember each of those scores? Would you remember them the next month? And the month after that? Would you immediately know which ones went up and which ones went down? And what if you trained for years? Could you remember all of the numbers, over time, and details about the sorts of training exercises you were doing whenever the numbers would rise or fall? Maybe you would. If so, your memory is absolutely commendable—astounding, in fact.

But most of us wouldn't be able to keep all of those numbers straight, not over the course of many months and certainly not over the span of several years.

Biomarker tracking isn't about knowing what your scores are today. It's about understanding where those numbers were when you began this journey, in relationship to where the numbers are now. It's also about coming to understand the factors that impact the numbers as they wax and wane over time—hopefully in directions that point to ever-improving health and less AFib.

All of this is to say that tracking actually means *tracking*. From the moment you get your first test, and for every test you take moving forward, you should keep a record of your numbers. Over time, this record, as part of your heart rhythm portfolio, will help you understand your numbers in context. It will help you build connections between, for instance, the amount of sleep you are getting and your levels of A1C,[30] or the ways in which exercise impacts your CRP count.[31]

It is true that some people can wage a good fight against atrial fibrillation without tracking their biomarkers. They can commit to eating an AFib diet, living a physically fit life, avoiding stress, and all of the other principles we have been discussing in this book. If they do these things, their biomarkers are almost sure to move in the right direction.

But back to our decathlon analogy: If you're not measuring your pole vault, would you inherently know the difference between 13 feet, 8 inches, and 13 feet, 7 inches? If you're not timing your sprint, will you be able to tell if you're doing 100 meters in 15.5 seconds or 15.4 seconds?

Now, if you're not a serious decathlete—if nothing whatsoever is on the line—then perhaps it doesn't matter. But if you're reading this book, there is almost certainly something on the line, because we're not talking about standing on a podium, about bragging rights, or even about personal pride.

We're talking about your life.

When the stakes are that high, small changes can really matter. If, for instance, your fasting blood glucose has always been in the low nineties for as long as you've been keeping track, but it suddenly jumps to the high nineties, you might not think much of it at first. Your doctor might not, either. After all, anything less than 100 mg/dL is considered normal and argues against diabetes. Indeed, it might not be anything more than a blip.

It might also be a clue that you need to spend some time thinking about what might have caused the jump. Are you eating more added sugars or processed carbohydrates? Have you put on a few extra pounds? Have you had an infection? Changed your medications? Take note of these possibilities while they are still fresh in your memory. There's no reason to panic, but there is good reason to pay a little closer attention.

To that end, if you or your doctor are infrequently checking for diabetes, which you know is highly correlated with AFib, and there has been a change—even one that didn't push you out of "normal"—that could be a good reason to take another look, a little sooner.

You don't need to overdo it. Just because you are getting close to the diabetes threshold doesn't mean you need an implantable glucose sensor. Also, don't test yourself into bankruptcy for any biomarker—work within your insurance benefits, your financial means, your personal preferences, and your doctor's recommendations.

It will take some time to identify some of the nuances at play in the interconnectedness between your life and your biomarkers. In the early months, and even through the first few years of doing this, it will be important to remember a common—but all too often ignored—warning about one of the most common health fallacies: correlation does not imply causation. Trying to link rising and falling numbers to a singular event in your life is a good path to madness.

But slowly, over time, you're going to notice that your biomarkers are indeed quite attuned to your lifestyle. You'll identify ways to move them—in some cases, there may be ways that work for you and perhaps no one else.

Would you like to be able to see these connections sooner rather than later? You're probably going to need a little help from a computer.

Mind you, we're not talking about heavy-on-the-math computer science. With nothing more than a simple app, you can start finding correlations that can help you optimize your life and keep your AFib at bay.

## GRAPHING SUCCESS

The best time to start tracking is right away. Building any habit can be hard work. And monitoring and recording your weight, sleep, exercise, stress, food, medications, and biomarkers is no small habit.

Do you have to track everything? Of course not. We would suggest focusing your efforts on where you need it the most. For example, if you've already optimized your weight, sleep, exercise, and food, but stress is the one thing you are still struggling with, then perhaps you might only track

HRV on a daily basis and do less frequent (but still periodic) checks on the others. But even if it's just one or two things right now, the sooner tracking becomes part of your life, the better.

On the other hand, "right away" isn't the right time to start trying to understand what your tracking data tells you—especially if you're making a lot of big changes to your life all at once, as most people do when they commit to stopping their AFib. This is a time in which your data will be very noisy.

Consider what Ajeet did when the smartwatch he received from a family member alerted him to the possibility that his heart rhythm might be atrial fibrillation.

"I sort of went into fix-it-all mode," Ajeet laughed. "I read everything I could, and so even before I could get in to see the doctor, I had joined a gym, worked on my diet, started doing some yoga and started monitoring my sleep. And, since I'm sort of obsessive, I decided to keep a spreadsheet of all of those things."

By the time he got in to see the doctor, just a few weeks later, his smartwatch was showing normal sinus rhythm, and that's what an EKG in the doctor's office showed, too. Perhaps the original indicators were wrong. Or perhaps he was simply paroxysmal and between events. Or perhaps the lifestyle changes he made had an immediate effect—but, if so, which ones? There was no way to know at that point.

If Ajeet had simply shrugged his shoulders and gone on with his life, he would be no better off when the AFib returned—as it eventually did. But because he had been keeping track, he was quickly able to identify a potential trigger.

"I was actually pretty proud of myself, because I really did do a good job of eating healthy and exercising every day," he said. "I was doing yoga every day, too. All of that stuff became my new normal."

But just as a big project came due at work a few months later, Ajeet's watch once again alerted him to an irregular heart rhythm. Fortunately, the AFib didn't last long before it stopped on its own. "At first I thought, 'Aha!

It's stress!' but honestly I wasn't feeling that stressed. I really loved the work I was doing. It was hard but it was really joyful."

But when Ajeet dove into his data, a different potential cause made itself known. His sleep-tracking app showed that he was getting quite a bit less REM sleep than normal. "Once I saw that, it really helped me build a better picture of what had been happening," he said. "I had been staying up a little later, working on my computer in bed, staring at that bright screen before I went to sleep, and even though I didn't at first perceive a big difference in the quality of my sleep, that seems to have been having an effect."

And of course, that late-night working also came with some late-night snacks and a bit of weight gain. His smartwatch shared the same story—his movement calories were down and his exercise time was down, while his sedentary time sitting at his desk was up. The drop in his heart rate variability confirmed all of the above. His heart was seeing higher loads of physical and emotional stress from lower-quality sleep, suboptimal eating, less physical activity, and an uptick in work-related stress. Basically, the brief AFib attack was his heart sounding the alarm that something needed to change.

After employing a few "countermeasures," including a new no-screens-in-the-bedroom policy, his sleep became normal again. As he was now sleeping again at night, the late-night snacks naturally stopped and the morning workouts resumed. While work didn't change much, his energy levels increased and his productivity during the day was up as well. The slight evening routine tweak was just enough to set into motion a cascade of changes that brought his HRV back up again. He now had the physical resilience he needed to continue with his rewarding, but also demanding, career.

Now, Ajeet has once again fallen into a routine—one that appears to be much healthier. That's good. After an initial period of "thrashing," trying everything he could to improve his health, his daily habits have once again become steady. That will make it easier in the future to see correlations between inputs (such as sleep, food, medications, stress, and exercise) and outputs (such as weight, biomarker scores, and time out of rhythm).

Do you want to make these potential correlations easier to see? It's time to get to know Karl Pearson—an English biostatistician and the namesake of the Pearson correlation, an easy way to indicate the potential extent to which two variables are related.

Now, at first, the "Pearson r" formula can look very intimidating . . .

$$r = \frac{n(\Sigma xy) - (\Sigma x)(\Sigma y)}{\sqrt{[n\Sigma x^2 - (\Sigma x)^2][n\Sigma y^2 - (\Sigma y)^2]}}$$

. . . but don't let that worry you, because you don't need to understand the equation itself. You only need to have reliably collected some data—generally one set of inputs and one set of outputs that were gathered over the same period.

When you plug those numbers into a Pearson correlation coefficient calculator (many versions of which are freely available online), the result is a scatterplot graph and an "r value."

A scatterplot that falls close to a straight, descending line will have a correlation close to –1, while a plot that falls close to a straight, ascending line will have a correlation close to 1. In either case, you have come upon a linear relationship—an indicator of a potential association between the two factors.

This is not causation. No matter what two variables you begin with, there are always a lot of other factors at play that might impact the relationship, one way or another. But what a linear relationship offers is the ability to focus your efforts on the parts of your life that have a better chance of impacting your AFib.

Let's say, for instance, that with a few months of daily data you find a strong correlation between your heart rate variability and the amount of time your heart is out of rhythm. In the same period, your exercise and sleep times have been constant and you see no relationship between the number of minutes you spend exercising or sleeping and your out-of-rhythm time. That absolutely doesn't make exercise and sleep unimportant, but in a world of limited time, resources, and energy, you might choose to spend the next month focusing on other ways to raise your HRV, such as lowering your actual and perceived stress (like with an evening walk with your spouse, a yoga class at the gym, or meditation) rather than adding extra minutes to your exercise or sleep routines. If you bring your stress down, and your out-of-rhythm time follows in kind, there's a good chance that you have indeed found one area of causation, and you can commit to making that area a priority in your life.

Even if you find a strong correlation indicative of a slide toward worsening health, it might not be enough to fix one part of it. By way of example, perhaps you've noticed that over recent years your blood pressure has been creeping steadily upward, while one of the exercise metrics you've been keeping, your average time in a daily mile run, is steadily going down. Now, maybe it's true that the cardiovascular benefit you were getting from running was helping keep your blood pressure down, but the problem here is that, at some point, we all slow down. The answer simply cannot be to train and train and train until you get you mile time down again. In this case, you'll want to look for multiple other ways to lower blood pressure that you *can* control, focus on optimizing those parts of your life, and watch closely to see if your efforts have an effect.

A scatterplot that looks like scattershot—little dots all over the place—will have a correlation of 0, meaning there is no linear relationship. This doesn't mean there is no relationship; if the scatterplot is curved, like a "U" or a "J," you may have found a nonlinear relationship. For instance, in plotting your daily minutes of exercise against your time out of rhythm, you might discover that up to 60 minutes of vigorous exercise a day is associated with less AFib, while more exercise than that is associated with more AFib. This, of course, can help you home in on an optimal time period to dedicate to exercise.

Remember that the impact of inputs from one day, week, or month might not have an effect on the outputs we measure on that same day, week, or month. The vitamin D you consume one month, for instance, might not have an apparent impact on biomarker scores in that same month, but might "show up" as potentially associated in the following month. Your intuition about these relationships will be a big helper in the search for correlations.

Of course, the search for X-Y relationships is endless, one that could drive you wild if you spend too much time searching for relationships that may not even exist. We have seen patients who have seemingly optimized everything in their lives but for whom AFib episodes still occur, quite randomly, with no apparent relationship to anything else. That's the way it goes, sometimes. But even if this is the case for you, our experience has also been that the more you can optimize your life, the fewer of these seemingly random AFib episodes you will probably have.

In other words, you definitely shouldn't wait to find a potential association before taking action. Even if the data isn't offering you any clues, keep moving toward a life of more exercise, less stress, better sleep, fewer medications, and lower body weight.

## TRACKING MUST BE EASY AND FUN

What separates patients who can maintain healthy lifestyles and beat AFib and those who can't? After long careers spent helping AFib patients live healthier lives that put and keep AFib in remission, we've learned that one of the most important differentiating factors is that successful patients are often those who find ways to make tracking easy and fun.

Why does it need to be easy? Because if this takes up time that you simply don't have, you're likely to quit. Let's face it: we're all busy. But if tracking becomes part of your routine, costing you nothing more than an extra minute here and an extra minute there, you're far more likely to keep it up. And this is where technology can really help.

With the right apps, tracking workouts can take either no time at all (because your smartwatch recognizes that you're engaged in vigorous activity) or just a few seconds (to tell the app what you did, how long you did it, and what intensity you did it at). With a few clicks, you can see your results in a graph that spans weeks, months, or many years.

When it comes to food and nutrition intake, once your app learns what foods you typically eat, entering each new meal or snack takes just a few seconds. And just like exercise apps, you can then review this data over whatever period you wish to see. Even better, these apps can alert you to an irregularity in nutrient intake if, at some point and without realizing it, you simply happen to fall deficient in your consumption of foods providing that nutrient.

Sleep apps can also be set to record your slumber, including total sleep time and REM, without requiring anything on your part. All you need to do is periodically review the data and add it to your portfolio.

Tracking stress can be completely stress-free, too. Even though the automatic background heart rate variability isn't as accurate as the manual checks, if you're looking at average HRV trends over weeks, months, and years, the occasional inaccurate measurement will be averaged out. If there is an acute stressor going on in your life, or you're getting low HRV numbers on the automatic checks, then you may want to do a manual HRV check to make sure it isn't damaging your heart, but this can be completed in just minutes.

Checking and tracking blood pressure rarely takes more than five minutes. But unless you're using a blood pressure machine that can also detect an irregular pulse, to track both AFib and blood pressure at the same time, you probably don't need to do it multiple times a day and, like most things, it can be checked with less frequency once your life has been optimized and your measurements are stable over time.

When it comes to the critical blood biomarkers, the periodicity with which you should test is going to be determined, in no small part, by your insurance and your financial means. But if you can get as many of these tests done at once as possible, you'll be saving yourself a lot of time in the long run. If your tests are completed within a hospital system, chances are good that your results will be maintained in a system that you can access with a password, and these systems increasingly offer the ability to graph and track your results with the click of a mouse.

Add it all up, and what does it take? Minutes a day. That's all. And the increased productivity that comes with better health and more energy will more than offset that investment of time.

But even when it's easy, we've found that patients are less likely to continue tracking if it isn't fun. This, too, is where apps can offer a big assist—by gamifying the process. Whether it's gold stars, a point system, or a friendly competition with others, games can make the process of tracking our health, and reaching our goals, more enjoyable.[32]

But, again, "enjoyable" is truly the key. Over the years, we've had more than a few patients who had to return their AFib-tracking smartwatches because they found themselves watching the watch all day long to see if their hearts were going into AFib or not. That's not adding fun, it's adding stress—and it could actually be counterproductive.

If you find that tracking makes you feel stressed or anxious, try starting with just a few things. Once you get the hang of tracking, you can add more over time. As you track more things that correlate with health, the reward of tracking will be magnified and it will become easier and more fun.

## YOUR HEART RHYTHM PORTFOLIO

Just as everyone comes to AFib in a different way, and everyone's fight against AFib will take a different shape, so too will everyone's heart rhythm portfolio look different.

For some people, a steady stream of automated data downloads will flow into a series of spreadsheets that have been built to track known and suspected correlations.

For others, the best choice will be an old-fashion daily journal that regularly includes their daily EKG results, along with weight, food, and exercise. Periodically, they'll update other metrics.

No matter what form your portfolio takes, however, it should have two essential qualities.

First, it should be something you can maintain with fidelity from day to day, month to month, and year to year. A very thorough portfolio does you no good at all if you keep it for a while but then regularly forget to keep it updated.

Second, it should be something that you can share with your doctor during a routine checkup. If it takes you twenty minutes just to explain how you're keeping your data, what variables you're tracking, and the intricate algorithms you've written to watch for this or that, you're not doing yourself or your doctor any good.

Aside from those two rules, though, the sky is the limit.

We've seen that some patients find spreadsheets pretty easy to fill out daily and with just a bit of computer knowledge (or help from a friend or relative who happens to be a whiz at such things). Automating a lot of inputs can be fairly easy, too.

Others enjoy keeping one or more apps on their phone: some that automatically update and others that take some input, but that can be accessed at any time of the day (as long as users remember to charge their batteries).

Still others love spreadsheets but prefer actual paper. For these patients, these old-school accounting methods are akin to doing a daily crossword puzzle.

Some patients really love journals, and keep their portfolios in the form of journals or notebooks.

So, what should your portfolio look like? It should look like a reflection of who you are, and tell a story about your lifelong dedication to controlling or even eliminating your AFib.

## NINE THINGS THAT EVERYONE SHOULD TRACK IN THEIR AFIB PORTFOLIO

| Things to Track | Goal |
| --- | --- |
| 1. EKG with smartphone/watch | Normal sinus rhythm 100 percent of the time |
| 2. Sleep | Seven to nine hours of high-quality sleep every night |
| 3. Exercise | Ten thousand steps and daily exercise to break a sweat |
| 4. Stress | HRV/SDNN of 50 ms or higher |

| 5. Weight | Maintain target weight or lose 0.5–1 pound per month if over target weight |
| 6. Food | Hit 100 percent of all vitamins/nutrients, work toward 100 g of fiber and 0 added sugars daily |
| 7. Meds | Safely minimize as many meds as possible |
| 8. Blood pressure | Below 130/80 at all times, ideally 110/70 without the need for blood pressure meds |
| 9. Biomarkers from chapter four | Optimize all ten AFib biomarkers—easy to track as it has likely already been done for you through your hospital's patient portal |

Chapter Nine

## ⎯⎯⎯⎯⎯ ⟋⎺⎺⟍ THE AFIB DIET ⟋⎺⎺⟍ ⎯⎯⎯⎯⎯

Why the best diet for your heart is one in which you
don't count calories and never feel hungry again

Anan had done just about everything right. For more than a year, he
had never missed a workout—a streak broken only by a bout of the
flu. He'd changed his travel schedule to reduce stress, spent more
time with his family, and found ways to improve his sleep. He'd undergone
an ablation. He had been monitoring his biomarkers, tracking his heart
rhythm with a smartwatch, and logging inputs and outputs with the attentiveness of a sports statistician. All of that had allowed him to get off all of
his AFib medications.

Most of all, perhaps, he'd committed to a diet that had helped him
bring down his weight by twenty pounds. But the problem was that Anan
was still overweight. And that, as you know, is a big risk factor for a return
of AFib.

To keep his AFib from coming back, we suggested, Anan probably needed to drop another twenty pounds, and perhaps even more.

"I just don't think I can," he said. "I'm committed to this new lifestyle but I'm always right on the edge of hungry and sometimes I'm really, really hungry. I don't think I can cut back even more."

Okay, let's freeze right there. Why in the world was Anan talking about cutting back? Why was he worried about being hungry? Those aren't experiences that people have to have in order to lose weight, and yet most people share these beliefs.

The messages most people have gotten about healthy dieting aren't helpful. In fact, they're dooming a lot of people to failure.

Whenever we discuss the AFib diet with patients, we are always asked, "Can I eat . . . ?" Now, if you have to ask if you can eat something, then there's a good chance you shouldn't, but, nonetheless, the answer is seldom a hard "no." There are no restricted foods on the AFib diet, because this way of eating isn't about limits. Rather, it's about lifestyle and choices. And, if you make the right choices, then you'll never be hungry.

The best part, though, is that this science-backed diet can play a big role in reversing AFib, sometimes without drugs and procedures. To make that happen, though, we can't just change the way we eat—we have to change the way we live. And, with this in mind, perhaps "diet" is a bit of a misnomer. Most people think diets are something people go on and off. Lifestyles, on the other hand, are something you hold onto for life. This is a lifestyle.

This lifestyle is specifically geared toward mitigating and counteracting the key causes of atrial fibrillation. As we'll describe in this chapter, it is based on how to eat (slow and steady, never to over-fullness, learning and avoiding triggers), what to eat (lots of veggies, fruits, and other plants, along with plenty of fiber), and what to avoid (all processed foods and anything that spikes your blood sugar).

Before we get to all of that, though, we should understand *why* it works. This is essential, because knowing why you're doing what you're doing helps align action to purpose.

So, to begin, let's talk about some of the different ways in which the causes of AFib can help point us in the direction of a food lifestyle that helps fix AFib.

## FOOD CLUES

There are two main places where fat is stored in the body: under your skin and around your internal organs. Of the two, that latter type—visceral fat—is by far the more dangerous, especially when it is found around the heart in the pericardial sac. And while an MRI or CT scan can give you a good idea of how much visceral fat you have, you don't actually need to go to those lengths. That's because studies show that waist circumference is strongly associated with visceral fat.[1]

The relationship is so close and tidy that it is nearly predictive. With this in mind, a way of eating designed to beat AFib should reduce your measured waist size. (This is not the same as pant size, as most clothing manufacturers have a reported "waist size" that is one to two inches below what it really should be to make you feel good about yourself and buy their product.) Everyone is different, but a good target is somewhere below thirty-five inches if you are a man, and thirty-two inches if you are a woman. These aren't perfect numbers, of course, but when researchers completed the cross-sectional study that led to the realization that your waist is a good stand-in for determining AFib risk, those were the measurements where a real difference was seen. An eating lifestyle that attacks AFib, then, should be one that includes foods that specifically combat visceral fat while optimizing nutrition.

Let's now talk a bit about reactive oxidants, or "free radicals." You can pick these up as by-products of your body's normal cellular metabolism as well as from pollution; this includes smoking and vaping, pesticides, heavy metals, processed foods, and fried foods. These chemicals have been shown to disrupt electrical pathways in the heart,[2] and electrical disruption, of course, is a core part of the definition of AFib.

With enough antioxidants in your diet, however, the overproduction of reactive oxidants can be stopped. One study of 800 people, for example, showed that those who got the most antioxidants from vitamins like C and E, and carotenoids from vegetables and fruit, were twice as likely to have their hearts go back to normal rhythm without drugs or procedures.[3] The same effect hasn't been seen in antioxidant supplements, though; there's something special about the way these foods deliver the goods. Therefore, any way of eating designed to put AFib into remission—and keep it there— should include many of these foods.

Those same foods, it turns out, are exceptionally protective against inflammation, which is a major cause of damaged heart cells and electrical pathways.[4] We've already discussed inflammation, so you know that one of the key reasons our bodies over-produce the substances usually employed to fight infection, illness, and injury is blood glucose spikes from sugar and flour[5] and from processed and fried foods.[6] So, getting plenty of foods that protect against inflammation, and avoiding those that cause it, will need to be a key element of the AFib diet.

Speaking of glucose spikes, for people who have AFib, who are at risk of AFib, or who have put it into remission and want to keep it there, the blood sugar roller-coaster ride that comes along with the way most people eat in the Western world is absolutely horrible for our heart health. You already know from earlier chapters that diabetes, with an accompanying high hemoglobin A1C, is a powerful risk factor for AFib. But long before you ever get to diabetes—which hopefully is never—meals that trigger blood sugar spikes may cause you to have blood sugar that runs ever so slightly on the higher end of normal, increasing your risk of an AFib attack.

In one study in rats, for instance, researchers found that blood sugar levels that went up and down throughout the day resulted in a lot more cardiac fibrosis and AFib[7]—two things you definitely want to avoid. Of course, you're not a rat, so it's important to note that human studies have pointed to the same conclusion. And while it would be hard, if not unethical, to manipulate human diets in the same way scientists can with model organisms like rats, human studies have shown that even if your blood sugar levels run slightly high-normal, but still well below diabetes or prediabetes levels, your AFib risk is nonetheless increased.[8] So with this in mind, the AFib diet also must be a low-glycemic diet.

Let's not forget the important role of ions for heart health. People who don't get enough potassium are four times more likely to suffer from atrial fibrillation.[9] Likewise, those who don't get enough magnesium are significantly more likely to develop AFib.[10] This makes plenty of sense, since low levels of ions like potassium and magnesium can hinder cells' ability to effectively send electrical signals. It also makes it easy to see why an AFib diet should be high in electrolytes from natural food sources. (Not sports drinks, as we discussed in chapter four.)

Perhaps the most historically overlooked driver of human health and sickness is the microbiome; indeed, the composition of our gut flora is important to the health of our hearts. Having the wrong balance of gut bacteria may lead to a spike in a cardiac toxic by-product called trimethylamine N-oxide, or TMAO, which, as mentioned in chapter three, has been shown to significantly increase your risk of atrial fibrillation.[11] The mechanisms through which TMAO damages the heart's electrical system aren't perfectly clear, but some studies have suggested that it could be harming the autonomic nervous system,[12] which controls heart rhythm, or directly by an inflammation process. However it happens, limiting foods that stimulate our gut bacteria to produce TMAO (animal-based proteins, processed foods, some energy drinks, and some supplements) should be another key goal of any anti-AFib diet.

Last, but not least, it has long been known that the more enlarged your atria are, the higher your risk of developing atrial fibrillation. And while some atrial enlargement may happen with age, foods like sugar, refined grains, and salt play a much bigger role through weight gain and hypertension.[13] A diet intended to defeat AFib should avoid these causes.

Okay, so now that we know what sorts of foods to emphasize and avoid, do we have everything we need to create a perfect AFib diet? Not quite. That's because the *way* we eat might be just as important as *what* we eat.

# WE ARE *HOW* WE EAT

It took a few years for Zoey to get to know her triggers. "I'd been pretty good at keeping track of what I eat," she said. "But I was ignoring a lot of other things. Once I realized what was triggering my AFib, it all seemed so clear, and I felt a bit foolish that I didn't recognize it earlier."

Like a lot of people with atrial fibrillation. Zoey had an overactive vagus nerve. As we've mentioned, the vagus nerve is a part of the parasympathetic nervous system, which controls heart rate, intestinal activity, and the muscles of the gastrointestinal tract. Studies show that overstimulation of the vagus nerve—like what happens when you eat too big of a meal—can trigger atrial fibrillation.[14] This may occur because an overfilled belly spikes acetylcholine levels, provoking heart cells in or near the pulmonary veins to fire, even when they're not supposed to.

"One day I had an episode, and it occurred to me that I'd just eaten a really big meal," Zoey said. "Then I started thinking about it, and I suddenly recognized that had happened before."

It's not just big meals that can trigger AFib. Small meals can do the same thing if those meals are eaten too fast. That's because fast eating results in more stomach stretching and a rapid blood glucose rise, both of which can cause an AFib attack.

Another culprit that might be a potent trigger: very cold foods. That's what a California research team learned when they reviewed the case of a young adult man who drank one of those sugary "slushed ice" drinks, the type you commonly find at gas station convenience stores. Just about everyone who has tried one of these drinks knows the sensation of "brain freeze," an intense, rapid-onset headache also known as sphenopalatine ganglioneuralgia. Brain freeze is caused by sudden temperature changes to the carotid artery and anterior cerebral artery, which are located near the back of the throat, and which feed blood to the brain. The man immediately began to suffer from both atrial fibrillation and brain freeze at the same time.[15] Researchers have theorized that the vagus nerve may be similarly stimulated.[16] This doesn't mean we need to avoid cold foods; we just need to be mindful of how we consume them. When it comes to smoothies, slow and steady wins the race.

We have also had many patients report to us over the years that sugar, fast food, foods with caffeine, processed foods, fried foods, or really spicy foods have also been atrial fibrillation triggers—not just contributors to the rising risk of getting AFib in the first place. Once again, all of these triggers probably have something to do with vagus nerve stimulation or glucose fluctuations.

If the way we eat can trigger AFib, can it also protect us against it? Yes. Slowing down the way we eat in general can speed up our pace toward losing weight. That's what researchers in Japan discovered when they studied the medical records of nearly 60,000 patients who had answered a health survey that included a question about how fast they eat. Self-reported slow eaters, it turned out, were significantly less likely to be overweight or clinically obese, irrespective of any other factor.[17] Since we know that extra pounds are a key driver of heart health, anyone trying to stop AFib should take a little extra time with each bite.

The same study included an interesting finding: regardless of how much someone ate overall, skipping dinner, once in a while, was associated with a lower chance of obesity. This is yet another piece of evidence in the rapidly growing evidence mountain showing the health benefits of intermittent fasting. The process of spending time away from food—skipping a meal or two consecutive meals a few times a week, for instance—is an exciting new area of research that a growing number of scientists believe may help control the process of biological aging.[18] If true, that wouldn't be a side benefit for those who are trying to reduce their risk of AFib because, as you'll recall, the risk of AFib increases with age or premature aging, as we showed in our telomere study of AFib patients.[19] But there's an important difference between age and aging; the first term can be marked in months and years, while the second term can only be seen in our biology.

Slowing down aging, then, is almost certainly going to have an impact on AFib. Even if it didn't, though, intermittent fasting seems to be helpful for optimizing blood glucose fluctuations and vagus nerve excitability. And while there aren't any published studies on this connection, our unpublished data of more than 300 patients showed a statistical trend toward a 20 to 40 percent reduction in atrial fibrillation among those who fasted at various times throughout the week, with periods of fasting as short as twelve hours. That's a time frame almost anyone can reach without much effort just by eating an early dinner and then getting a good night of sleep—or, as many people in the Japanese study did, skipping dinner and heading to bed. Others, particularly those who are trying to optimize their glucose metabolism and drop weight, likewise find it beneficial to skip dinner.[20]

However, as with any food advice, everyone's body functions a little differently. For example, a number of patients have reported to us over the years that skipping meals is tremendously stressful, or it causes them to overeat after the skipped meal. That's just trading one potential trigger for another. Still others need frequent small meals to help them lose weight or maintain a healthy weight. So while fasting is good for everyone to try, it might not be good for everyone to do.

There is one thing, however, that almost everyone can benefit from—and for most people, it's not only the easiest and most transformative change, but it's also the change that makes so many other changes possible.

## WE ARE WHAT WE DRINK

The Japanese have some of the lowest rates of atrial fibrillation on the planet.[21] Why? One clue might be the way they eat—a practice known as *hara hachi bu*, which stems from a Confucian teaching to only eat until you are 80 percent full.

This doesn't just curtail the consumption of extra calories. If you never fill your stomach beyond 80 percent, then you will never have to worry about excessive vagal stimulation from an overfilled belly, thus taking away a common AFib trigger.[22]

After a lifetime of eating to over-satiation, though, most people find it difficult to know when to stop. If you find yourself in that situation, the solution to your problem might be a few glasses of water away, especially if you drink them a bit before you eat.

Drinking water doesn't just fill space in your belly. It also helps satiate needs that many people mistake for hunger.[23] In fact, keeping well hydrated might be one of the best tricks for warding off the desire to eat. That's why simply drinking a glass of water about thirty minutes before each meal can be so powerful. It's enough time to let the water help you feel full while addressing the sensations often registered as hunger, but not so much time that the water will have passed out of your system.

It is important, though, that "water preloading" actually be done with water. Soda, energy drinks, coffee, tea, beer, wine, and fruit juices all have water in them, but water is the only liquid that can and should be drunk without limitation; you can drink water as much as you want. (This is all predicated on the words "within reason," of course. Going overboard by drinking more water than your body "asks" for can cause hyponatremia, a condition of dangerously diluted blood that is sometimes called water intoxication.[24])

A glass of water after dinner is a good way to help prevent snacking after your last meal—a real essential for losing weight, since your body doesn't use foods consumed before sleeping the same way as those you consume during the day, especially if you are staying in motion right up until you hit the sack. Having a small bottle of water on your bedside table can be a big help, too, if you're trying to overcome the common urge to jump out of bed for a snack.

Of course, too *much* water in the evening can interrupt your sleep cycle, which, as you know, is a big risk factor for AFib. If you're making extra trips to the restroom, and that's affecting the amount and quality of sleep you are getting, you'll want to drink less water right before bed. If you're keeping hydrated throughout the day, you won't need as much water at night to satiate your thirst and stave off your hunger.

There is one more time when water can be a huge help: if you're trying to extend an intermittent fast for a few hours. A lot of people find the easiest way to do this is to either skip breakfast or start your fast after an early dinner a day or two each week. This is a lot easier to do when you've got something in your stomach, and especially when you're not feeling dehydrated.

The bottom line on $H_2O$ probably won't surprise you: water is essential for life and should be consumed with that fact in mind. While a commonly cited estimate that three-quarters of Americans are "chronically dehydrated" might be overblown, most people could and should be drinking more water. The health benefits of adequate water consumption, after all, aren't in question whatsoever: it can play a tremendously positive role in energy intake, weight, performance, and functioning.[25] And if all that isn't enough to convince you, there's one more thing you should bear in mind: staying well hydrated can be an excellent tool in avoiding dehydration-induced AFib attacks.

With these concepts as background, along with the "food clues" we discussed earlier, we can now begin to build a diet that almost anyone can follow, that doesn't require people to go hungry, and that will help put AFib in the past.

Ready for that? Okay, let's set the table.

## VEGGIES, VEGGIES, VEGGIES

You probably knew this was coming. But don't feel bad if you didn't. Even though the copious merits of predominantly plant-based diets have been well studied, many people still don't realize how important vegetables are to nearly every aspect of their health. That particularly includes heart health because vegetables help us cut visceral fat and reduce inflammation—two key drivers of atrial fibrillation. Natural, plant-based foods are the cornerstone of the Mediterranean diet, which has been associated with lower AFib risk.[26]

So how many vegetables should you be eating each day? Let's turn that question around: How many veggies *can* you eat each day? Because when it comes to vegetables, there is almost no way to overdo it. In fact, if you are concerned about not getting enough to eat, veggies are the solution.

That bears repeating: veggies are the solution.

In fact, that bears capitalization: VEGGIES ARE THE SOLUTION.

On the AFib diet, you may eat as many vegetables as you wish. And the more the better. Munch on cauliflower all day long. Eat broccoli like it's going out of style. Chomp on carrots to your heart's content—your heart will, indeed, be content.

There is a caveat here: starchy vegetables, like potatoes, are not the solution. Drenching veggies with unhealthy oils like ranch salad dressing, cheeses, or processed sauces, is not the solution, either. The closer to zero as you can get when it comes to consuming starchy vegetables and unhealthy oils, the better off you will be.

But raw or lightly cooked veggies, in all their gloriously tasty and colorful combinations, are the key to weight loss without hunger.

What kinds of veggies? Aim to optimize your nutrients. Track your nutrient intake, so you can keep it fairly consistent over time while building good data about yourself. Unless you suffer from kidney failure, the more potassium- and magnesium-rich foods (like vegetables) you eat, the lower your chances of an AFib attack. The three most potassium- and magnesium-dense foods are spinach, Swiss chard, and beet greens. Veggies like broccoli, cabbage, asparagus, Brussels sprouts, and kale are also high in these nutrients, as are many fruits, beans, nuts, and seeds.

To make sure you get all the plant-based nutrients your body needs, you can track your micronutrients with a smartphone app. A simpler approach, however, is to eat as wide of a variety of colors as you can. Red from apples. Yellow from bananas. Orange from carrots. Green from spinach. Blue from blueberries. You get the idea. If your plate includes all the colors of the rainbow, you've probably hit on all the nutrients you need as well.

In most cases, fresher is better. The longer a food has been out of the ground, the fewer nutrients it will deliver to your body when you digest it. This is why flash-frozen organic frozen vegetables can also be a good option. Likewise, vegetables that have been overcooked lose some of the qualities that make them such a healthy choice. Raw, lightly steamed, broiled, or tastily sautéed veggies are all good choices. Of course, if you're on certain medications, you still need to be vigilant about avoiding vegetables that could interact poorly with those drugs. You'll recall, for instance, that warfarin thins the blood by blocking vitamin K. And since leafy greens are sky-high in this health-promoting vitamin, you'll completely overwhelm warfarin's capacity to block the vitamin. If you're still craving greens, speak to your doctor about switching to a newer blood thinner that does not work through blocking vitamin K. If that is not an option, eat a steady and regular amount of these vegetables and ask your doctor to adjust the warfarin dose to your diet.

Some people have a hard time with "just eat as many veggies as you want." They want more guidance in the form of specific quantities. Truly, your appetite should be your guide—eat until you are satiated. But, if you still need a way to visualize this, a good rule of thumb for vegetables is that they should cover two-thirds to three-quarters of your plate at every meal. Alternatively, you could shoot for at least five to six servings of vegetables daily.

As you're putting more vegetables into your daily diet, you might notice that you are indeed feeling hungry between meals. That's a feature, not a bug. Many of our patients find they need to eat smaller, more frequent meals when they increase their consumption of vegetables, especially if they don't replace unhealthy fats with healthy fats. There's a very simple solution to this problem: eat more veggies.

That's the case even for people whose brains are wired in such a way that they simply never feel full. This could be due to a genetic disposition or psychological factors.[27] Whatever the reason, though, veggies are still the solution—just use the "vegetable test." Is your brain telling you that you're hungry when you're pretty sure you shouldn't be? If you're truly hungry, you'll happily eat vegetables. If veggies don't sound good at the moment, that's not hunger you're feeling—it's something else.

Okay, got that? Eat veggies first and eat veggies most. That's easy enough, right? But what should be on the rest of the plate?

Lots of stuff, but let's start by talking about other plant-based foods.

## PLANT IT

Fruits are another key part of the AFib diet, although fruits should not be treated with the same "eat as much as you want" approach as vegetables.

That's because fruit, depending on the type, can spike blood glucose without offering the same rich complexity of vitamins and minerals that vegetables may deliver.

All things considered, your best bet when it comes to fruit is berries, which have minimal effects on blood glucose, have been associated with natural weight loss, and are packed with fiber. One to three servings of fruit each day is a reasonable target, with berries leading the way. Bananas, which you likely know are high in potassium, are another great fruit to have on your plate provided they aren't too ripe, which spikes blood glucose levels. And avocados, which are a great source of vitamins $B_6$, C, E, and K, and nutrients including folate, niacin, and riboflavin, are a smart addition to breakfasts, lunches, and dinners. Even tomatoes, also high in potassium and fiber, can be a great fruit to include in your diet.

Whatever fruit you eat, however, the best way to eat fruit is to eat as much of the entire fruit as possible, in as close to its natural state as possible. There is a big difference between orange juice, which is essentially just sugar water, and an orange, which retains the parts of the fruit that make the body work harder to digest it and deliver nutrients that are often discarded in the juicing process.

One special fruit to be aware of is grapefruit. Studies show that grapefruit lengthens the QT interval on an EKG.[28] That can be especially dangerous if you are on QT-prolonging AFib medications like sotalol, Tikosyn (dofetilide), Multaq (dronedarone), or amiodarone; antidepressants; or antibiotics. If you're unsure whether you should consume grapefruit in any form, check with your doctor or pharmacist.

Grains are problematic for most of our atrial fibrillation patients because of the strong role that refined grains play in diabetes and weight gain, but this doesn't mean you need to avoid grains. If you do choose to eat grains, stick with intact grains whenever possible—foods like quinoa and brown rice, which haven't been pulverized into flour. Many people believe that whole wheat and gluten-free flours are healthy, but these flours can also spike your blood glucose very quickly. If you can't live without bread, keep an eye open for flourless breads, which have long been available at health food stores and are increasingly stocked at mainstream supermarkets.

Nuts and seeds are another great plant-based food source, and a superior way to stave off feelings of hunger in between veggie-heavy meals, since studies show that eating these foods regularly helps to decrease your AFib risk.[29] Just a few almonds, a handful of pumpkin seeds, or a small helping of chia seeds can help deliver much-needed proteins, fiber, potassium, magnesium, and other nutrients, including plant-based fats, which have been shown to promote weight loss and prevent blood-glucose spikes. Olive oil and dark chocolate, both in moderation, are other plant-based fat-containing foods that have been shown to decrease AFib risk.[30] An added benefit of dark chocolate is that it also packs plenty of the AFib-suppressing minerals potassium and magnesium.[31]

Last but not least: legumes, including beans, chickpeas, lentils, soybeans, peanuts, and tamarinds, are safe to eat and likely will improve your AFib situation. As is the case with the other foods we've discussed so far, though, beans and lentils are best for you when they look like what they actually are: part of a plant.

## FIBER OPTICS

If hunger is a cruel enemy for people battling atrial fibrillation (and it is), then fiber is a very good friend. That's because fiber—the parts of plant-based foods that can't be completely broken down during digestion—increases the sense of feeling full by 39 percent, according to a review of forty-four published studies by University of Minnesota researchers.[32] This correspondingly decreases caloric intake. The more fiber you get, the less you will weigh. And the less you weigh, the less visceral fat you likely will be carrying, which in turn means less AFib. Researchers from the University of Helsinki have shown that fiber is also effective at preventing blood glucose spikes.[33]

What foods pack a lot of fiber? Plants of all sorts. (Meat doesn't have fiber.) In particular, vegetables, berries (especially raspberries), lentils, beans, peas, and chia seeds are all fantastic sources of fiber. And for dessert, some healthy dark chocolate—at least 70 percent cacao with few to no added sugars—is a great way to add even more fiber.

The result of eating lots of these foods? Less atrial fibrillation. Researchers have found a statistical trend of up to a 36 percent reduced risk of atrial fibrillation among people who eat plenty of fiber.[34] That study was based on a cohort of people who were topping out at about 27 grams of fiber a day—nowhere near the daily 100 to 150 grams of fiber that our Paleolithic ancestors and modern-day hunter-gathering peoples consume.[35] That's a good target for just about anyone, and even in our modern society, people who eat a veggie-heavy diet can usually get somewhere near 100 grams of fiber without needing fiber supplements.

## GO WILD ON THE MEAT

Thomas was first diagnosed with paroxysmal AFib when he was fifty-four, with a new episode coming about once per week and lasting about twenty-four hours. It was a busy time for him as he was taking his software company public through an initial stock offering. A year and a half later, though, his episodes had completely ceased, without any drugs or procedures.

How? Well, Thomas did make a lot of lifestyle changes. These all helped a little. But the big change came after he began a mostly plant-based diet, supplemented with wild meats. After that, Thomas said, he didn't have any further episodes—not a single one, even as he moved on to his next tech startup and another big dose of job-related stress.

"My cardiologist seems unimpressed and skeptical, but I know what I'm experiencing," Thomas said. "I believe I have found my proper medication in a mostly vegetable and wild meat diet."

Not everyone will experience a result like that, but if you can manage to eat a 100 percent all-natural diet, meaning that even your meat is wild game, it may be worth a try. As long as you're getting a healthy dose of all of the nutrients your body needs to function, you will almost certainly be healthier for it.

Thomas's diet, after all, closely replicated the way of eating of the Tsi-mane people, a hunter-gatherer tribe of the Bolivian lowlands who subsist on a diet of mostly vegetables supplemented with wild game and fish. They also have the lowest levels of heart disease ever recorded on this planet.[36] Not surprisingly, there is a near absence of atrial fibrillation and strokes among these people as well.

There is, no doubt, a confluence of reasons for the Tsimanes' remark-able heart health. They do not eat sugar or processed foods. They live a family-centered, technology-free, slow-paced life. They forage for food for seven hours a day while logging an average of 17,000 steps daily. Could there also be a partial genetic answer to this question? Most certainly.[37] But they also eat a lot of vegetables and wild meat.

Whatever the reason, studies of the Tsimane people teach us that meat isn't always bad for human health, as some would argue. While many stud-ies have found an association between meat consumption and risk of heart disease, heart disease–related death, and death in general, this is probably because most of these people were mostly eating processed or industrially raised meats in conjunction with other unhealthy lifestyle habits. The meat that the Tsimane consume, on the other hand, does not come from animals that are kept in small cages, packed into corrals, pumped full of antibiotics, slaughtered, packaged in plastic, and transported hundreds of miles to sit in a grocery store freezer case. As such, please do not make the mistake of concluding that because some people are able to consume meat without consequences to their hearts, everyone else can, too. That's particularly important when it comes to meats like hotdogs, bacon, and deli meats, which have been shown to contain known carcinogens.[38] These are not natural cuts of meat, but heavily processed meat products.

Most people, of course, can't eat like the Tsimane, and even a diet that mimics theirs can be difficult to achieve. Even Thomas acknowledges that his ability to access wild game was a matter of certain privilege—he had both the means and the connections to access that food source.

That doesn't mean you're out of luck, though. For most people, the easiest and healthiest source of animal protein will be fish—and not just any fish, but wild fish that also deliver a healthy dose of omega-3 fatty acids without an accompanying dose of mercury and PCBs. A handy way to remember which fish fit the bill is the acronym SMASH, which stands for salmon, mackerel, anchovies, sardines, and herring. Even these fish, though, can be problematic if they are cooked in unhealthy ways. Whatever benefits you might derive from a SMASH fish are quickly destroyed if that fish is fried, battered, or drenched in unhealthy sauces. Just as with vegetables and grains, when a piece of fish actually looks like a piece of fish, it's likely to be much better for you.

One study of nearly 5,000 people showed that regular fish eaters had a 31 percent decreased risk of atrial fibrillation. And while not every study has shown that fish protects against AFib (and, after decades of research, there is also no clear AFib benefit from fish oil, either[39]), there is no signal from these studies that SMASH fish, cooked in healthy ways, increases your AFib risk.[40]

And yet it is important to remember that fish, like other meat, also increases the production of TMAO. Thus, the association between fish eating and atrial fibrillation rates may be nonlinear, with a little bit being protective but a lot being dangerous. That's why, in the AFib diet, the equivalent of one or two servings of wild fish weekly is plenty.

Why "the equivalent"? Because, if you do choose to eat meat, one way of doing so while protecting your heart may be to adhere to the culinary principles of people from many Far East Asian countries, including Japan, China, and Korea, where very small portions of meat are used to flavor vegetable dishes. In a way of thinking, people in these cultures use meat like Westerners use veggies. Instead of a big salmon steak served with a small side of asparagus, for instance, think about a big plate of vegetables tossed with small morsels of salmon. With this way of eating, it is no wonder that obesity is almost nonexistent among people who eat traditional Far East Asian diets, with studies showing that the AFib rate among people who eat in this way is up to ten times lower than that of the United States.[41]

Whatever approach to meat you ultimately choose, as long as you are eating as naturally as possible and consuming small portions of wild meats and SMASH fish with copious amounts of vegetables, you probably won't increase your risk of cardiovascular disease, including AFib.

# BE NUTTY

If you were a voracious eater of almonds back in the middle part of the last century, people would probably think you were a little bit, well, nutty. Since the 1960s, though—and spurred on by the incredibly successful "a can a week, that's all we ask" campaign of the Blue Diamond brand—almond consumption has increased tenfold. Even then, a lot of people who were trying to lose weight avoided nuts because they are so high in fat and calories, even as medical studies consistently demonstrated that not all fats and calories are equal.

Today, almonds have overtaken peanuts as Americans' favorite nut. Despite the new American love affair with almonds, though, many other types of nuts haven't seen a similar increase in consumption. Yet many of the same benefits almonds offer are shared by walnuts, cashews, macadamias, pecans, Brazil nuts, and hazelnuts. (And, yes, these health benefits are present in that lovely legume that is always posing as a nut: the mighty peanut.)

Nuts are huge for weight loss. All of those healthy fats, protein, and fiber fill you up, after all, and may also offer a boost in metabolism.[42] According to one study, people who included almonds in their diets were able to lose 65 percent more weight than their non-almond-eating counterparts.[43] While that effect seems to be a bit of an outlier among other studies, the totality of the evidence suggests that nuts of all sorts either help reduce weight or, at the very least, don't contribute to weight gain—meaning they are a great way to add protein and healthy fats without the health consequences that come from eating excessive meat.

That's a conclusion supported by another research-backed fact about nuts: eating them every day lowers your risk of heart problems of all sorts, including atrial fibrillation.[44]

When eating nuts, however, it's important to avoid the gussied-up versions that have grown very popular in recent years, and that almost always include a heavy dose of salt, sugar, and preservatives that counteract the positive health benefits. If you need to flavor these treats, do it at home with a pinch of garlic, chili, or onion powder; a squirt of lemon juice; or a dash of hot sauce.

You might have noticed that we haven't spoken at all, yet, about what *not* to eat, and that might jump out at you because most diets start with prohibitions. But if you start by eating all of the things we've discussed so far, the likelihood that you'll want to eat anything else is drastically diminished. And that's like having the wind in your sails when you do meet the challenge of avoiding the foods that conspire to make AFib worse.

## PROCESSED ELIMINATION

In recent years, marketers who are tuned in to increasing consumer desire to eat better have worked hard to brand prepackaged foods as "healthy." They put these foods in muted green and brown boxes, proclaim organic credentials, and advertise "natural" sweeteners.

Marketing is a fascinating game—and there's nothing inherently wrong with trying to convince people to spend their money on Product A instead of Product B. The problem is that these gimmicks aren't just an attempt to get you to consider a different brand; they're an attempt to get you to choose a different kind of food.

Here's the truth: packaged foods, no matter how fancy manufacturers make them, are almost always processed foods—which use added chemicals as preservatives. Thus, it doesn't matter that their makers proclaim their healthiness. A label doesn't make something healthy.

How do you know that something is processed? It's simple: processed foods rarely look like the raw ingredients from which they were made, and are often cooked up with heavy doses of sugar and salt.

Most Americans get way too much sodium in their diets, and that's not because they're a little too liberal with the salt shaker—it's because processed foods are often swimming in salt. As we age, we need less salt in our diets to stay healthy. In particular, people over fifty need about one gram less sodium daily compared to younger people. Also, salt is added for taste, texture, and as a preservative in many common foods we purchase. And given that high-sodium diets may be a cause of AFib, the best option would be to dramatically reduce or even eliminate processed, packaged, or prepared foods.[45]

Of course, there are plenty of food products that don't even make an attempt to look healthy, like plastic-packaged cakes and cookies, freezer meals, and soft drinks. In some cases, it is an affront to good sense and human decency to even call these products "food." They might more accurately be called "food-like substances" or "Frankenfoods," as they have few if any nutritionally redeeming qualities.

From canned soups to boxed cereals to bottled sauces, processed foods are simply not good for us, and are absolutely detrimental to those who want to reduce their risk of AFib.

The same goes for fast food. There is little, if anything, you can get from a drive-through that can even passingly be called "healthy," let alone be considered safe to eat without increasing your risk of AFib. These foods are engineered to be "hyper-palatable," with mega-doses of sodium that increase blood pressure and fluid retention, plenty of sugar that spikes glucose, unhealthy oils that sabotage your cholesterol numbers, and lots of industrially produced and highly processed animal-based proteins that feed TMAO production.

Many fast-food restaurants have recently begun pushing toward plant-based proteins that are designed to taste and look very similar to animal proteins. While there may be a lot of merit to these experiments in new food sources, particularly in terms of the moral implications and environmental impact of meat consumption, these are laboratory-created foods. They are, by definition, heavily processed, and since they have been created to virtually mirror animal proteins, they may carry many of the same potential health implications. Long-term studies will help us better understand what those implications are, but it's important not to assume that "plant-based" means "eat as much as you want." These foods are not vegetables.

There's another heavily processed food that few people recognize is, in fact, a processed food—and it makes up a large part of a lot of people's diets. It's not immediately obvious, though, unless you take a walk around your market with an eye toward avoiding foods that don't look like the raw ingredients from which they were made. When you do that, a rather large section of the market often jumps right out: the bakery.

Most breads are heavily processed foods, often chock full of added ingredients intended to keep staling and molding at bay for as long as possible. And yet many people, especially those who recall being taught in elementary school that breads and cereals are an essential base to the food pyramid, have come to think of it as a very healthy part of a balanced diet.

The belief that bread is healthy for us is compounded by the Judeo-Christian concept of "daily bread," which suggests that bread isn't just something we want but rather something we need.

For what it's worth, though, many scholars who have taken deep linguistic dives into the Lord's Prayer have concluded that the Greek word *epiousios*, most commonly translated as "daily," might be better translated as "supersubstantial," rendering this Biblical passage less about literal food and rather about more transcendent needs. You don't have to go traipsing through the semasiological weeds, though, to understand that the breads that are most commonly available in modern supermarkets, and that are almost always made with processed flour, don't really resemble the bread that was served in Biblical times.

That form of bread was made of "wheat and barley, beans and lentils, millet and spelt," according to the writings of the Hebrew prophet Ezekiel. Indeed, if you feel you cannot live without bread, your best bet is sprouted-grain bread—often called Ezekiel bread—which is made from a variety of whole grains and legumes.

Most modern breads are a double whammy, though. Not only are they processed, that processing turns the key ingredient into something that is tremendously bad for people with atrial fibrillation: sugar.

## AVOID BLOOD SUGAR SPIKES

Brian was an MIT-trained chemical engineer and former professor who had reinvented himself as a serial entrepreneur. A life focused on his career, though, came at a consequence to his health: Brian suffered from diabetes, high blood pressure, a weight problem, and, yes, AFib.

It didn't take long for Brian to learn that carbohydrates—especially anything that has flour or added sugar—are a sure-fire way to send a person's blood sugar through the roof.

Nonstarchy veggies won't spike blood glucose levels. Fruits are pretty safe, too, in moderation, so long as you aren't eating tropical or overripe fruits. Berries are probably the best for nutrition and to keep your blood sugars in check. Legumes are also low glycemic. But when grains, even whole grains, are pulverized into fine powder, they can instantly be converted to sugar in the body—and at that point you might as well be chewing on candy.

After doing a lot of research, the "avoid sugar like the plague" part of the ketogenic diet seemed to Brian like a good way to get out of the mess he was in. Indeed, the principles of keto aren't a bad starting place for battling AFib, as a low-glycemic diet is essential to those for whom a ride on a blood sugar roller-coaster can be both a cause and trigger for arrhythmia.

Brian, who goes "all in" on pretty much everything he does, wasn't interested in the "soft keto" approach most people attempt by trying to limit carbs. He bought a ketone meter, which tests for chemicals that the liver produces when the body doesn't have enough insulin to turn sugar into energy, and made sure that every day, he reached this state of "ketosis," in which the body burns fat for energy because it lacks carbohydrates. Then he graphed his results with the sort of precision worthy of his engineering background. Truly, it was something to behold.

Some studies have linked low-carb diets to AFib,[46] but in our experience it is because people who quit carbs try to game the system with lots of foods that are unhealthy in other ways.

With copious amounts of vegetables and a moderate intake of berries paired with healthy fats, Brian's hypertension, diabetes, and extra pounds were gone within months. However, he found that his "true keto" diet depleted him of the potassium and magnesium he needed to fight his AFib. He also found that, contrary to what many people believe about the keto diet, too much meat actually kicked him out of ketosis. This makes sense, since when we get too much protein in our diets, our bodies convert the excess protein to sugar.

Brian dramatically increased his intake of low-glycemic potassium- and magnesium-rich vegetables, and cut back on the meat. And with that, he was home free. His medical problems disappeared, and the number of medications he takes each day went to zero.

## PUTTING IT ALL TOGETHER

Want to eat amazing food, never feel hungry, lose weight, and help your heart? All you've got to do is follow the AFib diet for two weeks. If you're like most people, that will be enough time for you to grow accustomed to this new way of eating, begin to break the physiological and psychological bonds that enslave humans to sugar, feel a measurable difference in energy, and help quiet your heart.

Does it seem like it might be hard to eat this way for fourteen days? For some people, it can be.

One of the chief concerns we hear, for instance, is that this way of eating could be a lot more expensive. And the truth is that it often does cost more, especially for people who live in food deserts, where affordable nutritious food can be harder to find. That's not of small consequence.

When researchers from the Harvard School of Public Health con- ducted a comprehensive examination of the prices of healthy versus less healthy food, however, they found that the healthiest diets cost about $1.50 more per day than the least healthy diets—a cost that is trivial compared to the healthcare costs associated with eating unhealthy foods.[47]

There is a time commitment at play here, too. It unquestionably takes less time to pop open a can of soup than it does to cook soup from scratch— and anyone who tells you otherwise probably doesn't realize just how much extra time they have on their hands.

Whether we're talking about time or money, it's important to recognize that this is an investment in both of those things. Like all of the other strategies in this book, the AFib diet asks you to do something now in exchange for a much better life down the line. And while that can easily be quantified in terms of time and money, too, the greatest returns are simply immeasurable.

For Meredith, the shift from "This is hard" to "This is worthwhile" to "This is so much better" took only a few weeks.

"It took some getting used to, for sure," Meredith said. "I used to absentmindedly grab things off the shelf at the grocery store without even considering what it would do to my heart, or pick something up from the drive-through on my way home from work, or completely disregard everything I knew about what was healthy, because I felt so hungry. Once these principles became part of my life, though, it was really simple. I never felt hungry. And I never want to go back."

What do fourteen days of meals in Meredith's life look like? They look like a whole lot of deliciousness.[48] Take a peek:

## Sunday

**Breakfast:** Smoothie (almond milk, peaches, vanilla, almond butter, hemp seeds, spinach, avocado). Water.

**Lunch:** Quinoa salad (celery, bell peppers, edamame, red onion). Water.

**Dinner:** Harvest soup (onion, vegetable bouillon, red lentils, carrots, squash, tomatoes) and salad (spinach, dried cranberries, almonds). Water. A square of stevia-sweetened dark chocolate.

## Monday

**Breakfast:** Quinoa crêpes with blueberries. Water.

**Mid-morning:** Coffee.

**Lunch:** Soup (navy beans, nutritional yeast, herbs, vegetable bouillon, carrots). Water.

**Afternoon:** Minimally ripened banana.

**Dinner:** Grilled tempeh topped with avocado, romaine lettuce, red onion, tomato, tahini, sesame oil, and soy sauce. Water.

## Tuesday

**Breakfast:** Almond butter on sprouted-grain bread topped with chia and flax seeds. Smoothie (cashew milk, blueberries, hemp seeds, spinach, kale, walnuts).

**Mid-morning:** Coffee.

**Lunch:** Sweet spice soup (sweet potato, butternut squash, onions, tomatoes, garlic, almond milk, nutmeg, cardamom). Water.

**Afternoon:** Celery with peanut butter and chia seeds.

**Dinner:** Stir-fry (peas, carrots, peppers, water chestnuts, bamboo shoots, broccoli, mushrooms) with peanut sauce (peanut butter, lime juice, rice vinegar, soy sauce, fish sauce, chili flakes) over brown rice. Water.

## Wednesday

**Fasting morning.** Water.

**Lunch:** Spring salad (spinach, arugula, red quinoa, chickpeas, dried cranberries, butternut squash, pumpkin seeds, almonds) with honey sesame dressing (white balsamic vinegar, tahini, olive oil, honey). Unsweetened iced tea and water.

**Afternoon:** Mango slices with chili powder and lime.

**Dinner:** Taco chili (lentils, pintos, black beans, tomatoes, corn, chili pepper, paprika, garlic powder, onion powder, coriander, cumin, cayenne, curry powder) topped with onion, avocado, and cilantro. Water.

**Dessert:** Fruit smoothie (apples, bananas, kale, hemp milk, orange juice).

## Thursday

**Breakfast:** Hazelnut smoothie (almond milk, hazelnuts, dates). Water.

**Mid-morning:** Coffee.

**Lunch:** Lemon-pepper cucumber sandwiches on sprouted-grain bread. Water.

**Afternoon:** Banana and peanut butter.

**Dinner:** Whole-grain rice with peas, carrots, and soy. Water.

## Friday

**Breakfast:** Steel-cut oats with strawberries, walnuts, and flaxseed. Water.

**Mid-morning:** Coffee.

**Lunch:** Kale salad with Caesar dressing (walnuts, white miso, olive oil, garlic, shallots, lemons, balsamic vinegar). Water.

**Afternoon:** Almonds.

**Dinner:** Baked salmon with quinoa and broccoli. White wine and water.

## Saturday

**Fasting morning.** Water.

**Lunch:** Southwest salad (black beans, corn, red onion, cherry tomatoes, red bell peppers, barley, lime juice, cilantro, balsamic vinegar). Unsweetened iced tea and water.

**Afternoon:** Cashews.

**Dinner:** Creamy vegetable curry (cauliflower, broccoli, yellow onion, curry powder, olive oil, chickpeas, tomatoes, green onion, peanuts, Greek yogurt). Water.

## Sunday

**Breakfast:** Peanut butter smoothie (almond milk, peanut butter, hemp seeds, avocado, spinach, dates). Coffee and water.

**Lunch:** Beets and greens (spring lettuce mix, beets, cherries, pumpkin seeds) with miso vinaigrette (miso, white balsamic vinegar, lime juice, olive oil, Dijon mustard). Water.

**Dinner:** Vegetables (onion, cauliflower, cabbage, pepper, zucchini, tofu) over creamy quinoa (quinoa, hummus, lime juice) with sliced avocado. Water.

## Monday

**Breakfast:** Breakfast hash (corn, sweet potato, bell peppers, carrots, apples). Coffee and water.

**Mid-morning:** Coffee.

**Lunch:** Mediterranean bowl (hummus, cucumber, tomatoes, sun-dried tomatoes, kalamata olives, red onion, pickles). Water.

**Afternoon:** Pumpkin seeds with curry powder and cayenne pepper.

**Dinner:** Moroccan-style sauté (cauliflower, yellow onion, garlic, chickpeas, vegetable bouillon, raisins, dates, toasted almonds, harissa, cinnamon, cumin, hummus). Water.

## Tuesday

**Breakfast:** Avocado slices on sprouted-grain toast. Water.

**Mid-morning:** Coffee.

**Lunch:** Hot and sour soup (vegetable bouillon, sriracha, peanut butter, soy sauce, collard greens, tofu, peanuts, pepper flakes). Water.

**Afternoon:** Bell pepper slices with hummus.

**Dinner:** Sautéed Brussels sprouts and cashews (Brussels sprouts, cashews, garlic, olive oil) with quinoa and green beans. Water.

## Wednesday

**Fasting morning.** Water.

**Lunch:** Almond butter and honey sandwich on sprouted-grain bread. Unsweetened iced tea and water.

**Afternoon:** Banana.

**Dinner:** Quinoa crêpes with asparagus and "nooch" (nutritional yeast sauce). Water.

**Dessert:** Pumpkin pie smoothie (almond milk, banana, avocado, pumpkin puree, cinnamon, ginger, nutmeg, allspice).

## Thursday

**Breakfast:** Quinoa breakfast porridge (quinoa, oat milk, cinnamon, vanilla, coconut flakes, dates, walnuts). Water.

**Mid-morning:** Coffee.

**Lunch:** Warm kale and onion salad with Asian dressing (liquid aminos, sesame oil, garlic, rice vinegar, vegetable bouillon). Water.

**Afternoon:** Mango slices with chili powder and lime.

**Dinner:** Sweet and sour potatoes (sweet potatoes, tomatoes, carrots, green peppers, mung beans, onion, lemon, olive oil, balsamic vinegar, Chinese five-spice blend, chili flakes, bouillon). Water.

## Friday

**Breakfast:** Steel-cut oats with blackberries, walnuts, chia seeds, and vanilla.

**Mid-morning:** Coffee.

**Lunch:** Rainbow chard smoothie (coconut water, mango, lemon, ginger, Swiss chard). Water.

**Afternoon:** Dried blueberries.

**Dinner:** Korean braised mackerel (mackerel, chili pepper, gochugaru red pepper flakes, chile paste, soy sauce, honey, garlic, ginger, daikon radish, onions) with kimchi and whole-grain rice.

## Saturday

**Fasting morning.** Water.

**Lunch:** Creamy savory quinoa (quinoa, garlic, onion, sweet potatoes, tomatoes, hemp milk, cardamom, nutmeg, cinnamon). Unsweetened iced tea and water.

**Afternoon:** Seaweed crackers.

**Dinner:** Burrito bowl (kale, black beans, avocado, "riced" cauliflower, tomatoes, lime, cayenne pepper, hot sauce, plain Greek yogurt).

**Dessert:** Cookie dough (whole-grain oats, cashew butter, vanilla, stevia-sweetened dark chocolate chips).

## FOOD IS THE BEST MEDICINE

There isn't just one way to eat "right," not even for those suffering from atrial fibrillation. After all, everyone who has ever been diagnosed with AFib has come to have this condition due to a slightly—and sometimes broadly—different set of risk factors from anyone else. Our genes are all different. So are our gut microbiomes. So are our lifestyles, including the factors affecting our lives that aren't easily changeable—such as where we live—but impact the diets we maintain.

Provided you are minimizing or avoiding any added sugars, flour, and processed foods, while maximizing vegetables, just about any diet can be a good diet for AFib. But if you've tried other paths, and haven't been able to lose enough weight, the AFib diet could be the thing you need to give your body the nutrients it needs while keeping away from the substances that have been proven to aggravate atrial fibrillation.

That's what Cassandra did. When we first met her, back in chapter one, the "super mom" was struggling to break her energy drink reliance and get more sleep. All things considered, her diet and exercise patterns were good, and so when she finally "got off the sauce," and began sleeping more, she figured the worst of her problems were over.

Indeed, her paroxysmal atrial fibrillation improved—with fewer episodes overall and triggered events that lasted a shorter time, too.

"That was better," she recalled. "But I wasn't content to settle for better. I wanted this to no longer be a part of my life."

After just two weeks on the AFib diet, Cassandra had noticed—and tracked—a significant reduction in her time out of rhythm. After two months, her episodes had nearly disappeared. And after two years of steadfast dedication to the diet, along with staying away from those no-good energy drinks, she could very safely say that she was not only no longer living with atrial fibrillation, but that her life was better than ever.

"In a way, I'm really thankful that I got AFib," she said. "It was really terrifying at first, and forced me to make a lot of changes that I honestly didn't want to make, maybe especially when it came to the way I ate, which I had always thought was pretty healthy."

But as a result of those changes, she said, "I don't worry about AFib anymore. In fact, I actually feel younger and healthier than I did even before I had AFib. I have more energy. I have more stamina."

At that point she paused and brushed away the tears that were welling under her eyes.

"I have more of everything," she said.

She's not alone.

## EATING FOR AFIB

### How to eat

1.  Stop eating before you feel full. Wait at least thirty minutes before snacking. Stop eating at least three hours before you go to bed.

2.  Stay well hydrated by drinking water. Limit other drinks and eliminate all sugar-sweetened drinks.

### What to eat

1.  Eat as many nonstarchy vegetables as you can. At least five servings each day. The more the better. Organic is preferable when possible.

2.  Eat nuts, seeds, and legumes daily. Intact grains can also be eaten daily if desired.

3.  Eat up to three servings of fruits each day. Berries and other low-glycemic fruits are best. Organic is preferable when possible.

4. Strive for a goal of 100 grams of fiber each day.

5. If you choose to consume meat, wild game and SMASH fish are best. Whenever possible, use meat as a flavor-adding element of a meal, rather than the main course.

## What not to eat

1. Stay away from fast, fried, and processed foods.

2. Avoid grains that have been pulverized into flour, which acts like added sugar in the body.

3. Avoid added sugars. If you need a treat, dark chocolate is best, especially if it has minimal to no added sugar.

## Chapter Ten

# ᴧᴧ MAKE IT STICK ᴧᴧ

### How everyone can make BLAST work for them, through seven easy lessons

After one hundred years, the human heart has beat about 4.2 billion times. At some point something is bound to go wrong, right?

Not necessarily.

One of the little-discussed attributes of centenarians everywhere is that they are usually in quite good health. In fact, they are often in significantly better health than people who are several decades younger. And this actually makes a lot of sense; in order to reach such an advanced age, you really must have been doing a few things right.

Even still, more than a quarter of centenarians in the United States have atrial fibrillation.[1]

In Spain and Denmark, it's about one in five.[2]

But there are places in the world in which the rate is much lower. One of these places is the village of Bapan, which straddles the breathtakingly

beautiful Panyang River in southern China. The rate of AFib among centenarians in this area of the world is less than one in twenty.[3]

Bapan is a place that has long been known in China for its remarkable
number of people who live past the age of one hundred. And almost all of
these elders come to the century mark in remarkable health. Some are still
working in the fields at that age.

Did the people in this part of the world simply win the genetic lottery?
Maybe. But initial genetic tests we have conducted on the centenarians in
Bapan have demonstrated that these individuals actually have quite a few
markers that generally indicate a *greater* risk of chronic diseases of all kinds.
Somehow, they've bucked the odds.

How? The lessons of Longevity Village can be distilled into seven basic
rules for better living:

1. Eat good food.
2. Master your mindset.
3. Build your place in a positive community.
4. Be in motion.
5. Find a rhythm.
6. Make the best of your environment.
7. Proceed with purpose.

These are more than simple platitudes. They're lessons in health that
are very much aligned with Western medical research, with the BLAST
approach to fighting AFib, and with the AFib diet.

You can read about the way the villagers of Bapan applied these lessons
to their lives in *The Longevity Plan: Seven Life-Transforming Lessons from
Ancient China*. One of the key points of that book, however, is that these
lessons do us no good if they can only be applied to life in a small village in
China. So, let's look at how they have been applied in the lives of several of
the world's most prominent survivors of atrial fibrillation. These individuals
have made it their life's work to help others fight AFib in the context of the
Western world's realities of life.

# EAT GOOD FOOD

Shannon Dickson was forty years old when he had his first experience with atrial fibrillation.

The year was 1991. In that precise moment, Shannon wasn't doing anything that you might typically expect to trigger an AFib episode. Much to the contrary, in fact.

"I was meditating, of all things," explained Shannon, the editor and a moderator of the website AFibbers.org, which has tens of thousands of active users and has been helping AFib patients for more than twenty years. "I was in the middle of a deep meditation. I was just as quiet and calm as you could possibly be, and all of a sudden it felt like I had just been unplugged and there was just like a free-floating feeling. And the next thing I knew, my heart was coming out of my chest."

Meditation is often part of an Eastern-informed regimen for reducing the incidence of AFib,[4] so Shannon's situation was certainly unusual. It's likely, of course, that the meditation itself wasn't a trigger at all; it just happened to be what he was doing when all of the other factors that were contributing to his condition came together to create an arrhythmic event.

In the years since that frightening first episode, Shannon has done a lot of work to identify the causes and triggers of his AFib, and has dedicated a substantial part of his life to helping others do the same. Over time, he has come to believe that "chasing every little possible trigger" is a strategy with diminishing returns. The better approach, he reckons, is a holistic one.

And that starts with good food—food that is supplying your body with the nutrients it needs and that you actually want to eat, rather than loading you up with anything detrimental.

"We tell people to eat better. To try to eat good, clean food, and cut out the junk food," he said. "I've been completely devoted to all of that, too."

For Shannon, that means a largely organic paleo and plant-based diet replete with fresh vegetables, plus some supplementation for nutrients that his body needs and isn't getting enough of, for whatever reason, such as magnesium, potassium, and vitamin $D_3$.

When it comes to potassium, for instance, Shannon gets almost all he needs from food, but keeps a bottle of potassium chloride tablets, just in case. "So if I ever have a real stressful day, like if it's real hot in Arizona in the middle of the summer and I've been out in the yard all day, I'll just take one to be safe."

There's nothing magical about a good diet. To the contrary, a good diet is scientific—a never-ending chemistry experiment aimed at ensuring your body has what it needs, when you need it, informed by the way you feel from day to day, and the information you're getting by tracking your heart and watching your biomarkers.

But a lifelong commitment to eating good food isn't always easy, particularly not in a world in which we are constantly being bombarded with opportunities to stray away from the foods that help keep our hearts in rhythm. Once AFib is gone for a bit, many patients have a tendency to start breaking the rules they've set for themselves.

You simply cannot afford to do that. Keeping AFib in remission takes a lifelong commitment to eating good food.

To survive and thrive in the midst of a world that is constantly telling you it's okay not to eat good food, you're going to need more than determination. You're going to need a new mindset.

## MASTER YOUR MINDSET

Atrial fibrillation doesn't just rob people of their normal heart rhythm. It saps them of their strength. It reduces the time and energy they have to engage in the things they love. And it makes the end seem nearer, often because the end is, in fact, nearer.

All too often, the result is pessimism and despondency. Researchers have shown that AFib patients often experience significant symptoms of depression,[5] and that these symptoms might actually aggravate their AFib symptoms[6]—a vicious cycle of the worst sort.

Mellanie True Hills can certainly understand. The e-business strategy consultant was at the top of her game in 2003, helping companies around the world embrace the paradigm-shifting power of information technology in a highly connected world. At just fifty-one years old, she had authored several books that had been translated into many languages, was a regular speaker at e-business conferences worldwide, and also consulted for companies that did high-tech manufacturing and automotive manufacturing.

"I was on the road all the time," she said, noting that she was working very long hours, traveling across time zones, and "on airplanes all the time."

Then, "after returning late one night from a business trip, the next morning I was in my home office going through emails when my heart skipped a beat and took off racing. I lay down on the sofa, and my husband came running over with the blood pressure cuff.

"It was warm weather and I was wearing shorts, and my husband noticed that my right leg was as white as snow. It felt cold, and I noticed that the vision in my right eye was blurry. At the emergency room, they said I'd had blood clots and a close call with a stroke from a condition called atrial fibrillation, which I had never heard of."

And, like many others, Mellanie's doctors told her the best way to combat her condition was medication, including beta-blockers and blood thinners, the latter of which left her body bruised all over. "It was embarrassing," she recalled.

And even with the drugs, Mellanie's symptoms weren't completely curtailed. "It really takes a physical toll on you," she said. "If you have paroxysmal AFib and you have an episode, when it's over with, you feel like a limp dishrag and all you can do is sleep. You're just totally wiped out, so it does take a physical toll. And it takes an emotional toll. You just feel this fear of 'When's the AFib beast going to strike again?' and 'When am I going to have to tell my family I can't go do something with them?' and 'Am I going to have to cancel out of something yet again?'"

Just as Mellanie was beginning to recognize that life as she knew it was over, she had a stroke of luck: she ran across an article about surgical ablation, featuring her own health plan provider. In a matter of weeks, she was in the operating room.

"Afterwards, I was AFib free," she said, "and I have been ever since."

Recognizing that many people are not nearly so fortunate as she was, Mellanie launched the website StopAfib.org, which now gets more than one million unique views each month. She also hosts AFib patient conferences and forums.

While Mellanie's surgical ablation helped put her heart back into rhythm, keeping it there has taken a commitment to lifestyle optimization. And it's very likely that the boundless optimism that had defined her life before AFib—and that she got a second dose of in the wake of her surgical ablation—has been a big contributing factor, too.

Optimism isn't simply something you can turn on and turn off. It is, however, something you can train yourself to improve upon. In a seminal paper on "optimism training" in the *Journal of Cognitive Psychotherapy*, published in 1996 and still much cited, the psychologists John Riskind, Christopher Sarampote, and Mary Ann Mercier described four research-based techniques for creating a more positive personal vision:

- Identifying pessimistic beliefs, such as "Wishful thinking is dangerous," and introducing optimistic beliefs, such as "Wishful thinking can temporarily remove obstacles to our ability to see alternative solutions."
- Engaging in positive visualization of the future.
- Finding silver linings, the meaningful moments that come of even the most miserable situations.
- Practicing "positive priming." For instance, intentionally starting the day with positive memories, good news stories, or a dose of comedy in order to increase the likelihood of thinking spontaneously of such happy things throughout the day.

If you want to send AFib into remission and keep it there, an optimistic mindset is a force multiplier. But it's a lot easier to be optimistic when you've got a team around you. So let's talk about that next.

## BUILD YOUR PLACE IN A POSITIVE COMMUNITY

You'll remember Debbe McCall from chapter eight, in which the meticulous health tracker recalled her dealings with "Dr. Fancypants."

You'd have a hard time finding three stronger self-advocates than Debbe, Mellanie, and Shannon, and yet each of these people felt compelled to build or help grow a community of support to help them in their health journey—and give them the opportunity to help others. That, of course, is the definition of community—people who you count on and who are counting on you. And if you're going to beat AFib, you're going to need that kind of support.

It's important to note that community can take on a variety of forms. If your goal is to BLAST your AFib into remission, for instance, and your immediate family members understand that goal and what it will take for you to get there—and are ready and willing to actively help, and even sacrifice to help you do it—then perhaps that's the only community you need.

Not everyone is that fortunate. It's not hard at all to find AFib patients who desperately want to eat better, but whose families only gather around dinners of pizza, fried chicken, or hamburgers. Stories abound of husbands who learn their wives need to exercise more to keep their hearts healthy, but won't get up from their own recliner to exercise with them. If you're in a situation like this, it's not that your family is bad—it's just that your family, for whatever reason, isn't in a good position to help you and become part of your health community. Fighting that will add stress and sorrow to your life, likely with limited benefit. Instead, you'll need to find your community elsewhere.

Friends and colleagues are another obvious place to look, but can also (and often) disappoint us. Friends might like to get together late at night over drinks—that's two potential AFib triggers in one meetup. Colleagues might like to gather for lunch in places where the only healthy thing on the menu is a glass of water.

The good news is that, as the groups facilitated by Debbe, Mellanie, and Shannon exhibit, you've got options—networks of people from around the world who know what it's like to go to battle with AFib. And not only can you easily find a group of fellow AFib fighters, but you can find a group with members who have similar experiences to yours.

Debbe's group, for instance, skews young and female. "Two-thirds are female and the average age is forty," she said, "so we're very young."

As a result, the questions posed on her forum are ones that, in other settings, might not be met with a knowledgeable answer, let alone an answer that comes from experience. "I'm dealing with, 'I want to have another baby. I work for UPS. I'm a firefighter, I'm a salesperson,'" Debbe said. "I've got completely different questions than, say, those that might be asked by the typical over-sixty-five-year-old man."

While your community should be one that respects your desire to reduce your AFib risk, it doesn't need to be an AFib community, per se. Your community could be a softball team, a religious study group, or a knitting club. The only real qualifications are that you should feel comfortable being yourself—meaning the lifestyle you must maintain to keep AFib away is respected and supported—and that you should feel as though your community needs you as much as you need it.

The health benefits of feeling connected to others, through whatever mechanism that connection is made, are hard to overstate. The feeling of connectedness has been demonstrated to be protective against stroke, and to increase heart health.[7] Why? That's harder to say. It could be that people who feel more socially isolated are also more likely to succumb to behaviors like smoking, drinking, and overeating that are likely to aggravate their risks. On the other hand, it could be that people who feel needed by a community have a greater incentive to eat good food, get great sleep, and avoid stressful situations.

Oh yes, and exercise.

# BE IN MOTION

Well into his late sixties—more than a quarter century after he was first diagnosed with atrial fibrillation—Shannon was still maintaining a routine that was keeping him healthy, happy, and in rhythm.

He spent part of every day in meditation. He ate lots of vegetables. He was committed to the community he had helped grow at AFibbers.org. And he got plenty of exercise.

That last part couldn't be more important. You know, of course, that exercise is a vital part of lifestyle optimization. What you might not realize is how easy it is to put more of it into your day with just one easy trick: simply substitute the word "exercise" with "motion."

To be clear, intense vigorous exercise—the kind that makes you sweat profusely and breathe hard—is important. But you actually don't need *a lot* of exercise like that. You might recall from our chapter on lifestyle optimization that just five or ten minutes of highly strenuous exercise is often enough. And too much extreme vigorous exercise—the sort that people get when they engage in a competitive endurance sport—can actually be an AFib trigger.

What you do need a lot of is the sort of exercise that simply gives your body a good dose of consistent, low-level physical stress. This is the sort that might make you breathe a little harder and break a sweat, but doesn't leave you gasping for air or your clothes soaked, and that raises your heart rate, but doesn't send it through the roof. Indeed, this is the sort of exercise you get by simply staying in motion.

If you work in an office building, staying in motion might mean committing to never taking the elevator. It could also mean organizing a walking group at lunchtime or putting a small set of exercise pedals under your desk. Even better, a standing treadmill desk can be a tremendously good investment for people who want to keep moving. It's true that it can take a few days to get used to working while walking, but research shows that people who use treadmill desks are no less productive than people who sit,[8] just healthier.

If you're retired, or simply a fan of a lot of great TV programs, then treadmills, exercise bikes, and elliptical machines can also offer a guilt-free way to watch your shows, taking an activity that is typically quite unhealthy[9] and turning it into something that is beneficial to your heart—giving "binge watching" a whole new meaning.

If you are an endurance athlete and have had your AFib ablated, you'll still need to be smart about the way you work out. Physical stress can increase the risk of atrial fibrillation, and the long-term repetitive effects of prolonged, high-intensity exercise can cause structural and electrical changes in the heart that promote AFib. In fact, almost anyone can go into AFib if their bodies are under severe stress—we've certainly seen this in very young, very healthy adults following a motor vehicle accident, surgery, or even a massive infection. The same thing can happen if you are severely dehydrated or electrolyte depleted, or have pushed yourself in a competition beyond what you have trained to do. But there are also a lot of other athletic endeavors that can feed your need for competition without putting you at risk for renewed AFib.

For most people, though, the problem isn't too much exercise. The problem is fitting in enough exercise in our busy modern world. The point of staying in motion is that the exercise you get doesn't need to happen during time you've intentionally dedicated to exercise. In fact, the more unintentional you can make it, the easier it will be to keep it up.

And yes, you've got to keep it up. To do that, you need to make it part of the rhythm of your life.

## FIND A RHYTHM

Atrial fibrillation is an excellent metaphor for life. When your heart is out of rhythm, it's almost always an indicator that some other part of your life is out of rhythm, too. That can be sleep, metabolism, medications, exercise, stress, or any of the other "probable causes" we discussed in chapter one. And, most likely, it's a combination of imbalances.

Once you find balance through the BLAST approach, the trick is to maintain it. And the best way to do that is to recognize that Sir Isaac Newton's First Law of Motion didn't just help lay down the foundation for classical mechanics; it also applies to your life.

Don't fret if you can't remember your middle-school physics class. Newton's First Law states that objects at rest will stay at rest, while objects in motion will stay in motion, unless acted upon by external forces.

We're not all that different than a meteoroid, flying through space. Once we get started moving in one direction, and get a little momentum behind us, we have a tendency to stay right on pace, and right on course. The problem is that the path we've been on, for a very long time, is usually the course that put us at risk for AFib in the first place. And, complicating matters, even once we've gotten into the habit of following good habits, the world is a never-ending gantlet of external forces conspiring to push us off course.

In the midst of this, how do we keep watching our biomarkers, maintaining a constant process of lifestyle optimization, and tracking as we go? One more metaphor is helpful.

Consider the original meaning of the word *gantlet*—a military exercise in which a soldier would have to run between two rows of men with sticks, each of whom would do their best to knock the soldier off balance. Who would be most likely to succeed at such a challenge? A very small soldier or a larger, muscular one? Of course it is the one with more muscles—more than would be necessary to run the same distance in less punishing circumstances.

Staying in rhythm is about creating so much momentum that all those external forces don't stand a chance of knocking you down. If your doctor says your body needs thirty minutes of moderate exercise a day, go for sixty—or even more on the weekends when you've got a little more time. If through tracking you learn that your heart is most likely to stay in rhythm when you meditate in the morning, practice that stress-relieving exercise in the evening, too. If your incidents of AFib stay low even if your biomarkers are a bit on the high or low side, keep working to bring those numbers into an even healthier range.

Build up these habits when times are good, when everything seems fine, and when it's been so long since your last AFib episode that you're starting to forget you were ever at risk. That way, when times are tougher, you'll have the momentum you need to carry you through the gantlet of life—without risking your life.

That's one of the philosophies that has helped Shannon come to appreciate the power of ablation. For eleven years after his diagnosis, he was controlling his AFib with lifestyle optimization alone, and had no interest in a procedure. "If anybody thought that I would get an ablation, I would just laugh at that point," he said. "I thought oh my gosh, I've got this whipped. This is not a big deal. I've now mastered my AFib."

Many people can indeed put an end to their AFib in this way. But Shannon had some additional factors to contend with: both his father and sister had passed away from AFib-related strokes. His very genes were one of the factors working to push him off balance. "And, lo and behold," he said, "it returned. It was like life said, 'Wait a minute, we're going to humble you a bit here.'"

If Shannon had gotten an ablation *and* committed to lifestyle optimization immediately following his diagnosis, would he have had the experience? That's very hard to say. He was just forty years old when he had his first episode, after all, and that tends to be a good time to try lifestyle optimization alone, because atrial remodeling tends to be less significant among younger people.

In any case, hindsight is twenty-twenty. What Shannon did *next* is a good example of the sort of momentum building that allows AFib survivors to find and keep the rhythm they need in their lives, so that they can enjoy the rhythm they need in their hearts. He got an ablation *and* he doubled down on lifestyle optimization, "and I've never had a single beat of AFib since that day."

Whether it's getting an ablation, jogging an extra few miles a week, focusing on a few additional biomarkers, or spending a little more time with your tracking data, anything you can do to go "above and beyond" in your effort to keep your life in rhythm will help you when AFib tries to push you off balance. And that's especially true when it comes to one of the biggest factors in AFib: the environment in which you live.

## MAKE THE BEST OF YOUR ENTIRE ENVIRONMENT

When we consider our environment, we often think of it as something very big and very hard to change. And it's true that there are a lot of things about the ecological and geographical conditions under which we live that, as individuals, we're close to helpless to do anything about.

That doesn't stop those conditions from impacting *us*, of course.

Take air pollution, for example. While our study showed that short-term spikes in the microscopic particulate matter known as PM2.5 don't increase the risk of atrial fibrillation,[10] longer-term exposure has consistently been associated with AFib.[11]

While many people initially picture dirty air when they think about pollution, that's not the only kind of pollution. Researchers have found that noise pollution—which has been shown to elevate stress in the human body—may also have a negative effect on people at risk of AFib.[12] If you have to deal with both noise and air pollution, because you live near a busy street or freeway, you might be in double jeopardy.[13]

And it's not just the air and the noise. Your work environment can play a tremendously important role in your health. Toxic work environments, work-related stress, and long hours have consistently been associated with atrial fibrillation.[14] Even your family environment can be an AFib risk factor if you're dealing with a child who is off course, marital discord, or the death of your spouse.[15] And if your work colleagues and family members surround themselves with a never-ending supply of junk food, your environmental challenges are doubly bad.

Up to this point we have only discussed the "external environment." But the environment within your own body can contribute to AFib risk, too. When we're not caring for our internal environment, by eating a mostly plant-based diet, it puts our health at risk in many ways. For instance, as we discussed in chapter nine, recent research suggests that TMAO production by the microbes living in your gut is an additional risk factor for atrial fibrillation.[16]

For people of significant privilege, the answer to such AFib environmental problems might seem simple: quit your job, move away from the city, avoid difficult family members, grow your own organic food, and live off the land in a meditative and blissful state. Nice and easy.

But this obviously isn't an option for most people. So what can you do to optimize your environment when you have a job, family, and other responsibilities that are all vying for your time? When the world isn't perfect? When you don't have unlimited resources?

Probably the best thing you can do is identify as many ways as possible to spend a little less time at work and a little more time in nature. That doesn't just mean taking a few camping trips in the summer, although that does sound nice. Rather, we're proposing finding ways to spend time with friends and family away from the pollution, noise, and job-related stress, if only for a little bit each day.

Nature doesn't need to be "the great outdoors." It could be a trip to a nearby park, a few minutes in a rooftop garden, or a little time walking along a riverfront or around a city lake. Indeed, studies show that the more time you spend in these kinds of environments, the lower your cardiovascular risk.[17]

Can you afford to make these big changes in your life? Can you structure your workday to avoid overtime, or work from home on some days? If not, are you in a position to consider changing jobs? What good does your current job do you, after all, if you can't go to work because you're in the hospital? And what good does all that overtime pay or end-of-the-year bonus do if you're spending it on AFib medications?

Could you move closer to your family, work, or nature to improve your chances of beating AFib? Would moving on to a new job that gave you more personal time help?

Sure, there are costs to making big life changes like that. But there is also a cost to not making these changes. After all, AFib patients "are the frequent fliers of the emergency room," Mellanie reminded us. "You have huge copays and those who don't have insurance get stuck for years paying off their medical costs. It's very expensive to have to keep going back and forth."

Almost every day, she said, someone is posting on her StopAFib forum about a lack of ability to pay for care. "Someone posted just a few minutes ago that she just got a bill for $3,000 for her cardioversion," Mellanie said. "She said, 'I can't pay it. I don't know what to do.' I hear it all the time."

But even still, let's not pretend this is an easy decision. It's not. Myriad factors impact the ability to change locations or jobs, not the least of which is a person's basic economic status.

Peri, for example, was in no position to leave her job as a factory worker. Besides, she truly loved her work and the people she worked with. The problem for her wasn't job stress or too many hours, but a hundred-minute round-trip commute that crowded out the most important things in life. All of this time in the car kept her from exercise, preparing healthy meals, and time with her family. Working from home wasn't an option, but she didn't want to move. She liked her neighborhood and the schools were good.

Because she could no longer ignore her health, something had to give. There simply weren't enough hours in the day for her to do everything. Either she needed a new job closer to home or she had to move. In the end she and her family decided that finding new employment closer to home was the best option, but they easily could have gone the other direction. A year later, she couldn't be sure she made the better of the two choices—there will always be "what ifs"—but she was positive that the choice she did make had impacted her health for the better.

Eliminating the long commute was a tremendous help. Not only was the stress of a long commute gone, but she had a lot more time to focus on her health and her family. She spent more time with her children at a park near their school and took evening walks with her husband.

"I'm not going to lie," she said. "I do miss my old job. I miss my friends there. But I was confused. I convinced myself that job was really essential to who I am. It wasn't. Being here for my family—healthy and happy—that's my purpose."

## PROCEED WITH PURPOSE

The nineteenth-century Unitarian clergyman George Washington Burnap was certainly not the first man to try to tell women how to live their lives, but the course of lectures he called "The Sphere and Duties of Woman" might have won the "mansplaining" award for the year 1848.

That shouldn't discount the quality of one particular piece of advice—what came to become his most famous quote (albeit one that has been attributed to many other people over the years). "The grand essentials of happiness in this life," he wrote, "are something to do, something to love, and something to hope for."

That's as true today as it was in the mid-1800s. It will be just as true tomorrow, too. And for anyone who wants to make the AFib Cure stick in their lives, it couldn't be more important.

When it comes to the connection between our minds and our health, purpose is powerful. Study after study has found an association of purpose in life with all kinds of better health outcomes—an effect that stands regardless of age, sex, education, or race. The feeling of purpose appears to be a universal tonic.[18]

Do you know what your purpose is? Do you know why you're engaged in this fight? If not, just answer these questions:

- What is something you would like to do better?
- Who is someone you'd like to love longer?
- What is something you're hoping for?

At the confluence of these answers is purpose—a reason to get up, every morning, and do the hard work it takes to apply the BLAST approach to your life. A reason to find the time and money to do those biomarker checks. A reason to engage in the rest-of-your-life effort to optimize your lifestyle. A reason to build up the courage it takes to talk to your doctor about ablation, if you haven't already done so. A reason to keep working toward a life free of medications and expensive copays. A reason to track your progress, step by step, pound by pound, heartbeat by heartbeat.

It's a lot. No one should tell you otherwise. Anyone offering simple solutions to atrial fibrillation is selling snake oil.

And yes, there's a lot of snake oil out there.

How do you know what's real and what's not? Well, we certainly hope you'll keep this book as a guide. And make sure you check out the resources that Mellanie True Hills provides at StopAfib.org, Shannon Dickson moderates at AFibbers.org, and Debbe McCall facilitates at the Atrial Fibrillation Support Forum on Facebook.

Beyond that, there's just one more thing to do: go take a look in the mirror.

That's the person who has the power to make this happen. And maybe it seems like a long and hard journey, but there are lots of people out there who have been where you are right now.

You can do this.

You truly can.

## THE LESSONS OF BAPAN

### Eat good food

- Follow a diet that results in weight loss and healthy weight maintenance without significant fluctuations.
- If the diet you're using isn't working to control weight and arrhythmic incidents, use the AFib diet.
- Avoid processed foods.

### Master your mindset

- Identify pessimistic beliefs and replace them with optimistic alternatives.

- Engage in positive visualization of the future.
- Begin each day with activities that promote positivity.

## Build your place in a positive community

- Ask family members and friends to help you reach your goals.
- Don't fight with unsupportive people. If they aren't essential to your life, say goodbye. If they are essential to your life, recognize that they simply aren't in a position to be supportive at this time.
- Seek alternative supportive communities, including those that are online.

## Be in motion

- Strive to be in motion for half of your waking hours.
- Engage in vigorous exercise for at least a few minutes, a few times each day.
- No matter where you start, build more motion and vigorous exercise into your life as you go.

## Find a rhythm

- Start with as much momentum as possible.
- Go over and above the minimum.
- In respect to your AFib-fighting habits, build a routine.

## Make the best of your environment

- Reduce your exposure to pollution of all kinds.
- Get into nature as much as possible.
- Seek work environments that eliminate stress and other health dangers.

## Proceed with purpose

- Consider why you are fighting AFib.
- Remind yourself of your purpose every day.

## Conclusion

# ⎯⎯⎯᭟᭝᭟ JUST THE BEGINNING ᭟᭝᭟⎯⎯⎯

### Why atrial fibrillation could be the best thing to ever happen to you

erhaps it might seem inappropriate, even gauche, to congratulate people on being diagnosed with atrial fibrillation. This is, after all, a condition that changes most people's lives for the worse, leaves them stuck on some rather heinous medications, and leads them down a steep road to greater and greater health problems. A third will suffer from stroke.[1] Those who live long enough will face an increased risk of dementia.[2] And, for the vast majority, traditional treatments won't lead to a meaningfully better long-term quality of life.[3]

But, if you have been diagnosed with AFib, congratulations.

If you have discovered that you are at an increased risk of AFib, congratulations.

If you have a loved one with AFib, and want to give them the gift of more good years of life, congratulations.

If you have AFib, and are sick and tired of the way your life is going, congratulations.

Because there is hope. And there is a path. Many people have taken this path before, and many more people are coming to learn about it now. It is a path to a better life—not just better than life is now, but potentially better than life has ever been.

The pounding and throbbing and breathlessness and exhaustion and fear that mark AFib are the signals that many people need to make significant lifestyle changes that improve their overall health. They are the body's warning sirens. Something has gone wrong, yes, but many more things are *about* to go wrong, if nothing is done. This is the moment to address the things that turned those sirens on, and to make the changes that can turn those sirens off—and keep them off for the rest of your life.

Sure, it's better to never have had to make those changes in the first place, but what's done is done. Your past is your past. Fix what is wrong now, and your future is your future. And, of the two, the future can be better.

And so, congratulations. This is your moment.

## PUTTING AFIB DOWN UNDER

As you have learned, the AFib Cure isn't a set of rules. It's a process of goals, decisions, assessments, and reevaluations. It's a lifetime commitment to health and happiness. It's also a process backed by a lot of very promising research, including a remarkable study by electrophysiologist Dr. Prash Sanders.

Sanders specializes in cardiac ablation at the University of Adelaide in Australia, which has a public access care system with generally good outcomes across the land. But, like any system, it has some downsides, too, one of which, at the time Sanders began his practice, was that ablation was covered inconsistently in different states and territories. Ironically, this was because nothing was left inside the body after the procedure. For years in Australia, reimbursement was mandatory for many implantable heart devices such as stents, pacemakers, and defibrillators—but not for ablation. The result was a very long waiting list to receive an ablation.

"As medications were no longer effective for these patients, there was nothing more I could offer them while they waited up to a year for their ablation procedure," Sanders explained.

While the patients waited, though, Sanders advised them to try a life-optimization strategy—a multidisciplinary approach that also included a weight-loss program. And recognizing this as an opportunity to gather data, the award-winning investigator followed them closely. "What I saw was that as my patients lost weight, there was a striking correlation to a reduction in atrial fibrillation symptoms," he said.

That led to a further study, in the prestigious *Journal of the American College of Cardiology*, confirming what Sanders had seen in his own patients. Remarkably, over five years, 46 percent of people who were able to drop a significant percentage of their body weight—an average of thirty-five pounds—pushed their AFib into remission to the point that they no longer needed drugs or an ablation.

But this group didn't *just* benefit from a tremendously reduced rate of AFib. When people lose weight, after all, their health tends to improve in other ways, too. Among the members of the group who had hypertension, systolic blood pressure dropped by eighteen points on average; that's more than twice the reduction achieved by the average blood pressure medication. Inflammation, as measured by C-reactive protein, dropped 76 percent; that's a tremendously important finding, since inflammation of the heart is one of the main causes of fibrosis or scarring, which ultimately leads to AFib.[4]

LDL cholesterol, which significantly increases the risk of heart disease, dropped 16 percent. Triglyceride levels, which have been linked to atrial fibrillation, heart attacks, and strokes, dropped by 31 percent. And there was an 18 percent improvement in the dilation and thickness of their hearts, as measured by an echocardiogram. In other words, their hearts actually transformed into much healthier and better-functioning organs.

And, in what was perhaps the best indicator that addressing the problems that cause AFib will positively impact other diseases, 88 percent of the people in the group who had diabetes pushed that disease into remission by getting their hemoglobin A1C back down to the normal range by losing weight.

Perhaps not surprisingly, given their tremendous health improvements, the self-reported sense of well-being among patients in this group improved an average of 200 percent. No antidepressant in the world has demonstrated an effect as powerful as that.

And that's just with weight loss. When you combine these effects with the improvements that come from better attentiveness and monitoring of biomarkers, other lifestyle optimization changes like stress reduction and better sleep, the life-changing power of a cardiac ablation for those who need it, a reduction in a dependency on drugs, and a lifetime commitment to tracking, the result isn't just better health.

It could be a cure.

## LIFE AT ONE HUNDRED

Will everyone who follows the BLAST strategy put their AFib into complete remission and keep it there forever? It would be irresponsible to say such a thing. The older a person is and the longer they have had AFib, the harder it can be to reach remission.

But that doesn't mean that these people don't have hope for a better life or that they have no hope for a cure. Much to the contrary, in fact. Anyone who follows the guidelines in this book can realize a tremendous improvement in their quality of life, even if their AFib isn't completely eradicated. And no one, at any age, should believe that remission is impossible.

Remember Jake, the accountant from chapter seven, who was in his early eighties when he decided he'd had enough drugs and wanted to take control of whatever years he had left?

At the time of this writing, Jake is in his early nineties and still doing volunteer work. He's still drug free, and he's still AFib free.

"Even before I was diagnosed with AFib, I used to believe that life at one hundred years old would be miserable and then, once I did get AFib, life at that age wasn't even conceivable," he said. "And now, one hundred is just around the corner, and I'm actually looking forward to it. I truly am."

Another AFib survivor, Robert, still has a long time to go before he reaches the age of one hundred, but he has no doubts he'll get there. That wasn't always his perspective, though. Shortly after retiring, his heart began to flutter.

"I had felt the symptoms of AFib before," he said, "but it had always seemed to resolve itself. This time something told me I needed to get to the hospital. A few minutes later, I was lying in the emergency room, undergoing stabilizing treatment. The drug therapy didn't work so they moved on to shock therapy."

The cardioversion worked in two ways, Robert said. "It got my heart regulated and it also convinced me that I didn't want to do that again."

Under the guidance of a doctor, he began to implement the strategies detailed in this book.

Now in his sixties, Robert's AFib is in remission, and he's living a life that is better than he ever could have imagined.

"I just completed a bicycle event where I rode 140 miles in one day," he recently reported. "When I finished I felt I had enough energy to ride another sixty. I feel great with more energy. This way of living has truly made a difference. My goal is still to leave this world at a good age over one hundred with my hair on fire at Mach 4 speed, making a contribution until I die, and never looking back with regrets."

That's Gavrilo's plan, too. When you first met him in the opening pages of this book, he was twenty-seven years old and had just learned of his genetic abnormality through a home DNA genetic test. As part of this test, he learned that he had gs275, meaning that one copy of each of the two AFib single-nucleotide polymorphisms tested were defective. This genetic defect gave him a nearly 50 percent chance of developing AFib and put him at high risk for blood clots and strokes.

He's thirty now. Three years doesn't offer much of an indication of whether the strategies in this book will prevent him from ever getting AFib. It is often said that our genes are not our destiny, and this is true: Gavrilo could have gone his whole life, just the way things were going, and never have gotten AFib.

But even if that were true, Gavrilo said, he would not regret dedicating himself to the process of biomarker monitoring, lifestyle optimization, and wellness tracking.

"I'll be doing this for the rest of my life," he said. "And I know it's a long way away, but I feel like one hundred healthy years isn't crazy these days. And, who knows, maybe I'll go on even longer."

Gavrilo has plenty of reason to feel confident.

"Because of these changes, I've dropped thirty pounds, which puts me at the weight I was a decade ago," he said. "My blood pressure was a little high for someone of my age; that's fallen now to a very normal range. My CRP and A1C got better and better for the first eighteen months, and have stabilized from there. I sleep better than I ever have, I know exactly what I'm putting into my body, and I know how much exercise I'm getting each day, right down to the step. And because I wear this watch, I've got confidence that if anything does ever start to go wrong, I'll likely know about it before anything crazy and scary happens."

All of that is giving Gavrilo a lot of hope for the future. And this is a good time for that sort of perspective, he figures, "because my wife is pregnant, and we're going to have twins. It's a boy and a girl. Leo and Gabriela. And people keep telling me, you know, you can never be ready for parenthood. But in my heart, everything feels right."

## WHAT LIES AHEAD

This book includes the stories of a lot of *other* people.

There was Angelica, who beat her stress by changing her "side hustle." There was Laura, whose goal to put her AFib into remission was driven by her desire to get back on the ski slopes with her children. There were

Shannon, Debbe, and Mellanie, who have all beaten AFib and made it their life's work to help others who are living with this condition. And there were others, too, who came into the world of AFib from a variety of backgrounds, and who wanted desperately to ensure this terrible condition didn't come to *define* their lives.

Now is the time when you decide what your story will be. Are you willing to stop, and possibly even reverse, atrial fibrosis from developing? Will you commit to biomarker monitoring? Will you optimize your lifestyle? Will you begin the work it takes to reduce and ultimately stop any unnecessary medications? Will you begin the lifelong process of tracking your wellness to make sure improvements don't slide away as the years go by?

If all of that is part of your story, then there is absolutely no reason why you cannot dream big right now. The years ahead can be your best years yet.

The beat can go on.

And on.

And on.

---

*We want to hear from you. While we can't treat your AFib by email, we do want to know what you think about this book, and we'd love to hear your stories. Please feel free to reach out to us via email at john@drjohnday.com and TJaredBunch@gmail.com. You can also follow us on Twitter at @drjohndayMD and @tjaredbunch.*

# ACKNOWLEDGMENTS

We are deeply grateful to the many people who have helped us take care of our patients and assisted our research over the last three decades. This book represents everything we have learned.

First, our thanks to our families for their love and support, not only in the writing of this book, but also in our lifelong quest to eradicate atrial fibrillation.

Second, to our patients: Everything we have learned about how to beat atrial fibrillation has come from you. Your faith and trust in us are humbling and inspiring.

Third, thanks to our physician and research colleagues in the atrial fibrillation world, as well as the nurses and other team members within our own hospitals and clinics over the years. The search for an atrial fibrillation cure is a team sport, and we are all on this journey together.

Fourth, a special thanks to our literary agent, Trena Keeting, and the fantastic team at BenBella Books for their belief in the healing message of this book. It has been a wonderful experience to partner with you on this book.

# NOTES

## Introduction

1. Lloyd-Jones, D., Wang, T., Leip, E., et al. (2004). Lifetime risk for development of atrial fibrillation: The Framingham Heart Study. *Circulation*.
2. Mou, L., Norby, F., Chen, L., et al. (2018). Lifetime risk of atrial fibrillation by race and socioeconomic status: ARIC Study (Atherosclerosis Risk in Communities). *Circulation: Arrhythmia and Electrophysiology*.
3. Chugh, S., Havmoeller, R., Narayanan, K., et al. (2014). Worldwide epidemiology of atrial fibrillation: A Global Burden of Disease 2010 Study. *Circulation*.
4. Delaney, J., Yin, X., Fontes, J., et al. (2018). Hospital and clinical care costs associated with atrial fibrillation for Medicare beneficiaries in the Cardiovascular Health Study and the Framingham Heart Study. *SAGE Open Medicine*.
5. Stewart, S., Murphy, N., Walker, A. et al. (2004). Cost of an emerging epidemic: An economic analysis of atrial fibrillation in the UK. *Heart*.
6. Carlquist, J., Knight, S., Cawthon, R., et al. (2016). Shortened telomere length is associated with paroxysmal atrial fibrillation among cardiovascular patients enrolled in the Intermountain Heart Collaborative Study. *Heart Rhythm*.
7. Benjamin, E., Virani, S., Callaway, C., et al. (2018). Heart disease and stroke statistics—2018 update: A report from the American Heart Association. *Circulation*.
8. The stories in this book are based on interactions and treatments with diagnosed AFib patients; in some cases names and other biographical details have been changed to protect their confidentiality and their families'. The life circumstances and outcomes these example patients have experienced, though, are absolutely representative of patients seen by Dr. Day and Dr. Bunch.
9. Bassand, J., Virdone, S., Goldhaber, S., et al. (2019). Early risks of death, stroke/systemic embolism, and major bleeding in patients with newly diagnosed atrial fibrillation. *Circulation*.
10. Gardarsdottir, M., Sigurdsson, S., Aspelund, T., et al. (2018). Atrial fibrillation is associated with decreased total cerebral blood flow and brain perfusion. *EP Europace*.
11. Gaita, F., Corsinovi, L., Anselmino, M., et al. (2013). Prevalence of silent cerebral ischemia in paroxysmal and persistent atrial fibrillation and correlation with cognitive function. *Journal of the American College of Cardiology*.
12. Galenko, O., Jacobs, V., Knight, S., et al. (2019). Circulating levels of biomarkers of cerebral injury in patients with atrial fibrillation. *American Journal of Cardiology*.

13. Conen, D., Rodondi, N., Müller, A., et al. (2019). Relationships of overt and silent brain lesions with cognitive function in patients with atrial fibrillation. *Journal of the American College of Cardiology.*

## Chapter One

1. Chen, Y., Xu, S., & Bendahhou, S. (2003). KCNQ1 gain-of-function mutation in familial atrial fibrillation. *Science.*
2. Carlquist, J., Knight, S., Cawthon, R., et al. (2016). Shortened telomere length is associated with paroxysmal atrial fibrillation among cardiovascular patients enrolled in the Intermountain Heart Collaborative Study. *Heart Rhythm.*
3. Ogunsua, A., Shaikh, A., Ahmed, M., & McManus, D. (2015). Atrial fibrillation and hypertension: Mechanistic, epidemiologic, and treatment parallels. *Methodist DeBakey Cardiovascular Journal.*
4. Vasan, R., Beiser, A., Seshadri, S., et al. (2002). Residual lifetime risk for developing hypertension in middle-aged women and men: The Framingham Heart Study. *JAMA.*
5. Gurven, M., Blackwell, A., Rodríguez, D., et al. (2012). Does blood pressure inevitably rise with age? Longitudinal evidence among forager-horticulturalists. *Hypertension.*
6. Day, J., Day, J., & LaPlante, M. (2017). *The Longevity Plan: Seven Life-Transforming Lessons from Ancient China.* Harper.
7. Emara, M. & Saadet, A. (1986). Transient atrial fibrillation in hypertensive patients with thiazide induced hypokalaemia. *Postgraduate Medical Journal*; Robertson, J. (1984). Diuretics, potassium depletion and the risk of arrhythmias. *European Heart Journal.*
8. van der Hooft, C., Heeringa, J., van Herpen, G., et al. (2004). Drug-induced atrial fibrillation. *Journal of the American College of Cardiology.*
9. Wehber, A. & Hirsh, J. (2016). New onset atrial fibrillation after initiating amphetamine-dextroamphetamine therapy for ADHD: A case report. *Case Reports in Internal Medicine.*
10. Schaer, B., Schneider, C., Jick, S., et al. (2010). Risk for incident atrial fibrillation in patients who receive antihypertensive drugs: A nested case-control study. *Annals of Internal Medicine.*
11. Bunch, T., Anderson, M., May, H., et al. (2009). Relation of bisphosphonate therapies and risk of developing atrial fibrillation. *American Journal of Cardiology.*
12. Smith, M., May, H., Bair, T., et al. (2011). Abstract 14699: Vitamin D excess is significantly associated with risk of atrial fibrillation. *Circulation.*
13. Abdulla, J. & Nielsen, J. (2009). Is the risk of atrial fibrillation higher in athletes than in the general population? A systematic review and meta-analysis. *EP Europace.*
14. Turagam, M., Flaker, G., Velagapudi, P., et al. (2015). Atrial fibrillation in athletes: Pathophysiology, clinical presentation, evaluation and management. *Journal of Atrial Fibrillation.*
15. Aagaard, P., Sharma, S., McNamara, D., et al. (2019). Arrhythmias and adaptations of the cardiac conduction system in former National Football League players. *Journal of the American Heart Association.*
16. Elliott, A., Maatman, B., Emery, M., & Sanders, P. (2017). The role of exercise in atrial fibrillation prevention and promotion: Finding optimal ranges for health. *Heart Rhythm.*
17. Ng, M., Fleming, T., Robinson, M., et al. (2014). Global, regional, and national prevalence of overweight and obesity in children and adults during 1980–2013: A systematic analysis for the Global Burden of Disease Study 2013. *Lancet.*
18. Bunch, T., May, H., Bair, T., & Day, J. (2016). Long-term influence of body mass index on cardiovascular events after atrial fibrillation ablation. *Journal of Interventional Cardiac Electrophysiology.*
19. Stritzke, J., Markus, M., Duderstadt, S., et al. (2009). The aging process of the heart: Obesity is the main risk factor for left atrial enlargement during aging: The MONICA/KORA study. *Journal of the American College of Cardiology.*

20. Echouffo-Tcheugui, J., Shrader, P., Thomas, L., et al. (2017). Care patterns and outcomes in atrial fibrillation patients with and without diabetes: ORBIT-AF registry. *Journal of the American College of Cardiology.*

21. Saito, S., Teshima, Y., Fukui, A., et al. (2014). Glucose fluctuations increase the incidence of atrial fibrillation in diabetic rats. *Cardiovascular Research.*

22. Zhuang, X., Zhang, S., Zhou, H., et al. (2019). U-shaped relationship between carbohydrate intake proportion and incident atrial fibrillation. *Journal of the American College of Cardiology.*

23. Krijthe, B., Heeringa, J., Kors, J., et al. (2013). Serum potassium levels and the risk of atrial fibrillation. *International Journal of Cardiology.*

24. Khan, A., Lubitz, S., Sullivan, L., et al. (2013). Low serum magnesium and the development of atrial fibrillation in the community: The Framingham Heart Study. *Circulation.*

25. Anderson, J., Jacobs, V., May, H., et al. (2019). Free thyroxine within the normal reference range predicts risk of atrial fibrillation. *Journal of Cardiovascular Electrophysiology.*

26. Thompson, J., Nitiahpapand, R., Bhatti, P., & Kourliouros, A. (2015). Vitamin D deficiency and atrial fibrillation. *International Journal of Cardiology.*

27. Voskoboinik, A., Kalman, J., & Kistler, P. (2018). Caffeine and arrhythmias: Time to grind the data. *Journal of the American College of Cardiology: Clinical Electrophysiology.*

28. Nettleton, J., Lutsey, P., Wang, Y., et al. (2009). Diet soda intake and risk of incident metabolic syndrome and type 2 diabetes in the Multi-Ethnic Study of Atherosclerosis (MESA). *Diabetes Care.*

29. Conen, D., Chiuve, S., Everett, B., et al. (2010). Caffeine consumption and incident atrial fibrillation in women. *American Journal of Clinical Nutrition.*

30. Mattioli, V. & Facc Fesc, A. (2014). Beverages of daily life: Impact of caffeine on atrial fibrillation. *Journal of Atrial Fibrillation*; Di Rocco, J., During, A., Morelli, P., et al. (2011). Atrial fibrillation in healthy adolescents after highly caffeinated beverage consumption: Two case reports. *Journal of Medical Case Reports.*

31. Dr. Day has this same variant.

32. Meredith, S., Juliano, L., Hughes, J., & Griffiths, R. (2013). Caffeine use disorder: A comprehensive review and research agenda. *Journal of Caffeine Research.*

33. Larsson, D., Drca, N., & Wolk, A. (2014). Alcohol consumption and risk of atrial fibrillation: A prospective study and dose-response meta-analysis. *Journal of the American College of Cardiology.*

34. Voskoboinik, A., Wong, G., Lee, G., et al. (2019). Moderate alcohol consumption is associated with atrial electrical and structural changes: Insights from high-density left atrial electroanatomic mapping. *Heart Rhythm.*

35. Burton, R., & Sheron, N. (2018). No level of alcohol consumption improves health. *The Lancet.*

36. Stranges, S., Tigbe, W., Gómez-Olivé, F., et al. (2012). Sleep problems: An emerging global epidemic? Findings from the INDEPTH WHO-SAGE study among more than 40,000 older adults from 8 countries across Africa and Asia. *Sleep.*

37. Centers for Disease Control and Prevention. (2008). Perceived insufficient rest or sleep among adults—United States, 2008. *Morbidity and Mortality Weekly Report.*

38. Sheehan, C., Frochen, S., Walsemann, S., & Ailshire, J. (2019). Are U.S. adults reporting less sleep?: Findings from sleep duration trends in the National Health Interview Survey. *Sleep.*

39. Choi, D., Chun, S., Lee, S., et al. (2018). Association between sleep duration and perceived stress: Salaried worker in circumstances of high workload. *International Journal of Environmental Research and Public Health.*

40. Lee, H., Kim, T., Baek, Y., et al. (2017). The trends of atrial fibrillation-related hospital visit and cost, treatment pattern and mortality in Korea: 10-year nationwide sample cohort data. *Korean Circulation Journal.*

41. Christensen, M., Dixit, S., Dewland, T., et al. (2018). Sleep characteristics that predict atrial fibrillation. *Heart Rhythm.*

42. Christensen, M., Dixit, S., Dewland, T., et al. (2018). Sleep characteristics that predict atrial fibrillation. *Heart Rhythm.*

43. Tung, P. & Anter, E. (2016). Atrial fibrillation and sleep apnea: Considerations for a dual epidemic. *Journal of Atrial Fibrillation.*

44. Kayrak, M., Gul, E., Aribas, A., et al. (2013). Self-reported sleep quality of patients with atrial fibrillation and the effects of cardioversion on sleep quality. *Pacing and Clinical Electrophysiology.*

45. Nakamoto, K. (1965). Psychogenic paroxysmal cardiac arrhythmias. Contents of mental events, age and patterns of arrhythmias. *Japanese Circulation Journal.*

46. Svensson, T., Kitlinski, M., Engström, G., & Melander, O. (2017). Psychological stress and risk of incident atrial fibrillation in men and women with known atrial fibrillation genetic risk scores. *Scientific Reports.*

47. Legallois, D., Gomes, S., Pellissier, A., & Milliez, P. (2013). Medical emotional stress-induced atrial fibrillation: My own personal experience. *International Journal of Cardiology.*

48. Graff, S., Fenger-Grøn, M., Christensen, B., et al. (2016). Long-term risk of atrial fibrillation after the death of a partner. *Open Heart.*

49. Wandell, P., Carlsson, A., Gasevic, D., et al. (2018). Socioeconomic factors and mortality in patients with atrial fibrillation—a cohort study in Swedish primary care. *European Journal of Public Health.*

50. Fransson, E., Stadin, M., Nordin, M., et al. (2015). The association between job strain and atrial fibrillation: Results from the Swedish WOLF study. *Biomed Research International.*

51. Fransson, E., Nordin, M., Magnusson Hanson, L., & Westerlund, H. (2018). Job strain and atrial fibrillation—results from the Swedish Longitudinal Occupational Survey of Health and meta-analysis of three studies. *European Journal of Preventive Cardiology.*

52. Lampert, R., Jamner, L., Burg, M., et al. (2014). Triggering of symptomatic atrial fibrillation by negative emotion. *Journal of the American College of Cardiology.*

53. Fenger-Grøn, M., Vestergaard, M., Pedersen, H., et al. (2019). Depression, antidepressants, and the risk of non-valvular atrial fibrillation: A nationwide Danish matched cohort study. *European Journal of Preventive Cardiology.*

54. Lubitz, S., Yin, X., Rienstra, M., et al. (2015). Long-term outcomes of secondary atrial fibrillation in the community: The Framingham Heart Study. *Circulation.*

55. Penrod, E. (January 9, 2018). Utah's air quality is sickening, even killing locals year-round, new research suggests. *Salt Lake Tribune.*

56. Shao, Q., Liu, T., Korantzopoulus, P., et al. (2016). Association between air pollution and development of atrial fibrillation: A meta-analysis of observational studies. *Heart & Lung.*

57. Bunch, T., Horne, B., Asirvatham, S., et al. (2011). Atrial fibrillation hospitalization is not increased with short-term elevations in exposure to fine particulate air pollution. *Pacing and Clinical Electrophysiology.*

58. Watanabe, I. (2018). Smoking and risk of atrial fibrillation. *Journal of Cardiology.*

59. Groh, C., Vittinghoff, E., Benjamin, E., et al. (2019). Childhood tobacco smoke exposure and risk of atrial fibrillation in adulthood. *Journal of the American College of Cardiology.*

60. Groh, C., Faulkner, M., Getabecha, S., et al. (2019). Patient-reported triggers of paroxysmal atrial fibrillation. *Heart Rhythm.*

61. Bunch, T., Day, J., Anderson, J., et al. (2008). Frequency of *Helicobacter pylori* seropositivity and C-reactive protein increase in atrial fibrillation in patients undergoing coronary angiography. *American Journal of Cardiology.*

62. Bunch, T., Weiss, J., Crandall, B., et al. (2010). Atrial fibrillation is independently associated with senile, vascular, and Alzheimer's dementia. *Heart Rhythm.*

63. Rahman, F., Ko, D., & Benjamin, E. (2016). Association of atrial fibrillation and cancer. *JAMA Cardiology.*

64. O'Neal, W., Lakoski, S., Qureshi, W., et al. (2015). Relation between cancer and atrial fibrillation (from the Reasons for Geographic and Racial Differences in Stroke Study). *The American Journal of Cardiology*.

65. Bunch, T., Weiss, J., Crandall, B., et al. (2010). Atrial fibrillation is independently associated with senile, vascular, and Alzheimer's dementia. *Heart Rhythm*.

## Chapter Two

1. Piccini, J., Hammill, B., Sinner, M., et al. (2012). Incidence and prevalence of atrial fibrillation and associated mortality among Medicare beneficiaries, 1993–2007. *Circulation*.

2. Curran, J. (2008). The Yellow Emperor's classic of internal medicine. *BMJ: British Medical Journal*.

3. Lip, G. & Beevers, D. (1995). ABC of atrial fibrillation. History, epidemiology, and importance of atrial fibrillation. *British Medical Journal*.

4. Nattel, S., Allessie, M., & Haissaguerre, M. (2002). Spotlight on atrial fibrillation—the 'complete arrhythmia.' *Cardiovascular Research*.

5. Goette, A., Honeycutt, C., & Langberg, J. (1996). Electrical remodeling in atrial fibrillation. Time course and mechanisms. *Circulation*.

6. Li, D., Fareh, S., Leung, T., & Nattel, S. (1999). Promotion of atrial fibrillation by heart failure in dogs: Atrial remodeling of a different sort. *Circulation*.

7. Wijffels, M., Kirchhof, C., Dorland, R., et al. (1995). Atrial fibrillation begets atrial fibrillation: A study in awake chronically instrumented goats. *Circulation*.

8. Caldeira, D., David, C., & Sampaio, C. (2012). Rate versus rhythm control in atrial fibrillation and clinical outcomes: Updated systematic review and meta-analysis of randomized controlled trials. *Archives of Cardiovascular Diseases*.

9. Fauchier, L., Villejoubert, O., & Clementy, N. (2016). Causes of death and influencing factors in patients with atrial fibrillation. *American Journal of Medicine*.

10. Avitall, B., Bi, J., Mykytsey, A., & Chicos, A. (2008). Atrial and ventricular fibrosis induced by atrial fibrillation: Evidence to support early rhythm control. *Heart Rhythm*.

11. Segura, A., Frazier, O., & Buja, L. (2014). Fibrosis and heart failure. *Heart Failure Review*.

12. Day, T., May, H., Afshar, K., et al. (2019). Mechanisms of improved mortality following ablation: Does ablation restore beta-blocker benefit in atrial fibrillation/heart failure? *Cardiology Clinics*.

13. Haque, M., Sartelli, M., McKimm, J., & Abu Bakar, M. (2018). Health care-associated infections—an overview. *Infection and Drug Resistance*.

14. Kim, M., Johnston, S., & Chu, B. (2011). Estimation of total incremental health care costs in patients with atrial fibrillation in the United States. *Circulation: Cardiovascular Quality and Outcomes*.

15. Friedant, A., Gouse, B., Boehme, A., et al. (2015). A simple prediction score for developing a hospital-acquired infection after acute ischemic stroke. *Journal of Stroke and Cerebrovascular Diseases*.

16. Bunch, T., Day, J., Anderson, J., et al. (2008). Frequency of Helicobacter pylori seropositivity and C-reactive protein increase in atrial fibrillation in patients undergoing coronary angiography. *American Journal of Cardiology*.

17. Hadi, H., Alsheikh-Ali, A., Mahmeed, W., & Suwaidi, J. (2010). Inflammatory cytokines and atrial fibrillation: Current and prospective views. *Journal of Inflammation Research*; Crandall, M., Horne, B., Day, J., Bunch, T., et al. (2009). Atrial fibrillation and CHADS2 risk factors are associated with highly sensitive C-reactive protein incrementally and independently. *Pacing and Clinical Electrophysiology*.

18. Altman, L. (April 24, 1994). The 37th president. The last days: Disabled, yet retaining control over his care. *New York Times*.
19. Kannel, W., Wolf, P., Benjamin, E., & Levy, D. (1998). Prevalence, incidence, prognosis, and predisposing conditions for atrial fibrillation: Population-based estimates. *American Journal of Cardiology*.
20. Jacobs, V., May, H., Bair, T., et al. (2019). The impact of repeated cardioversions for atrial fibrillation on stroke, hospitalizations, and catheter ablation outcomes. *Journal of Atrial Fibrillation*.
21. Bunch, T., Galenko, O., Graves, K., et al. (2019). Atrial fibrillation and dementia: Exploring the association, defining risks and improving outcomes. *Arrhythmia & Electrophysiology Review*.
22. Blum, S., Kuehne, M., Rodondi, N., et al. (2018). Prevalence of silent vascular brain lesions among patients with atrial fibrillation and no known history of stroke. *European Heart Journal*.
23. Morimatsu, M., Hirai, S., Muramatsu, A., & Yoshikawa, M. (1975). Senile degenerative brain lesions and dementia. *Journal of the American Geriatrics Society*.
24. Bunch, T., Weiss, J., Day, J., et al. (2010). Atrial fibrillation is independently associated with senile, vascular, and Alzheimer's dementia. *Heart Rhythm*.
25. Boyle, P., Buchman, A., Wilson, R., et al. (2012). Effect of purpose in life on the relation between Alzheimer disease pathologic changes on cognitive function in advanced age. *Archives of General Psychiatry*.
26. Everson, S., Kaplan, G., & Goldberg, D. (1997). Hopelessness and 4-year progression of carotid atherosclerosis. The Kuopio Ischemic Heart Disease Risk Factor Study. *Arteriosclerosis, Thrombosis, and Vascular Biology*.
27. Shi, M., Wang, X., Bian, Y., & Wang, L. (2015). The mediating role of resilience in the relationship between stress and life satisfaction among Chinese medical students: A cross-sectional study. *BMC Medical Education*.
28. Boyle, P., Barnes, L., Buchman, A., & Bennett, D. A. (2009). Purpose in life is associated with mortality among community-dwelling older persons. *Psychosomatic Medicine*.
29. Koizumi, M., Ito, H., Kaneko, Y., & Motohashi, Y. (2008). Effect of having a sense of purpose in life on the risk of death from cardiovascular diseases. *Journal of Epidemiology*.
30. Lim, A. (2019). Thanos and the population bomb. *IPP Review*.
31. Day, J., Day, J., & LaPlante, M. (2017). *The Longevity Plan: Seven Life-Transforming Lessons from Ancient China*. Harper.

## Chapter Three

1. Bunch, T., May, H., Bair, T., et al. (2013). Increasing time between first diagnosis of atrial fibrillation and catheter ablation adversely affects long-term outcomes. *Heart Rhythm*.
2. O'Connor, A. (February 3, 2015). New York attorney general targets supplements at major retailers. *New York Times*.
3. January, C., Wann, L., Calkins, H., et al. (2019). 2019 AHA/ACC/HRS focused update of the 2014 AHA/ACC/HRS guideline for the management of patients with atrial fibrillation: A report of the American College of Cardiology/American Heart Association Task Force on Clinical Practice Guidelines and the Heart Rhythm Society. *Journal of the American College of Cardiology*.
4. Johnson, D., Day, J., Mahapatra, S., & Bunch, T. (2012). Adverse outcomes from atrial fibrillation: Mechanisms, risks, and insights learned from therapeutic options. *Journal of Atrial Fibrillation*.
5. Gaddum, G. (1956). Gleb Anrep. *Biographical Memoirs of Fellows of the Royal Society*.
6. Fischer, J. & Ganellin, C. (2005). *Analogue-Based Drug Discovery*. John Wiley & Sons.
7. Hudak, J., Banitt, E., & Schmid, J. (1984). Discovery and development of flecainide. *American Journal of Cardiology*.
8. Hodges, M., Haugland, J., Granrud, G., et al. (1982). Suppression of ventricular ectopic depolarizations by flecainide acetate, a new antiarrhythmic agent. *Circulation*.

9. Loring, Z., Holmes, D., Matsouaka, R., Day, J., et al. (pending publication). Get with the guidelines: Atrial fibrillation: Procedural patterns and safety of atrial fibrillation ablation.

10. Frabetti, L., Marchesini, B., Capucci, A., et al. (1986). Antiarrhythmic efficacy of propafenone: Evaluation of effective plasma levels following single and multiple doses. *European Journal of Clinical Pharmacology.*

11. Jones, R., Brace, S., & Vander Tuin, E. (1995). Probable propafenone-induced transient global amnesia. *Annals of Pharmacotherapy.*

12. Reiffel, J., Camm, A., Belardinelli, L., et al. (2015). The HARMONY Trial: Combined ranolazine and dronedarone in the management of paroxysmal atrial fibrillation: Mechanistic and therapeutic synergism. *Circulation: Arrhythmia and Electrophysiology.*

13. Verma, A., Kalman, J., & Callans, D. (2017). Treatment of patients with atrial fibrillation and heart failure with reduced ejection fraction. *Circulation.*

14. Van Gelder, I., Groenveld, H., Crijns, H., et al. (2010). Lenient versus strict rate control in patients with atrial fibrillation. *New England Journal of Medicine.*

15. Lopes, R., Rordorf, R., De Ferrari, G., et al. (2018). Digoxin and mortality in patients with atrial fibrillation. *Journal of the American College of Cardiology.*

16. Currie, G., Wheat, J., & Kiat, H. (2011). Pharmacokinetic considerations for digoxin in older people. *The Open Cardiovascular Medicine Journal.*

17. Jacobs, V., May, H., Bair, T., Day, J., & Bunch, T. (2017). Long-term aspirin does not lower risk of stroke and increases bleeding risk in low-risk atrial fibrillation ablation patients. *Journal of Cardiovascular Electrophysiology.*

18. Healey, J., Connolly, S., Gold, M., et al. (2012). ASSERT Investigators. Subclinical atrial fibrillation and the risk of stroke. *New England Journal of Medicine.*

19. Stahmann, M. & Huebner, C. (1941). Studies on the hemorrhagic sweet clover disease. *Journal of Biological Chemistry.*

20. Aguilar, M. & Hart, R. (2005). Oral anticoagulants for preventing stroke in patients with non-valvular atrial fibrillation and no previous history of stroke or transient ischemic attacks. *Cochrane Database of Systematic Reviews.*

21. Jones, M., McEwan, P., Morgan, C., et al. (2005). Evaluation of the pattern of treatment, level of anticoagulation control, and outcome of treatment with warfarin in patients with non-valvar atrial fibrillation: A record linkage study in a large British population. *Heart.*

22. Pirmohamed, M., James, S., Meakin, S., et al. (2004). Adverse drug reactions as cause of admission to hospital: Prospective analysis of 18 820 patients. *BMJ (Clinical research edition).*

23. Andrews, J., Psaltis, P., Bayturan, O., et al. (2018). Warfarin use is associated with progressive coronary arterial calcification: Insights from serial intravascular ultrasound. *JACC Cardiovascular Imaging*; Gu, Z., Zhou, L., Shen, L., et al. (2018). Non-vitamin K antagonist oral anticoagulants vs. warfarin at risk of fractures: A systematic review and meta-analysis of randomized controlled trials. *Frontiers in Pharmacology.*

24. Ng, K., Shestakovska, O., Connolly, S., et al. (2016). Efficacy and safety of apixaban compared with aspirin in the elderly: A subgroup analysis from the AVERROES trial. *Age and Ageing.*

25. Bunch, T., May, H., Bair, T., et al. (2016). Atrial fibrillation patients treated with long-term warfarin anticoagulation have higher rates of all dementia types compared with patients receiving long-term warfarin for other indications. *Journal of the American Heart Association.*

26. Jacobs, V., May, H., Day, J., et al. (2016). Long-term population-based cerebral ischemic event and cognitive outcomes of direct oral anticoagulants compared with warfarin among long-term anticoagulated patients for atrial fibrillation. *American Journal of Cardiology.*

27. January, C., Wann, L., Calkins, H., et al. (2019). 2019 AHA/ACC/HRS focused update of the 2014 AHA/ACC/HRS guideline for the management of patients with atrial fibrillation: A report of the American College of Cardiology/American Heart Association task force on clinical practice guidelines and the Heart Rhythm Society in collaboration with the Society of Thoracic Surgeons. *Circulation.*

28. Golive, A., May, H., Bair, T., et al. (2017). The population-based long-term impact of anticoag-ulant and antiplatelet therapies in low-risk patients with atrial fibrillation. *American Journal of Cardiology.*

29. Bunch, T., May, H., Bair, T., et al. (2013). Atrial fibrillation ablation patients have long-term stroke rates similar to patients without atrial fibrillation regardless of CHADS2 score. *Heart Rhythm*; Bunch, T., Crandall, B., Weiss, J., et al. (2011). Patients treated with catheter ablation for atrial fibrillation have long-term rates of death, stroke, and dementia similar to patients without atrial fibrillation. *Journal of Cardiovascular Electrophysiology.*

30. Bhatt, A. & Jani, V. (2011). The ABCD and ABCD2 scores and the risk of stroke following a TIA: A narrative review. *ISRN Neurology*; Fox, K., Lucas, J., Pieper, K., et al. (2017). Improved risk stratification of patients with atrial fibrillation: An integrated GARFIELD-AF tool for the predic-tion of mortality, stroke and bleed in patients with and without anticoagulation. *BMJ Open.*

31. Graves, K., May, H., Knowlton, K., et al. (2018). Improving CHA 2 DS 2-VASc stratification of non-fatal stroke and mortality risk using the Intermountain Mortality Risk Score among patients with atrial fibrillation. *Open Heart.*

32. Granger, C., Alexander, J., McMurray, J., et al. (2011). Apixaban versus warfarin in patients with atrial fibrillation. *New England Journal of Medicine.*

33. Golive, A., May, H., Bair, T., et al. (2017). The population-based long-term impact of anticoag-ulant and antiplatelet therapies in low-risk patients with atrial fibrillation. *American Journal of Cardiology.*

34. Lip, G. (2011). Implications of the CHA2DS2-VASc and HAS-BLED scores for thromboprophy-laxis in atrial fibrillation. *The American Journal of Medicine.*

35. Anter, E., Jessup, M., & Callans, D. (2009). Atrial fibrillation and heart failure: Treatment consid-erations for a dual epidemic. *Circulation.*

36. Schmiegelow, M., Pedersen, O., Køber, L., et al. (2011). Incidence of atrial fibrillation in patients with either heart failure or acute myocardial infarction and left ventricular dysfunction: A cohort study. *BMC Cardiovascular Disorders.*

37. DiNicolantonio, J., O'Keefe, J., & Wilson, W. (2018). Subclinical magnesium deficiency: A prin-cipal driver of cardiovascular disease and a public health crisis. *Open Heart.*

38. Khan, A., Lubitz, S., Sullivan, L., et al. (2012). Low serum magnesium and the development of atrial fibrillation in the community: The Framingham Heart Study. *Circulation.*

39. Bara, M., Guiet-Bara, A., & Durlach, J. (1993). Regulation of sodium and potassium pathways by magnesium in cell membranes. *Magnesium Research.*

40. Ho, K., Sheridan, D., & Paterson, T. (2007). Use of intravenous magnesium to treat acute onset atrial fibrillation: A meta-analysis. *Heart.*

41. Ho, K., Sheridan, D., & Paterson, T. (2007). Use of intravenous magnesium to treat acute onset atrial fibrillation: A meta-analysis. *Heart.*

42. Abbasi, B., Kimiagar, M., Sadeghniiat, K., et al. (2012). The effect of magnesium supplementation on primary insomnia in elderly: A double-blind placebo-controlled clinical trial. *Journal of Research in Medical Sciences: The Official Journal of Isfahan University of Medical Sciences.*

43. Krijthe, B., Heeringa, J., Kors, J., et al. (2013). Serum potassium levels and the risk of atrial fibril-lation: The Rotterdam Study. *International Journal of Cardiology.*

44. Chen, H., McGowan, E., Ren, N., et al. (2018). Nattokinase: A promising alternative in preven-tion and treatment of cardiovascular diseases. *Biomark Insights.*

45. Smith, M., Christensen, N., Wang, S., et al. (2010). Warfarin knowledge in patients with atrial fibrillation: Implications for safety, efficacy, and education strategies. *Cardiology.*

46. Thompson, J., Nitiahpapand, R., Bhatti, P., et al. (2015). Vitamin D deficiency and atrial fibrilla-tion. *International Journal of Cardiology.*

47. Smith, M., May, H., Bair, T., et al. (2011). Abstract 14699: Vitamin D excess is significantly asso-ciated with risk of atrial fibrillation. *Circulation.*

48. Martino, A., Pezzi, L., Magnano, R., et al. (2016). Omega 3 and atrial fibrillation: Where are we? *World Journal of Cardiology.*
49. Sharma, A., Fonarow, G., Butler, J., et al. (2016). Coenzyme Q10 and heart failure. *Circulation: Heart Failure.*
50. Deichmann, R., Lavie, C., & Andrews, S. (2010). Coenzyme Q10 and statin-induced mitochondrial dysfunction. *Ochsner Journal.*
51. Zhao, Q., Kebbati, A., Zhang, Y., et al. (2015). Effect of coenzyme Q10 on the incidence of atrial fibrillation in patients with heart failure. *Journal of Investigative Medicine: The Official Publication of the American Federation for Clinical Research.*
52. Dastan, F., Talasaz, A., Mojtahedzadeh, M., et al. (2017). Randomized trial of carnitine for the prevention of perioperative atrial fibrillation. *Seminars in Thoracic and Cardiovascular Surgery.*
53. DiNicolantonio, J., Lavie, C., Fares, H., et al. (2013). L-carnitine in the secondary prevention of cardiovascular disease: Systematic review and meta-analysis. *Mayo Clinic Proceedings.*
54. Vallance, H. D., Koochin, A., Rosen-Heath, A., et al. (2018). Marked elevation in plasma trimethylamine-N-oxide (TMAO) in patients with mitochondrial disorders treated with oral L-carnitine. *Molecular Genetics and Metabolism Reports.*
55. Tang, W. H., Wang, Z., Levison, B., et al. (2013). Intestinal microbial metabolism of phosphatidylcholine and cardiovascular risk. *New England Journal of Medicine*; Svingen, G., Zuo, H., Ueland, P., et al. (2018). Increased plasma trimethylamine-N-oxide is associated with incident atrial fibrillation. *International Journal of Cardiology.*
56. Ballegooijen, A. J. & Beulens, J. W. (2017). The role of vitamin K status in cardiovascular health: Evidence from observational and clinical studies. *Current Nutrition Reports.*
57. Nagata, C., Wada, K., Tamura, T., et al. (2016). Dietary soy and natto intake and cardiovascular disease mortality in Japanese adults: The Takayama Study. *The American Journal of Clinical Nutrition.*
58. Holubarsch, C., Colucci, W., Meinertz, T., et al. (2008). The efficacy and safety of Crataegus extract WS 1442 in patients with heart failure: The SPICE Trial. *European Journal of Heart Failure.*
59. Müller, A., Linke, W., & Klaus, W. (1999). Crataegus extract blocks potassium currents in guinea pig ventricular cardiac myocytes. *Planta Medica.*
60. Ewing, L., Skinner, C., Quick, C., et al. (2019). Hepatotoxicity of a cannabidiol-rich cannabis extract in the mouse model. *Molecules.*

## Chapter Four

1. Hulka, B., Wilcosky, T., & Griffith, J. (1990). *Biological Markers in Epidemiology.* Oxford University Press.
2. FDA-NIH Biomarker Working Group. (2016). *BEST (Biomarkers, EndpointS, and other Tools) Resource.* US Food and Drug Administration.
3. Morel, C., McClure, L., & Edwards S., et al. (2016). *Ensuring innovation in diagnostics for bacterial infection: Implications for policy.* European Observatory on Health Systems and Policies.
4. Crandall, M., Horne, D., Day, J., et al. (2009). Atrial fibrillation and CHADS2 risk factors are associated with highly sensitive C-reactive protein incrementally and independently. *Pacing and Clinical Electrophysiology.*
5. Harada, M., Van Wagoner, D., & Nattel, S. (2015). Role of inflammation in atrial fibrillation pathophysiology and management. *Circulation Journal: Official Journal of the Japanese Circulation Society.*
6. Sanches, F., Avesani, C., Kamimura, M., et al. (2008). Waist circumference and visceral fat in CKD: A cross-sectional study. *American Journal of Kidney Disease.*

7. Baek, Y., Yang, P., Kim, T., et al. (2017). Associations of abdominal obesity and new-onset atrial fibrillation in the general population. *Journal of the American Heart Association*.

8. Bohne, L., Johnson, D., Rose, R., et al. (2019). The association between diabetes mellitus and atrial fibrillation: Clinical and mechanistic insights. *Frontiers in Physiology*.

9. Dublin, S., Glazer, N., Smith, N., et al. (2010). Diabetes mellitus, glycemic control, and risk of atrial fibrillation. *Journal of General Internal Medicine*; Benjamin, E., Levy, D., Vaziri, S., et al. (1994). Independent risk factors for atrial fibrillation in a population-based cohort: The Framingham heart study. *JAMA*.

10. Saito, S., Teshima, Y., Fukui, A., et al. (2014). Glucose fluctuations increase the incidence of atrial fibrillation in diabetic rats. *Cardiovascular Research*.

11. Sun, Y. & Hu, D. (2010). The link between diabetes and atrial fibrillation: Cause or correlation? *Journal of Cardiovascular Disease Research*.

12. Rutter, M., Parise, H., Benjamin, E., et al. (2003). Impact of glucose intolerance and insulin resistance on cardiac structure and function: Sex-related differences in the Framingham heart study. *Circulation*.

13. Schmid, H., Forman, L., Cao, X., et al. (1999). Heterogeneous cardiac sympathetic denervation and decreased myocardial nerve growth factor in streptozotocin-induced diabetic rats: Implications for cardiac sympathetic dysinnervation complicating diabetes. *Diabetes*.

14. Fangel, M., Nielsen, P., Kristensen, J., et al. (2019). Glycemic status and thromboembolic risk in patients with atrial fibrillation and type 2 diabetes mellitus. *Circulation. Arrhythmia and Electrophysiology*.

15. Hall, S., Shackelton, R., Rosen, R., & Araujo, A. (2010). Sexual activity, erectile dysfunction, and incident cardiovascular events. *The American Journal of Cardiology*.

16. Hijioka, N., Kamioka, M., Matsumoto, Y., et al. (2019). Clinical impact of insulin resistance on pulmonary vein isolation outcome in patients with paroxysmal atrial fibrillation. *Journal of Cardiovascular Electrophysiology*.

17. Nakamoto, K. (1965). Psychogenic paroxysmal cardiac arrhythmias. Contents of mental events, age and patterns of arrhythmias. *Japanese Circulation Journal*.

18. Traube, E. & Coplan, N. (2011). Embolic risk in atrial fibrillation that arises from hyperthyroidism. *Texas Heart Institute Journal*.

19. Zhang, Y., Dedkov, E. I., Teplitsky, D., et al. (2013). Both hypothyroidism and hyperthyroidism increase atrial fibrillation inducibility in rats. *Circulation: Arrhythmia and Electrophysiology*.

20. Kolettis, T. M. & Tsatsoulis, A. (2012). Subclinical hypothyroidism: An overlooked cause of atrial fibrillation? *Journal of Atrial Fibrillation*; Sawin, C. (2002). Subclinical hyperthyroidism and atrial fibrillation. *Thyroid*.

21. Anderson, J., Jacobs, V., May, H., et al. (2019). Free thyroxine within the normal reference range predicts risk of atrial fibrillation. *Journal of Cardiovascular Electrophysiology*.

22. Intermountain Healthcare. (November 10, 2018). New Intermountain study shows overtreating patients for hypothyroidism could raise their risk of stroke. *Intermountain Healthcare*.

23. Pearce, E. (2014). Is iodine deficiency reemerging in the United States? *AACE Journals*.

24. Rosenthal, E. (June 2, 2012). Let's (not) get physicals. *New York Times*.

25. The normal/healthy ranges for all of the CMP biomarkers in this section come from a convenient chart published by the International Waldenstrom's Macroglobulinemia Foundation, a patient-founded and patient-led nonprofit organization dedicated to supporting individuals affected by Waldenstrom's macroglobulinemia and to advancing the search for a cure. List accessed on May 31, 2020, at https://www.iwmf.com/sites/default/files/docs/bloodcharts_cmp(1).pdf.

26. Krijthe, B., Heeringa, J., Kors, J., et al. (2013). Serum potassium levels and the risk of atrial fibrillation: The Rotterdam Study. *International Journal of Cardiology*.

27. Khan, A., Lubitz, S., Sullivan, L., et al. (2012). Low serum magnesium and the development of atrial fibrillation in the community: The Framingham Heart Study. *Circulation*.

28. Dibaba, D., Xun, P., & He, K. (2014). Dietary magnesium intake is inversely associated with serum C-reactive protein levels: Meta-analysis and systematic review. *European Journal of Clinical Nutrition*.

29. Rosanoff, A. (2005). Magnesium and hypertension. *Clinical Calcium*.

30. Franczyk, B., Gluba-Brzózka, A., Ciałkowska-Rysz, A., et al. (2016). The problem of atrial fibrillation in patients with chronic kidney disease. *Current Vascular Pharmacology*.

31. Makar, G., Weiner, M., Kimmel, S., et al. (2008). Incidence and prevalence of abnormal liver associated enzymes in patients with atrial fibrillation in a routine clinical care population. *Pharmacoepidemiology and drug safety*.

32. Alonso, A., Ying, X., Roetker, N., et al. (2014). Blood lipids and the incidence of atrial fibrillation: The Multi-Ethnic Study of Atherosclerosis and the Framingham Heart Study. *Journal of the American Heart Association*.

33. Qi, Z., Chen, H., Wen, Z., et al. (2017). Relation of low-density lipoprotein cholesterol to ischemic stroke in patients with nonvalvular atrial fibrillation. *The American Journal of Cardiology*.

34. Cunha, K., Frinchaboy, P., Souto, D., et al. (2016). Chemical abundance gradients from open clusters in the Milky Way disk: Results from the APOGEE survey. *Astronomische Nachrichten*.

35. Zhang, Z., Yang, Y., Ng, C., et al. (2016). Meta-analysis of vitamin D deficiency and risk of atrial fibrillation. *Clinical Cardiology*.

36. Thompson, J., Nitiahpapand, R., Bhatti, P., & Kourliouros, A. (2015). Vitamin D deficiency and atrial fibrillation. *International Journal of Cardiology*.

37. Smith, M., May, H., Bair, T., et al. (2011). Vitamin D excess is significantly associated with risk of atrial fibrillation. *Circulation*.

38. Buxbaum, J. & Furgerson, W. (1970). Atrial fibrillation in severe anemia. *JAMA*.

39. Puurunen, M., Kiviniemi, T., Nammas, W., et al. (2014). Impact of anaemia on clinical outcome in patients with atrial fibrillation undergoing percutaneous coronary intervention: Insights from the AFCAS registry. *BMJ Open*.

40. Horne, B., Muhlestein, J., Bennett, S., et al. (2018). Extreme erythrocyte macrocytic and microcytic percentages are highly predictive of morbidity and mortality. *JCI Insight*.

41. Mikkelsen, L., Nordestgaard, B., Schnohr, P., et al. (2019). Increased ferritin concentration and risk of atrial fibrillation and heart failure in men and women: Three studies of the Danish general population including 35799 individuals. *Clinical Chemistry*; Lowe, G. D., Jaap, A. J., & Forbes, C. D. (1983). Relation of atrial fibrillation and high haematocrit to mortality in acute stroke. *Lancet*.

42. Naji, F., Suran, D., Kanic, V., et al. (2010). High homocysteine levels predict the recurrence of atrial fibrillation after successful electrical cardioversion. *International Heart Journal*.

43. Zhang, C., Cai, Y., Adachi, M. T., et al. (2001). Homocysteine induces programmed cell death in human vascular endothelial cells through activation of the unfolded protein response. *Journal of Biological Chemistry*.

44. Marcus, J., Sarnak, M., & Menon, V. (2007). Homocysteine lowering and cardiovascular disease risk: Lost in translation. *Canadian Journal of Cardiology*.

45. Weber, M. & Hamm, C. (2006). Role of B-type natriuretic peptide (BNP) and NT-proBNP in clinical routine. *Heart (British Cardiac Society)*.

46. Hijazi, Z., Lindbäck, J., Alexander, J., et al. (2016). The ABC (age, biomarkers, clinical history) stroke risk score: A biomarker-based risk score for predicting stroke in atrial fibrillation. *European Heart Journal*.

47. McCarthy, C., Yousuf, O., Alonso, A., et al. (2017). High-sensitivity troponin as a biomarker in heart rhythm disease. *American Journal of Cardiology*.

48. Sollaci, L. B. & Pereira, M. G. (2004). The introduction, methods, results, and discussion (IMRAD) structure: A fifty-year survey. *Journal of the Medical Library Association*.

## Chapter Five

1. Spaeth, A., Dinges, D., & Goel, N. (2013). Effects of experimental sleep restriction on weight gain, caloric intake, and meal timing in healthy adults. *Sleep.*
2. Genuardi, M., Ogilvie, R., Saand, A., et al. (2019). Association of short sleep duration and atrial fibrillation. *CHEST.*
3. National Sleep Foundation (2018). 2018 Sleep in America poll: Sleep prioritization and personal effectiveness. *Sleep Health: Journal of the National Sleep Foundation.*
4. Kayrak, M., Gul, E., Aribas, A., et al. (2013). Self-reported sleep quality of patients with atrial fibrillation and the effects of cardioversion on sleep quality. *Pacing and Clinical Electrophysiology.*
5. National Sleep Foundation (2014). 2014 Sleep in America poll: Sleep in the modern family. *Sleep Health: Journal of the National Sleep Foundation.*
6. Tassa, P. & Muzet, A. (2000). Sleep inertia. *Sleep Medicine Review.*
7. Gooley, J., Chamberlain, K., Smith, K., et al. (2011). Exposure to room light before bedtime suppresses melatonin onset and shortens melatonin duration in humans. *Journal of Clinical Endocrinology and Metabolism.*
8. Gooley, J., Rajaratnam, S., Brainard, G., et al. (2010). Spectral responses of the human circadian system depend on the irradiance and duration of exposure to light. *Science Translational Medicine.*
9. National Sleep Foundation (2014). 2014 Sleep in America poll: Sleep in the modern family. *Sleep Health: Journal of the National Sleep Foundation.*
10. Kennedy, M. (December 24, 2015). How do successful people's sleep patterns compare to the average American? NPR.org.
11. Burkhart, K. & Phelps, J. (2009). Amber lenses to block blue light and improve sleep: A randomized trial. *Chronobiology International.*
12. Cornelius, M., El-Sohemy, A., Kabagambe, E., & Campos, H. (2006). Coffee, CYP1A2 genotype, and risk of myocardial infarction. *JAMA.*
13. Yang, A., Palmer, A., & de Wit, H. (2010). Genetics of caffeine consumption and responses to caffeine. *Psychopharmacology.*
14. Cornelius, M., et al. (2006).
15. Stone, B. (1980). Sleep and low doses of alcohol. *Electroencephalography and Clinical Neurophysiology.*
16. Colrain, I., Nicholas, C., & Baker, F. (2014). Alcohol and the sleeping brain. *Handbook of Clinical Neurology.*
17. Christensen, M., Dixit, S., Dewland, T., et al. (2018). Sleep characteristics that predict atrial fibrillation. *Heart Rhythm.*
18. GBD 2016 Alcohol Collaborators (2018). Alcohol use and burden for 195 countries and territories, 1990–2016: A systematic analysis for the Global Burden of Disease Study 2016. *Lancet.*
19. Larsson, S., Drca, N., & Wolk, A. (2014). Alcohol consumption and risk of atrial fibrillation: A prospective study and dose-response meta-analysis. *Journal of the American College of Cardiology.*
20. Voskoboinik, A., Kalman, J., De Silva, A., et al. (2020). Alcohol abstinence in drinkers with atrial fibrillation. *New England Journal of Medicine.*
21. Haghayegh, S., Khoshnevis, S., Smolensky, M., et al. (2019). Before-bedtime passive body heating by warm shower or bath to improve sleep: A systematic review and meta-analysis. *Sleep Medicine Reviews.*
22. Nam, S. & Stewart, K. Research presented at the American Heart Association Scientific Sessions on November 6, 2012: Predictors of sleep quality improvement among overweight or obese individuals: a randomized controlled trial.
23. Dopp, J., Reichmuth, K., & Morgan, B. (2007). Obstructive sleep apnea and hypertension: Mechanisms, evaluation, and management. *Current Hypertension Reports.*
24. Lin, C., Davidson, T., & Ancoli-Israel, S. (2008). Gender differences in obstructive sleep apnea and treatment implications. *Sleep Medicine Reviews.*

25. Deng, F., Raza, A., & Guo, J. (2018). Treating obstructive sleep apnea with continuous positive airway pressure reduces risk of recurrent atrial fibrillation after catheter ablation: A meta-analysis. *Sleep Medicine.*

26. Abbasi, B., Kimiagar, M., Sadeghniiat, K., et al. (2012). The effect of magnesium supplementation on primary insomnia in elderly: A double-blind placebo-controlled clinical trial. *Journal of Research in Medical Sciences.*

27. Dolezal, B., Neufeld, E., Boland, D., et al. (2017). Interrelationship between sleep and exercise: A systematic review. *Advances in Preventive Medicine.*

28. National Sleep Foundation. *How Exercise Impacts Sleep Quality.* https://www.sleepfoundation.org /articles/how-exercise-impacts-sleep-quality.

29. Jin, P. (1992). Efficacy of tai chi, brisk walking, meditation, and reading in reducing mental and emotional stress. *Journal of Psychosomatic Research.*

30. Grønli, J., Byrkjedal, I., & Bjorvatn, B. (2016). Reading from an iPad or from a book in bed: The impact on human sleep. A randomized controlled crossover trial. *Sleep Medicine.*

31. Stunkard, A. & McLaren-Hume, M. (1959). The results of treatment for obesity: A review of the literature and report of a series. *American Medical Association Archives of Internal Medicine.*

32. Mann, T., Tomiyama, A. J., Westling, E., et al. (2007). Medicare's search for effective obesity treatments: Diets are not the answer. *The American Psychologist.*

33. Jamaly, S., Carlsson, L., Peltonen, M., et al. (2016). Bariatric surgery and the risk of new-onset atrial fibrillation in Swedish obese subjects. *Journal of the American College of Cardiology.*

34. Donnellan, E., Wazni, O., Kanj, M., et al. (2019). Outcomes of atrial fibrillation ablation in morbidly obese patients following bariatric surgery compared with a nonobese cohort. *Circulation: Arrhythmia and Electrophysiology.*

35. Lindeberg, S., Jonsson, T., Granfeldt, Y., et al. (2007). Palaeolithic diet improves glucose tolerance more than a Mediterranean-like diet in individuals with ischaemic heart disease. *Diabetologia*; Dashti, H., Mathew, T., Hussein, T., et al. (2004). Long-term effects of a ketogenic diet in obese patients. *Experimental & Clinical Cardiology.*

36. Dill-McFarland, K., Tang, Z., Kemis, J., et al. (2019). Close social relationships correlate with human gut microbiota composition. *Scientific Reports.*

37. Hill, J., Wyatt, H., Phelan, S., & Wing, R. (2005). The National Weight Control Registry: Is it useful in helping deal with our obesity epidemic? *Journal of Nutritional Educational Behavior.*

38. Kaviani, S., vanDellen, M., & Cooper, J. (2019). Daily self-weighing to prevent holiday-associated weight gain in adults. *Obesity.*

39. The Obesity Society. (May 23, 2019). New strategy for preventing holiday weight gain. *ScienceDaily.*

40. Bunch, T., May, H., Bair, T., et al. (2016). Long-term influence of body mass index on cardiovascular events after atrial fibrillation ablation. *Journal of Interventional Cardiac Electrophysiology.*

41. Bunch, T., et al. (2016). Long-term influence of body mass index.

42. Lee, H., Choi, E., Han, K., et al. (2019). Bodyweight fluctuation is associated with increased risk of incident atrial fibrillation. *Heart Rhythm.*

43. Donnelly, J., Blair, S., Jakicic, J., et al. (2009). Appropriate physical activity intervention strategies for weight loss and prevention of weight regain for adults. *Medicine & Science in Sports & Exercise.*

44. Franz, M., VanWormer, J., Crain, A., et al. (2007). Weight-loss outcomes: A systematic review and meta-analysis of weight-loss clinical trials with a minimum 1-year follow-up. *Journal of the American Dietetic Association.*

45. Catenacci, V., Ogden, L., Stuht, J., et al. (2008). Physical activity patterns in the National Weight Control Registry. *Obesity.*

46. Catenacci, V., et al. (2008).

47. Lee, I., Shiroma, E., Kamada, M., et al. (2019). Association of step volume and intensity with all-cause mortality in older women. *JAMA Internal Medicine.*

48. Lee, D., Pate, R., Lavie, C., et al. (2014). Leisure-time running reduces all-cause and cardiovascular mortality risk. *Journal of the American College of Cardiology.*

49. Fothergill, E., Guo, J., Howard, L., et al. (2016). Persistent metabolic adaptation 6 years after "The Biggest Loser" competition. *Obesity.*

50. American College of Cardiology. (March 7, 2019). E-cigarettes linked to heart attacks, coronary artery disease and depression. *American College of Cardiology.*

51. Office of the United States Surgeon General. (1988). *The Health Consequences of Smoking: Nicotine Addiction.*

52. Richardson, S., Shaffer, J., Falzon, L., et al. (2012). Meta-analysis of perceived stress and its association with incident coronary heart disease. *The American Journal of Cardiology.*

53. Epel, E., Blackburn, E., Lin, J., et al. (2004). Accelerated telomere shortening in response to life stress. *Proceedings of the National Academy of Sciences of the United States of America.*

54. Lampert, R., Jamner, L., Burg, M., et al. (2014). Triggering of symptomatic atrial fibrillation by negative emotion. *Journal of the American College of Cardiology.*

55. Fransson, E., Nordin, M., Magnusson Hanson, L., & Westerlund, H. (2018). Job strain and atrial fibrillation—results from the Swedish Longitudinal Occupational Survey of Health and meta-analysis of three studies. *European Journal of Preventive Cardiology.*

56. Mishel, L. (2018). *Uber and the Labor Market: Uber Drivers' Compensation, Wages, and the Scale of Uber and the Gig Economy.* Economic Policy Institute.

57. Johnston, W. & Davey, G. (1997). The psychological impact of negative TV news bulletins: The catastrophizing of personal worries. *British Journal of Psychology.*

58. Schneiderman, N., Ironson, G., & Siegel, S. (2005). Stress and health: Psychological, behavioral, and biological determinants. *Annual Review of Clinical Psychology.*

59. Shusterman, V. & Lampert, R. (2013). Role of stress in cardiac arrhythmias. *Journal of Atrial Fibrillation.*

60. Lampert, R., Burg, M., Brandt, C., et al. (2008). Impact of emotions on triggering of atrial fibrillation. *Circulation.*

61. Mirer, M., Duncan, M., & Wagner, M. (2018). Taking it from the team: Assessments of bias and credibility in team-operated sports media. *Newspaper Research Journal.*

62. Shaer, M. (April 2014). What emotion goes viral the fastest? *Smithsonian Magazine.*

63. Fierberg, E. (January 10, 2018). I quit social media for a month—and it was the best choice I've ever made. *Business Insider.*

64. Lampert, R., Jamner, L., Burg, M., et al. (2014). Triggering of symptomatic atrial fibrillation by negative emotion. *Journal of the American College of Cardiology.*

65. Keller, A., Litzelman, K., Wisk, L., et al. (2012). Does the perception that stress affects health matter? The association with health and mortality. *Health Psychology.*

66. O'Neal, W., Qureshi, W., Judd, S., et al. (2015). Perceived stress and atrial fibrillation: The reasons for geographic and racial differences in stroke study. *Annals of Behavioral Medicine.*

67. Lakkireddy, D., Atkins, D., & Pillarisetti, J. (2013). Effect of yoga on arrhythmia burden, anxiety, depression, and quality of life in paroxysmal atrial fibrillation: The YOGA My Heart Study. *Journal of the American College of Cardiology.*

## Chapter Six

1. Davies, M. & Hollman, A. (2002). Werner Forssmann. *Heart.*

2. Sugumar, H., Prabhu, S., Voskoboinik, A., et al. (2019). Atrial remodeling following catheter ablation for atrial fibrillation-mediated cardiomyopathy: Long-term follow-up of CAMERA-MRI study. *JACC: Clinical Electrophysiology.*

3. Kuck, K., Brugada, J., Fürnkranz, A., et al. (2016). Cryoballoon or radiofrequency ablation for paroxysmal atrial fibrillation. *New England Journal of Medicine.*

4. Reddy, V., Neuzil, P., Koruth, J., et al. (2019). Pulsed field ablation for pulmonary vein isolation in atrial fibrillation. *Journal of the American College of Cardiology*.

5. Zei, P. & Soltys, S. (2017). Ablative radiotherapy as a noninvasive alternative to catheter ablation for cardiac arrhythmias. *Current Cardiology Reports*.

6. Haldar, S., Kahn, H. R., Boyalla, V., et al. (2020). Catheter ablation vs. thoracoscopic surgical ablation in long-standing persistent atrial fibrillation: CASA-AF randomized controlled trial. *European Heart Journal*.

7. Swaans, M., Post, M., Rensing, B., et al. (2012). Ablation for atrial fibrillation in combination with left atrial appendage closure: First results of a feasibility study. *Journal of the American Heart Association*.

8. Bunch, T. & Day, J. (2017). Is left atrial appendage isolation a pyrrhic victory in the effort to treat atrial fibrillation? *Journal of Thoracic Disease*.

9. Hrabia, J., Pogue, E., Zayachkowski, A., et al. (2018). Left atrial compliance: An overlooked predictor of clinical outcome in patients with mitral stenosis or atrial fibrillation undergoing invasive management. *Advances in Interventional Cardiology/Postępy w Kardiologii Interwencyjnej*.

10. Lee, C., Kim, J., Jung, S., et al. (2014). Left atrial appendage resection versus preservation during the surgical ablation of atrial fibrillation. *Annals of Thoracic Surgery*.

11. Wilber, D. (2018). Neurohormonal regulation and the left atrial appendage: Still more to learn. *Journal of the American College of Cardiology*.

12. Gramlich, M., Maleck, C., Marquardt, J., et al. (2019). Cryoballoon ablation for persistent atrial fibrillation in patients without left atrial fibrosis. *Journal of Cardiovascular Electrophysiology*.

13. Verma, A., Jiang, C., Betts, T., et al. (2015). Approaches to catheter ablation for persistent atrial fibrillation. *New England Journal of Medicine*.

14. Thiyagarajah, A., Kadhim, K., Lau, D., et al. (2019). Feasibility, safety, and efficacy of posterior wall isolation during atrial fibrillation ablation. *Circulation: Arrhythmia and Electrophysiology*; Sutter, J., Lokhnygina, Y., Daubert, J., et al. (2019). Safety and efficacy outcomes of left atrial posterior wall isolation compared to pulmonary vein isolation and pulmonary vein isolation with linear ablation for the treatment of persistent atrial fibrillation. *American Heart Journal*.

15. Sugumar, H., Prabhu, S., Voskoboinik, A., et al. (2019). Atrial remodeling following catheter ablation for atrial fibrillation-mediated cardiomyopathy: Long-term follow-up of CAMERA-MRI study. *JACC: Clinical Electrophysiology*.

16. Bunch, T., Crandall, B., Weiss, J., et al. (2011). Patients treated with catheter ablation for atrial fibrillation have long-term rates of death, stroke, and dementia similar to patients without atrial fibrillation. *Journal of Cardiovascular Electrophysiology*.

17. Park, J., Yang, P., Bae, H., et al. (2019). Five-year change in the renal function after catheter ablation of atrial fibrillation. *Journal of the American Heart Association*.

18. Marrouche, N., Brachmann, J., Andresen, D., et al. (2018). Catheter ablation for atrial fibrillation with heart failure. *New England Journal of Medicine*.

19. Packer, D., Mark, D., Robb, R., et al. (2019). Effect of catheter ablation vs antiarrhythmic drug therapy on mortality, stroke, bleeding, and cardiac arrest among patients with atrial fibrillation: The CABANA Randomized Clinical Trial. *JAMA*.

20. Kirchhof, P., Camm, A. J., Goette, A., et al. (2020). Early rhythm-control therapy in patients with atrial fibrillation. *New England Journal of Medicine*.

21. Shah, S., Moosa, P., Fatima, M., et al. (2018). Atrial fibrillation and heart failure—results of the CASTLE-AF trial. *Journal of Community Hospital Internal Medicine Perspectives*.

22. Wilson, D. (March 17, 2009). Fix a health problem or live with it? *New York Times*.

23. Darby, A. E. (2016). Recurrent atrial fibrillation after catheter ablation: Considerations for repeat ablation and strategies to optimize success. *Journal of Atrial Fibrillation*.

24. Silva, M., Kilpatrick, N., & Craig, J. (2019). Genetic and early-life environmental influences on dental caries risk: A twin study. *Pediatrics*.

25. Bunch, T., May, H., Bair, T., et al. (2013). Increasing time between first diagnosis of atrial fibrillation and catheter ablation adversely affects long-term outcomes. *Heart Rhythm*.

26. Bunch, T. & Day, J. (2015). Adverse remodeling of the left atrium in patients with atrial fibrillation: When is the tipping point in which structural changes become permanent? *Journal of Cardiovascular Electrophysiology.*

27. Kirchhof, P., Camm, A. J., Goette, A., et al. (2020). Early rhythm-control therapy in patients with atrial fibrillation. *The New England Journal of Medicine.*

28. Packer, D., Mark, D., Robb, R., et al. (2019). Effect of catheter ablation vs antiarrhythmic drug therapy on mortality, stroke, bleeding, and cardiac arrest among patients with atrial fibrillation: The CABANA Randomized Clinical Trial. *JAMA.*

29. Bunch, T., May, H., Bair, T., et al. (2015). The impact of age on 5-year outcomes after atrial fibrillation catheter ablation. *Journal of Cardiovascular Electrophysiology.*

30. Chelu, M., King, J., Kholmovski, E., et al. (2018). Atrial fibrosis by late gadolinium enhancement magnetic resonance imaging and catheter ablation of atrial fibrillation: 5-year follow-up data. *Journal of the American Heart Association*; Jiang, P., Yang, F., Wu, J., et al. (2018). Left atrial low-voltage areas: A powerful predictor in paroxysmal atrial fibrillation recurrence after catheter ablation? *International Journal of Cardiology.*

31. Kornej, J., Hindricks, G., Shoemaker, M., et al. (2015). The APPLE score: A novel and simple score for the prediction of rhythm outcomes after catheter ablation of atrial fibrillation. *Clinical Research in Cardiology: Official Journal of the German Cardiac Society.*

32. Kornej, J., et al. (2015).

33. Calkins, H., Hindricks, G., Cappato, R., et al. (2017). 2017 HRS/EHRA/ECAS/APHRS/SOLAECE expert consensus statement on catheter and surgical ablation of atrial fibrillation. *Heart Rhythm.*

34. Deshmukh, A., Patel, N., Pant, S., et al. (2013). In-hospital complications associated with catheter ablation of atrial fibrillation in the United States between 2000 and 2010: Analysis of 93801 procedures. *Circulation.*

35. Williamson, A. & Feyer, A. (2000). Moderate sleep deprivation produces impairments in cognitive and motor performance equivalent to legally prescribed levels of alcohol intoxication. *Occupational and Environmental Medicine.*

36. Wright, M., Phillips-Bute, B., Mark, J., et al. (2006). Time of day effects on the incidence of anesthetic adverse events. *Quality & Safety in Health Care.*

37. Smith, T., Darling, E., & Searles, B. (2011). 2010 survey on cell phone use while performing cardiopulmonary bypass. *Perfusion.*

38. De Pooter, J., Strisciuglio, T., El Haddad, M., et al. (2019). Pulmonary vein reconnection no longer occurs in the majority of patients after a single pulmonary vein isolation procedure. *JACC: Clinical Electrophysiology.*

39. Hendriks, J., Tieleman, R., Vrijhoef, H., et al. (2019). Integrated specialized atrial fibrillation clinics reduce all-cause mortality: Post hoc analysis of a randomized clinical trial. *EP Europace.*

40. Malasana, G., Day, J., Weiss, J., et al. (2011). A strategy of rapid cardioversion minimizes the significance of early recurrent atrial tachyarrhythmias after ablation for atrial fibrillation. *Journal of Cardiovascular Electrophysiology.*

## Chapter Seven

1. Piccini, J., Allred, J., Bunch, T., et al. (2020). HRS white paper on atrial fibrillation centers of excellence: Rationale, considerations, and goals. *Heart Rhythm.*

2. Hendriks, J., Tieleman, R., Vrijhoef, H., et al. (2019). Integrated specialized atrial fibrillation clinics reduce all-cause mortality: *Post hoc* analysis of a randomized clinical trial. *EP Europace.*

3. Jani, B., Nicholl, B., McQueenie, R., et al. (2017). Multimorbidity and co-morbidity in atrial fibrillation and effects on survival: Findings from UK Biobank cohort. *EP Europace.*

4. Avery, A., Langley-Evans, S., Harrington, M., & Swift, J. (2016). Setting targets leads to greater long-term weight losses and "unrealistic" targets increase the effect in a large community-based

commercial weight management group. *Journal of Human Nutrition and Dietetics*; DeWalt, D., Davis, T., Wallace, A., et al. (2009). Goal setting in diabetes self-management: Taking the baby steps to success. *Patient Education and Counseling*.

5. Aliot, E., Capucci, A., Crijns, H., et al. (2011). Twenty-five years in the making: Flecainide is safe and effective for the management of atrial fibrillation. *Europace*.

6. Graudal, N., Galløe, A., Garred, P., et al. (1998). Effects of sodium restriction on blood pressure, renin, aldosterone, catecholamines, cholesterols, and triglyceride: A meta-analysis. *JAMA*.

7. DiNicolantonio, J. & Lucan, S. (2014). The wrong white crystals: Not salt but sugar as aetiological in hypertension and cardiometabolic disease. *Open Heart*.

8. Arroll, B. & Beaglehole, R. (1992). Does physical activity lower blood pressure: A critical review of the clinical trials. *Journal of Clinical Epidemiology*.

9. Siebenhofer, A., Jeitler, K., Berghold, A., et al. (2011). Long-term effects of weight-reducing diets in hypertensive patients. *The Cochrane Database of Systematic Reviews*.

10. Whelton, S., Hyre, A., Pedersen, B., et al. (2005). Effect of dietary fiber intake on blood pressure: A meta-analysis of randomized, controlled clinical trials. *Journal of Hypertension*.

11. Appel, L., Moore, T., Obarzanek, E., et al. (1997). A clinical trial of the effects of dietary patterns on blood pressure. *New England Journal of Medicine*.

12. Kapil, V., Milsom, A., Okorie, M., et al. (2010). Inorganic nitrate supplementation lowers blood pressure in humans: Role for nitrite-derived NO. *AHA: Hypertension*.

13. Bedi, U. & Arora, R. (2007). Cardiovascular manifestations of posttraumatic stress disorder. *Journal of the National Medical Association*.

14. Bunch, T., Crandall, B., Weiss, J., et al. (2011). Patients treated with catheter ablation for atrial fibrillation have long-term rates of death, stroke, and dementia similar to patients without atrial fibrillation. *Journal of Cardiovascular Electrophysiology*.

15. Proietti, R., AlTurki, A., Biase, L., et al. (2018). Anticoagulation after catheter ablation of atrial fibrillation: An unnecessary evil? A systematic review and meta-analysis. *Journal of Cardiovascular Electrophysiology*.

16. Bunch, T., May, H., Bair, T., et al. (2017). Five-year impact of catheter ablation for atrial fibrillation in patients with a prior history of stroke. *Journal of Cardiovascular Electrophysiology*; Bunch, T., May, H., Bair, T., et al. (2013). Atrial fibrillation ablation patients have long-term stroke rates similar to patients without atrial fibrillation regardless of CHADS2 score. *Heart Rhythm*; Bunch, T., Crandall, B., Weiss, J., et al. (2011). Patients treated with catheter ablation for atrial fibrillation have long-term rates of death, stroke, and dementia similar to patients without atrial fibrillation. *Journal of Cardiovascular Electrophysiology*.

17. Calkins, H., Hindricks, G., Cappato, R., et al., (2018) 2017 HRS/EHRA/ECAS/APHRS/SOLAECE expert consensus statement on catheter and surgical ablation of atrial fibrillation. *Europace*.

18. Bunch, T., Crandall, B., Weiss, J., et al. (2009). Warfarin is not needed in low-risk patients following atrial fibrillation ablation procedures. *Journal of Cardiovascular Electrophysiology*.

19. Granger, C., Alexander, J., McMurray, J., et al. (2011). Apixaban versus warfarin in patients with atrial fibrillation. *New England Journal of Medicine*.

20. Granger, C., et al. (2011).

21. Golive, A., May, H., Bair, T., et al. (2017). The population-based long-term impact of anticoagulant and antiplatelet therapies in low-risk patients with atrial fibrillation. *American Journal of Cardiology*.

22. Berg, D., Ruff, C., Jarolim, P., et al. (2018). Performance of the ABC scores for assessing the risk of stroke or systemic embolism and bleeding in patients with atrial fibrillation in ENGAGE AF-TIMI 48. *Circulation*; Oldgren, J., Hijazi, Z., Lindback, J., et al. (2016). External validation of the biomarker-based ABC-stroke risk score for atrial fibrillation. *Journal of the American College of Cardiology*.

23. Bunch, T. (2019). When it comes to the left atrial appendage, first do no harm. *Heart Rhythm*.

24. Rosenblatt, Z., Gianni, C., & Al-Ahmad, A. (2020). Ultrasound-guided deployment of Vascade vascular closure devices. *Heart Rhythm*.

25. Perret-Guillaume, C. & Wahl, D. (2004). Low-dose warfarin in atrial fibrillation leads to more thromboembolic events without reducing major bleeding when compared to adjusted-dose—a meta-analysis. *Thrombosis and Haemostasis*.

26. Tauzin-Fin, P., Ragnaud, J., Bendriss, P., et al. (1989). Comparative study of 2 antibiotic prophylaxis regimens in endoscopic prostatic surgery. *Pathologie-biologie*.

27. Borne, R., O'Donnell, C., Turakhia, M., et al. (2017). Adherence and outcomes to direct oral anticoagulants among patients with atrial fibrillation: Findings from the Veterans Health Administration. *BMC Cardiovascular Disorders*.

28. Neale, T. (June 25, 2019). Anticoagulation on demand? The pill-in-the-pocket approach to A-Fib treatment. *TCTMD/The Heartbeat*.

29. Hernandez, I., He, M., Brooks, M., et al. (2019). Adherence to anticoagulation and risk of stroke among Medicare beneficiaries newly diagnosed with atrial fibrillation. *American Journal of Cardiovascular Drugs*.

30. Passman, R., Leong-Sit, P., Andrei, A., et al. (2015). Targeted anticoagulation for atrial fibrillation guided by continuous rhythm assessment with an insertable cardiac monitor: The Rhythm Evaluation for Anticoagulation with Continuous Monitoring (REACT.COM) Pilot Study. *Journal of Cardiovascular Electrophysiology*; Waks, J., Passman, R., Matos, J., et al. (2018). Intermittent anticoagulation guided by continuous atrial fibrillation burden monitoring using dual-chamber pacemakers and implantable cardioverter-defibrillators: Results from the Tailored Anticoagulation for Non-Continuous Atrial Fibrillation (TACTIC-AF) Pilot Study. *Heart Rhythm*; Martin, D., Bersohn, M., Waldo, A., et al. (2015). Randomized trial of atrial arrhythmia monitoring to guide anticoagulation in patients with implanted defibrillator and cardiac resynchronization devices. *European Heart Journal*; Zado, E., Pammer, M., Parham, T., et al. (2019). "As needed" nonvitamin K antagonist oral anticoagulants for infrequent atrial fibrillation episodes following atrial fibrillation ablation guided by diligent pulse monitoring: A feasibility study. *Journal of Cardiovascular Electrophysiology*.

31. Steinhaus, D., Zimetbaum, P., Passman, R., et al. (2016). Cost effectiveness of implantable cardiac monitor-guided intermittent anticoagulation for atrial fibrillation: An analysis of the REACT .COM Pilot Study. *Journal of Cardiovascular Electrophysiology*.

32. Brambatti, M., Connolly, S., Gold, M., et al. (2014). Temporal relationship between subclinical atrial fibrillation and embolic events. *Circulation*.

33. Turner, J., Lyons, A., Shah, R., et al. (2020). Accuracy of patient identification of electrocardiogram-verified atrial arrhythmias. *JAMA Network Open*.

34. Huizar, J., Ellenbogen, K., Tan, A., et al. (2019). Arrhythmia-induced cardiomyopathy: JACC state-of-the-art review. *Journal of the American College of Cardiology*.

35. Camm, A., Lip, G., De Caterina, R., et al. (2012). Focused update of the ESC guidelines for the management of atrial fibrillation. *European Heart Journal*.

36. Granger, C., Alexander, J., McMurray, J., et al. (2011). Apixaban versus warfarin in patients with atrial fibrillation. *New England Journal of Medicine*.

## Chapter Eight

1. Rho, R. & Page, R. (2005). Asymptomatic atrial fibrillation. *Progress in Cardiovascular Diseases*.

2. Vasamreddy, C., Dalal, D., Dong, J., et al. (2006). Symptomatic and asymptomatic atrial fibrillation in patients undergoing radiofrequency catheter ablation. *Journal of Cardiovascular Electrophysiology*.

3. Klemm, H., Ventura, R., Rostock, T., et al. (2006). Correlation of symptoms to ECG diagnosis following atrial fibrillation ablation. *Journal of Cardiovascular Electrophysiology*.

4. Lee, D., Pate, R., Lavie, C., et al. (2014). Leisure-time running reduces all-cause and cardiovascular mortality risk. *Journal of the American College of Cardiology*.

5. Lee, I., Shiroma, E., Kamada, M., et al. (2019). Association of step volume and intensity with all-cause mortality in older women. *JAMA Internal Medicine*.

6. Agarwal, S., Norby, F., Whitsel, E., et al. (2017). Cardiac autonomic dysfunction and incidence of atrial fibrillation: Results from 20 years follow-up. *Journal of the American College of Cardiology*.

7. Hernando, D., Roca, S., Sancho, J., et al. (2018). Validation of the Apple Watch for heart rate variability measurements during relax and mental stress in healthy subjects. *Sensors*.

8. Khushhal, A., Nichols, S., Evans, W., et al. (2017). Validity and reliability of the Apple Watch for measuring heart rate during exercise. *Sports Medicine International Open*.

9. Shaffer, F. & Ginsberg, J. (2017). An overview of heart rate variability metrics and norms. *Frontiers in Public Health*.

10. Agarwal, S., Norby, F., Whitsel, E., et al. (2017). Cardiac autonomic dysfunction and incidence of atrial fibrillation: Results from 20 years follow-up. *Journal of the American College of Cardiology*.

11. Zwan, J., Vente, W., Huizink, A., et al. (2015). Physical activity, mindfulness meditation, or heart rate variability biofeedback for stress reduction: A randomized controlled trial. *Applied Psychophysiology and Biofeedback*.

12. Jackowska, M., Dockray, S., Endrighi, R., et al. (2012). Sleep problems and heart rate variability over the working day. *Journal of Sleep Research*.

13. Cheng, Y., Huang, Y., & Huang, W. (2019). Heart rate variability as a potential biomarker for alcohol use disorders: A systematic review and meta-analysis. *Drug and Alcohol Dependence*.

14. Routledge, F., Campbell, T., McFetridge-Durdle, J., et al. (2010). Improvements in heart rate variability with exercise therapy. *The Canadian Journal of Cardiology*.

15. Mourot, L., Bouhaddi, M., Perrey, S., et al. (2004). Decrease in heart rate variability with overtraining: Assessment by the Poincaré Plot Analysis. *Clinical Physiology and Functional Imaging*.

16. Donoho, C., Seeman, T., Sloan, R., & Crimmins, E. M. (2015). Marital status, marital quality, and heart rate variability in the MIDUS cohort. *Journal of Family Psychology*.

17. Järvelin-Pasanen, S., Sinikallio, S., & Tarvainen, M. (2018). Heart rate variability and occupational stress-systematic review. *Industrial Health*.

18. Mellman, T., Bell, K., Abu-Bader, S., et al. (2018). Neighborhood stress and autonomic nervous system activity during sleep. *Sleep*.

19. Young, H. & Benton, D. (2018). Heart-rate variability: A biomarker to study the influence of nutrition on physiological and psychological health? *Behavioural Pharmacology*.

20. Kim, J., Park, Y., Cho, K., et al. (2005). Heart rate variability and obesity indices: Emphasis on the response to noise and standing. *Journal of the American Board of Family Practice*.

21. Li, S., Liu, Y., Liu, J., et al. (2010). Almond consumption improved glycemic control and lipid profiles in patients with type 2 diabetes mellitus. *Metabolism: Clinical and Experimental*.

22. Lichtman, S., Pisarska, K., Berman, E., et al. (1992). Discrepancy between self-reported and actual caloric intake and exercise in obese subjects. *New England Journal of Medicine*.

23. Chipponi, J., Bleier, J., Santi, M., et al. (1982). Deficiencies of essential and conditionally essential nutrients. *American Journal of Clinical Nutrition*.

24. Threapleton, D., Greenwood, D., Evans, C., et al. (2013). Dietary fibre intake and risk of cardiovascular disease: Systematic review and meta-analysis. *The British Journal of Medicine*.

25. van der Hooft, C., Heeringa, J., van Herpen, G., et al. (2004). Drug-induced atrial fibrillation. *Journal of the American College of Cardiology*.

26. Thyagarajan, B., Alagusundaramoorthy, S., & Agrawal, A. (2015). Atrial fibrillation due to over the counter stimulant drugs in a young adult. *Journal of Clinical and Diagnostic Research*.

27. Steinberg, D., Bennett, G., Askew, S., et al. (2015). Weighing everyday matters: Daily weighing improves weight loss and adoption of weight control behaviors. *Journal of the Academy of Nutrition and Dietetics*.

28. Wing, R. & Hill, J. (2001). Successful weight loss maintenance. *Annual Review of Nutrition*.

29. Aronow, W. (2017). Hypertension associated with atrial fibrillation. *Annals of Translational Medicine*.

30. Knutson, K., Ryden, A., Mander, B., et al. (2006). Role of sleep duration and quality in the risk and severity of type 2 diabetes mellitus. *Archives of Internal Medicine*.

31. Nunes, R., Araújo, F., Correia, G., et al. (2013). High-sensitivity C-reactive protein levels and treadmill exercise test responses in men and women without overt heart disease. *Experimental and Clinical Cardiology*.

32. Schoech, D., Boyas, J., Black, B., et al. (2013). Gamification for behavior change: Lessons from developing a social, multiuser, web-tablet based prevention game for youths. *Journal of Technology in Human Services*.

## Chapter Nine

1. Sanches, F., Avesani, C., Kamimura, M., et al. (2008). Waist circumference and visceral fat in CKD: A cross-sectional study. *American Journal of Kidney Diseases*.

2. Violi, F., Pastori, D., Pignatelli, P., & Loffredo, L. (2014). Antioxidants for prevention of atrial fibrillation: A potentially useful future therapeutic approach? A review of the literature and meta-analysis. *Europace*.

3. Mattioli, A., Miloro, C., Pennella, S., et al. (2013). Adherence to Mediterranean diet and intake of antioxidants influence spontaneous conversion of atrial fibrillation. *Nutrition, Metabolism and Cardiovascular Diseases*.

4. Hu, Y., Chen, Y., Lin, Y., & Chen, S. (2015). Inflammation and the pathogenesis of atrial fibrillation. *Nature Reviews Cardiology*.

5. Blaak, E., Antoine, J., Benton, D., et al. (2012). Impact of postprandial glycaemia on health and prevention of disease. *Obesity Reviews*.

6. Myles, I. (2014). Fast food fever: Reviewing the impacts of the Western diet on immunity. *Nutrition Journal*.

7. Saito, S., Teshima, Y., Fukui, A., et al. (2014). Glucose fluctuations increase the incidence of atrial fibrillation in diabetic rats. *Cardiovascular Research*.

8. Latini, R., Staszewsky, L., Sun, J., et al. (2013). Incidence of atrial fibrillation in a population with impaired glucose tolerance: The contribution of glucose metabolism and other risk factors. A post hoc analysis of the Nateglinide and Valsartan in Impaired Glucose Tolerance Outcomes Research trial. *American Heart Journal*.

9. Krijthe, B., Heeringa, J., Kors, J., et al. (2013). Serum potassium levels and the risk of atrial fibrillation: The Rotterdam Study. *International Journal of Cardiology*.

10. Khan, A., Lubitz, S., Sullivan, L., et al. (2013). Low serum magnesium and the development of atrial fibrillation in the community: The Framingham Heart Study. *Circulation*.

11. Svingen, G., Zuo, H., & Ueland, P. (2018). Increased plasma trimethylamine-N-oxide is associated with incident atrial fibrillation. *International Journal of Cardiology*.

12. Yu, L., Meng, G., Huang, B., et al. (2018). A potential relationship between gut microbes and atrial fibrillation: Trimethylamine N-oxide, a gut microbe-derived metabolite, facilitates the progression of atrial fibrillation. *International Journal of Cardiology*.

13. Patel, D., Lavie, C., Milani, R., et al. (2009). Clinical implications of left atrial enlargement: A review. *The Ochsner Journal*.

14. Carpenter, A., Frontera, A., Bond, R., et al. (2015). Vagal atrial fibrillation: What is it and should we treat it? *International Journal of Cardiology*.

15. Lugovskaya, N. & Vinson, D. (2016). Paroxysmal atrial fibrillation and brain freeze: A case of recurrent co-incident precipitation from a frozen beverage. *American Journal of Case Reports*.

16. Robinson, J. & Snyder, C. (2016). Cold-induced, swallow-related atrial fibrillation in an adolescent. *Journal of Innovations in Cardiac Rhythm Management*.

17. Hurst, Y. & Fukuda, H. (2018). Effects of changes in eating speed on obesity in patients with diabetes: A secondary analysis of longitudinal health check-up. *BMJ Open*.

18. Weir, H., Yao, P., Huynh, F., et al. (2017). Dietary restriction and AMPK increase lifespan via mitochondrial network and peroxisome remodeling. *Cell Metabolism*.

19. Carlquist, J., Knight, S., Cawthon, R., Bunch, T., et al. (2016). Shortened telomere length is associated with paroxysmal atrial fibrillation among cardiovascular patients enrolled in the Intermountain Heart Collaborative Study. *Heart Rhythm*.

20. Takahashi, M., Ozaki, M., Kang, M., et al. (2018). Effects of meal timing on postprandial glucose metabolism and blood metabolites in healthy adults. *Nutrients*.

21. Chugh, S., Havmoeller, R., Narayanan, K., et al. (2014). Worldwide epidemiology of atrial fibrillation: A Global Burden of Disease 2010 Study. *Circulation*.

22. van den Berg, M., Hassink, R., Baljé-Volkers, C., et al. (2003). Role of the autonomic nervous system in vagal atrial fibrillation. *Heart*.

23. McKiernan, F., Houchins, J., & Mattes, R. (2008). Relationships between human thirst, hunger, drinking, and feeding. *Physiology & Behavior*.

24. Whitfield, A. (2006). Too much of a good thing? *British Journal of General Practice*.

25. Popkin, B., D'Anci, K., & Rosenberg, I. (2010). Water, hydration and health. *Nutrition Reviews*.

26. Mattioli, A., Miloro, C., Pennella, S., et al. (2013). Adherence to Mediterranean diet and intake of antioxidants influence spontaneous conversion of atrial fibrillation. *Nutrition, Metabolism, and Cardiovascular Diseases*.

27. Fawcett, K. & Barroso, I. (2010). The genetics of obesity: FTO leads the way. *Trends in Genetics*.

28. Chorin, E., Hochstadt, A., Granot, Y., et al. (2019). Grapefruit juice prolongs the QT interval of healthy volunteers and patients with long QT syndrome. *Heart Rhythm*.

29. Larsson, S., Drca, N., Björck, M., et al. (2018). Nut consumption and incidence of seven cardiovascular diseases. *Heart*.

30. Martínez-González, M., Toledo, E., Arós, F., et al. (2014). Extravirgin olive oil consumption reduces risk of atrial fibrillation: The PREDIMED (prevención con dieta Mediterránea) Trial. *Circulation*; Mostofsky, E., Johansen, M., Tjønneland, A., et al. (2017). Chocolate intake and risk of clinically apparent atrial fibrillation: The Danish Diet, Cancer, and Health Study. *Heart*.

31. Katz, D., Doughty, K., & Ali, A. (2011). Cocoa and chocolate in human health and disease. *Antioxidants & Redox Signaling*.

32. Clark, M. & Slavin, J. (2013). The effect of fiber on satiety and food intake: A systematic review. *Journal of the American College of Nutrition*.

33. Ylönen, K., Saloranta, C., & Kronberg-Kippilä, C. (2003). Associations of dietary fiber with glucose metabolism in nondiabetic relatives of subjects with type 2 diabetes: The Botnia Dietary Study. *Diabetes Care*.

34. Shen, J., Johnson, V., Sullivan, L., et al. (2010). Dietary factors and incident atrial fibrillation: The Framingham Heart Study. *The American Journal of Clinical Nutrition*.

35. Eaton, S., Konner, M., & Shostak, M. (1988). Stone agers in the fast lane: Chronic degenerative diseases in evolutionary perspective. *American Journal of Medicine*.

36. Kaplan, H., Thompson, R., Trumble, B., et al. (2017). Coronary atherosclerosis in indigenous South American Tsimane: A cross-sectional cohort study. *Lancet*.

37. Vasunilashorn, S., Finch, C., Crimmins, E., et al. (2011). Inflammatory gene variants in the Tsimane, an indigenous Bolivian population with a high infectious load. *Biodemography and Social Biology*.

38. Bouvard, V., Loomis, D., Guyton, K., et al. (2015). Carcinogenicity of consumption of red and processed meat. *The Lancet Oncology*.

39. Martino, A., Pezzi, L., Magnano, R., et al. (2016). Omega 3 and atrial fibrillation: Where are we? *World Journal of Cardiology*.

40. Gronroos, N., Chamberlain, A., Folsom, A., et al. (2012). Fish, fish-derived n-3 fatty acids, and risk of incident atrial fibrillation in the Atherosclerosis Risk in Communities (ARIC) Study. *Plos One*; Mozaffarian, D., Psaty, B., Rimm, E., et al. (2004). Fish intake and risk of incident atrial fibrillation. *Circulation*; Shen, J., Johnson, V., Sullivan, L., et al. (2010). Dietary factors and incident atrial fibrillation: The Framingham Heart Study. *American Journal of Clinical Nutrition*.

41. Chugh, S., Havmoeller, R., Narayanan, K., et al. (2013). Worldwide epidemiology of atrial fibrillation: A global burden of disease 2010 study. *Circulation*.

42. Tan, S., Dhillon, J., & Mattes, R. (2014). A review of the effects of nuts on appetite, food intake, metabolism, and body weight. *American Journal of Clinical Nutrition*.

43. Abazarfard, Z., Salehi, M., & Keshavarzi, S. (2014). The effect of almonds on anthropometric measurements and lipid profile in overweight and obese females in a weight reduction program: A randomized controlled clinical trial. *Journal of Research in Medical Sciences*.

44. Kris-Etherton, P. (2014). Walnuts decrease risk of cardiovascular disease: A summary of efficacy and biologic mechanisms. *Journal of Nutrition*.

45. Pääkkö, T., Perkiömäki, J., Silaste, M., et al. (2018). Dietary sodium intake is associated with long-term risk of new-onset atrial fibrillation. *Annals of Medicine*.

46. Zhang, S., Zhuang, X., Lin, X., et al. (2019). Low-carbohydrate diets and risk of incident atrial fibrillation: A prospective cohort study. *Journal of the American Heart Association*.

47. Rao, M., Afshin, A., Singh, G., et al. (2013). Do healthier foods and diet patterns cost more than less healthy options? A systematic review and meta-analysis. *BMJ Open*.

48. Like many people around the world, Meredith has become a devotee of the recipes that *Longevity Plan* co-author Jane Day shares on the website of her husband and co-author, John Day. Many of Meredith's meals are based on these recipes, which you can find at https://drjohnday.com /recipes-jane/.

## Chapter Ten

1. Rabuñal-Rey, R., Monte-Secades, R., Gomez-Gigirey, A., et al. (2012). Electrocardiographic abnormalities in centenarians: Impact on survival. *BMC Geriatrics*.

2. Martínez-Sellés, M., García de la Villa, B., Cruz-Jentoft, A., et al. (2015). Centenarians and their hearts: A prospective registry with comprehensive geriatric assessment, electrocardiogram, echocardiography, and follow-up. *American Heart Journal*; Rasmussen, S., Andersen-Ranberg, K., Dahl, J., et al. (2019). Diagnosing heart failure in centenarians. *Journal of Geriatric Cardiology*.

3. Mo, Y., Liang, J., & Lu, Z. (2010). Electrogram analysis of 198 patients with extreme longevity in Bama County. *Guangxi Medical Journal*.

4. Kanmanthareddy, A., Reddy, M., Ponnaganti, G., et al. (2015). Alternative medicine in atrial fibrillation treatment—Yoga, acupuncture, biofeedback and more. *Journal of Thoracic Disease*.

5. Thrall, G., Lip, G., Carroll, D., & Lane, D. (2007). Depression, anxiety, and quality of life in patients with atrial fibrillation. *Chest*.

6. Charitakis, E., Barmano, N., Walfridsson, U., & Walfridsson, H. (2017). Factors predicting arrhythmia-related symptoms and health-related quality of life in patients referred for radiofrequency ablation of atrial fibrillation: an observational study (the SMURF Study). *JACC Clinical Electrophysiology*.

7. Valtorta, N., Kanaan, M., Gilbody, S., et al. (2016). Loneliness and social isolation as risk factors for coronary heart disease and stroke: Systematic review and meta-analysis of longitudinal observational studies. *Heart*.

8. Gilson, N., Hall, C., Renton, A., et al. (2017). Do sitting, standing, or treadmill desks impact psychobiological indicators of work productivity? *Journal of Physical Activity and Health*.

9. Garcia, J., Duran, A., Schwartz, J., et al. (2019). Types of sedentary behavior and risk of cardiovascular events and mortality in blacks: The Jackson Heart Study. *Journal of the American Heart Association*.

10. Bunch, T., Horne, B., Asirvatham, S., et al. (2011). Atrial fibrillation hospitalization is not increased with short-term elevations in exposure to fine particulate air pollution. *Pacing and*

*Clinical Electrophysiology*; Dixit, S., Pletcher, M., Vittinghoff, E., et al. (2015). Secondhand smoke and atrial fibrillation: Data from the Health eHeart Study. *Heart Rhythm.*

11. Shao, Q., Liu, T., Korantzopoulos, P., et al. (2016). Association between air pollution and development of atrial fibrillation: A meta-analysis of observational studies. *Heart & Lung.*

12. Monrad, M., Sajadieh, A., Christensen, J., et al. (2016). Residential exposure to traffic noise and risk of incident atrial fibrillation: A cohort study. *Environment International.*

13. Monrad, M., et al. (2016).

14. Mahmoodi, B. & Boersma, L. (2017). Do long working hours predispose to atrial fibrillation? *European Heart Journal*; Kivimäki, M., Nyberg, S., Batty, G., et al. (2017). Long working hours as a risk factor for atrial fibrillation: A multi-cohort study. *European Heart Journal.*

15. Svensson, T., Kitlinski, M., Engström, G., et al. (2017). Psychological stress and risk of incident atrial fibrillation in men and women with known atrial fibrillation genetic risk scores. *Scientific Reports*; Graff, S., Fenger-Grøn, M., Christensen, B., et al. (2016). Long-term risk of atrial fibrillation after the death of a partner. *Open Heart.*

16. Yu, L., Meng, G., Huang, B., et al. (2018). A potential relationship between gut microbes and atrial fibrillation: Trimethylamine N-oxide, a gut microbe-derived metabolite, facilitates the progression of atrial fibrillation. *International Journal of Cardiology.*

17. Twohig-Bennett, C. & Jones, A. (2018). The health benefits of the great outdoors: A systematic review and meta-analysis of greenspace exposure and health outcomes. *Environmental Research.*

18. Boyle, P., Barnes, L., Buchman, A., & Bennett, D. A. (2009). Purpose in life is associated with mortality among community-dwelling older persons. *Psychosomatic Medicine.*

## Conclusion

1. Son, M., Lim, N., Kim, H., & Park, H. (2017). Risk of ischemic stroke after atrial fibrillation diagnosis: A national sample cohort. *PloS One.*

2. de Bruijn R., Heeringa, J., Wolters, F., et al. (2015). Association between atrial fibrillation and dementia in the general population. *JAMA Neurology.*

3. Ha, A., Breithardt, G., Camm, A., et al. (2014). Health-related quality of life in patients with atrial fibrillation treated with rhythm control versus rate control: Insights from a prospective international registry (Registry on Cardiac Rhythm Disorders Assessing the Control of Atrial Fibrillation: RECORD-AF). *Circulation: Cardiovascular Quality and Outcomes.*

4. Crandall, M., Horne, B., Day, J., Bunch, T., et al. (2009). Atrial fibrillation and CHADS2 risk factors are associated with highly sensitive C reactive protein incrementally and independently. *Pacing and Clinical Electrophysiology.*

# INDEX

# ABOUT THE AUTHORS

**John D. Day, MD,** graduated from medical school at Johns Hopkins University. He did his residency and cardiac electrophysiology fellowship training at Stanford University. Dr. Day is a cardiologist/electrophysiologist at St. Mark's Hospital in Salt Lake City, Utah, where he leads the cardiac and vascular services for the mountain states division hospitals for HCA Healthcare, the largest healthcare provider in the United States. He previously served as president of the Heart Rhythm Society and is the immediate past president of the Utah chapter of the American College of Cardiology. He is recognized as an international thought leader on atrial fibrillation management. Dr. Day is board certified in cardiology and cardiac electrophysiology. He has published more than one hundred manuscripts, abstracts, and book chapters and regularly lectures both nationally and internationally on heart rhythm disorders. Dr. Day is the former editor-in-chief of the *Journal of Innovations in Cardiac Rhythm Management*. In 2017, Dr. Day published *The Longevity Plan: Seven Life-Transforming Lessons from Ancient China* (HarperCollins). *The Longevity Plan* was an Amazon number-one best-seller, was named one of the best books of 2017 by the *Huffington Post*, and won the Nautilus Book Award Gold Medal for the best book of 2017.

**T. Jared Bunch, MD,** is the founding editor of the *HeartRhythm Case Reports* journal and is active in the Heart Rhythm Society. During his residency at Mayo Clinic in Rochester, Minnesota, he received the Outstanding

Achievement Award and the Resident Research Award from the Department of Medicine, and the Donald J. Feist Primary Care Clinic Award for Clinical Excellence. He completed his fellowship in cardiovascular diseases and electrophysiology at the Mayo Clinic and received the Mayo Brothers Distinguished Fellowship Award for clinical care of patients and the Donald C. Balfour Award for meritorious research. He served as an assistant professor of medicine at the Mayo Clinic from 2003 to 2007. After his fellowship, he joined the cardiovascular team at Intermountain Heart Institute and directed heart rhythm research and received the Physician Researcher of the Year for the Intermountain Healthcare System in 2014 and 2017. In 2019, he joined the faculty at the University of Utah School of Medicine as a professor of medicine and currently serves as the medical director of Heart Rhythm Services at the University of Utah. Dr. Bunch is on the editorial boards of the *Heart Rhythm Journal*, *Journal of Cardiovascular Electrophysiology*, *Heart*, *American Heart Journal*, *JACC Clinical Electrophysiology*, and the *Journal of Innovations in Cardiac Rhythm Management*.

**Matthew D. LaPlante** is an associate professor of journalism at Utah State University, where he teaches news reporting, narrative nonfiction writing, and crisis reporting. He has reported from more than a dozen nations, including Iraq, Cuba, Ethiopia, and El Salvador, and his work has appeared in the *Washington Post, Los Angeles Daily News*, CNN.com, and numerous other publications. LaPlante is the author of *Superlative: The Biology of Extremes* and cowriter of several books on the intersection of scientific discovery and society.